T.F. Lüscher M. Turina
E. Braunwald (Eds.)

Coronary Artery Graft Disease

Mechanisms and Prevention

With 159 Figures, Some in Colour

Springer-Verlag
Berlin Heidelberg New York
London Paris Tokyo
Hong Kong Barcelona
Budapest

Professor Dr. med. THOMAS F. LÜSCHER
Abteilung Kardiologie, Inselspital
3010 Bern
Switzerland

Professor Dr. med. MARKO TURINA
Herz-Gefäßchirurgie, Universitätsspital
8091 Zürich
Switzerland

Professor Dr. med. EUGENE BRAUNWALD
Department of Medicine
Harvard University and
Brigham and Women's Hospital
Boston, MA 02115-6195
USA

Cover drawing reprinted with permission from Mayo Clinic Proceedings 61:3–8 (1986)

ISBN-13:978-3-642-78639-6 e-ISBN-13:978-3-642-78637-2
DOI: 10.1007/978-3-642-78637-2

Library of Congress Cataloging-in-Publication Data. Coronary artery graft disease: mechanism and prevention / T. Luscher, M Turina, E. Braunwald, eds. p. cm. Includes bibliographical references and index 1.
Coronary artery bypass—Complications. 2. Graft rejection. I. Luscher, Thomas F (Thomas Felix) II. Turina, Marko. III. Braunwald, Eugene, 1929- [DNLM: 1 Coronary Disease—therapy. 2. Coronary Artery Bypass—adverse effects. 3. Graft Rejection—prevention & control. WG 300 C81965 1994] RD598 35.C67C685 1994 617.4'120592 —dc20 DNLM/DLC for Library of Congress 94-16135

Softcover reprint of the hardover 1st edition 1994

Typesetting: Best-set Typesetter Ltd., Hong Kong
SPIN: 10134330 23/3130/SPS – 5 4 3 2 1 0 – Printed on acid-free paper

Preface

In 1969, Rene Favaloro published his landmark paper entitled "*Saphenous vein graft in the surgical treatment of coronary artery disease: operative technique*", which changed the care of patients with ischemic heart disease and the speciality of cardiovascular surgery forever. Since then, the use of coronary artery bypass grafting has relieved intractable angina pectoris in millions of patients worldwide and prolonged survival in countless others.

Despite the emergence and popularity of percutaneous transluminal coronary angioplasty and related techniques, coronary artery bypass surgery remains firmly entrenched as the only revascularization technique that has been demonstrated to improve the natural history of coronary artery disease. An increasing number of candidates for this operation are, in fact, now patients who have previously undergone angioplasty or bypass surgery. As a consequence, the total number of surgical revascularizations continues to rise steadily both in the United States and in Europe.

Even when it is successful technically, however, coronary artery bypass surgery is not a curative procedure. One major problem is coronary graft disease, a series of interrelated complications, some of which may commence at operation and others which continue for decades; all of them ultimately negate the benefit of the procedure, however. This book deals with the most important complications of the most important cardiovascular operation. Fortunately, the enormous advances in vascular pathobiology made in the past 15 years have shed much light on this problem and have pointed to its potential prevention and management. Approaches include the preoperative selection of the conduit(s) to be employed and their intraoperative handling, and the early and late postoperative care of the patient. We have learned that blood vessels are complex, living organs rather than simple mechanical conduits, that arteries differ considerably from veins when used for coronary bypass, and that the endothelium is an active tissue that influences profoundly both the fluidity of the blood and the tone and growth of the underlying smooth muscle.

The understanding of the cellular and molecular mechanisms involved in bypass graft disease may set the stage for more specific therapeutic interventions in the future which may help to prolong the patency and function of implanted grafts.

Assessment of the grafts, of course, is essential in the postoperative patient. While coronary arteriography remains the gold standard for the recognition of graft disease, a variety of noninvasive methods – radionuclide scintigraphy, duplex ultrasonography, magnetic resonance imaging, positron emission tomography and angiography – can all provide valuable information regarding the status of the graft and of both the viability and function of the myocardium that it perfuses. When considering reoperation in patients with diseased grafts, it is essential to evaluate the quality of salvageable myocardium perfused by diseased grafts and native vessels.

Management of the patient with coronary grafts may be divided into two phases. Prevention of graft disease, which should be applied to all patients, currently involves the use of antiplatelet drugs, vigorous control of lipid abnormalities, and strict smoking cessation. In patients with established graft disease, percutaneous transluminal angioplasty, sometimes aided by intraluminal stents, is often helpful. When these measures fail or are not suitable, reoperation – despite its higher risk – may be in order. Heart transplantation always remains a last resort for patients with severe graft disease, but it is an effective last resort since the long-term outcome has improved substantially in recent years.

It is fitting, therefore, that as we celebrate the silver anniversary of coronary artery bypass surgery, we re-examine this important operation and describe approaches that may protect the many patients who have already undergone it and the even larger number who will do so in the future.

Bern, Switzerland
Zürich, Switzerland
Boston, USA

THOMAS F. LÜSCHER
MARKO TURINA
EUGENE BRAUNWALD

Contents

The Problem

Surgical Aspects

Diagnosis of Graft Failure

Pharmacological Intervention

Revascularization Strategies

List of Contributors

AMANN, F.W., PD Dr., Abteilung Kardiologie, Department für Innere Medizin, Universitätsspital Zürich, 8091 Zürich, Schweiz

ANGELINI, G.D., M.D., Department of Cardiac Surgery, Bristol Royal Infirmary, Bristol BS2 8HW, UK

DE BONO, D.P., Department of Cardiology, University of Leicester, Clinical Sciences Wing, Glenfield General Hospital, Leicester LE3 9QP, UK

BUSER, P.T., M.D., Division of Cardiology, University Hospital, Petersgraben, 4031 Basel, Switzerland

CHESBRO, J.H., M.D., Division of Cardiology, Massachusetts General Hospital, Harvard Medical School, Boston, MA 02115, USA

DREXEL, H., PD Dr., Abteilung Kardiologie, Department für Innere Medizin, Universitätsspital Zürich, 8091 Zürich, Schweiz

FUSTER, V., M.D., Ph.D., Chief, Cardiac Unit, Massachusetts General Hospital, BUL 105, Fruit Street, Boston, MA 02114, USA

GOTTLIEB, S.O., M.D., FACC, Johns Hopkins University School of Medicine, Midatlantic Cardiovascular Consultants, P.A., GBMC Pavilion, Suite 408, 6585 North Charles Street, Baltimore, MD 21204, USA

GRONDIN, C.M., M.D., Professor of Surgery, Case Western Reserve University, Cleveland, OH 44104, USA

HAUSMANN, H., M.D., Zentrum Innere Medizin, Abteilung Kardiologie, Hochschule Hannover, Konstanty-Gutschow-Str. 8, 30625 Hannover, Germany

HESS, O.M., M.D., Professor of Medicine, Department of Medicine, Cardiology University Hospital, 8091 Zurich, Switzerland

HIGGINS, C.B., Department of Radiology, MRI Section, University of California, San Francisco, CA 94143, USA

HOLLMAN, J., M.D., Department of Cardiology, Ochsner Clinic of Baton Rouge, 16777 Medical Center Drive, Baton Rouge, LA 70816, USA

JAKOB, M., M.D., Division of Cardiology, University Hospital, 8091 Zurich, Switzerland

JANG, I.K., M.D., Ph.D., Assistant Professor of Medicine, Massachusetts General Hospital, BUL 105, Fruit Street, Boston, MA 02114, USA

KRAYENBÜHL, H.P., M.D.†, Professor of Cardiology, Medical Policlinic, University Hospital, 8091 Zurich, Switzerland

LEWIS, D.A., Department of Surgery and Physiology, 9 Guggenheim Building, Mayo Clinic and Foundation, Rochester, MN 55905, USA

LICHTLEN, P.R., Prof. Dr., Zentrum Innere Medizin, Abteilung Kardiologie, Hochschule Hannover, Konstanty-Gutschow-Str. 8, 30625 Hannover, Germany

LOOP, F.D., M.D., The Cleveland Clinic Foundation, 9500 Euclid Avenue, Cleveland, OH 44195, USA

LÜSCHER, T.F., M.D., Professor of Medicine, Cardiology, University Hospital, 3010 Bern, Switzerland

MEYER, B.J., M.D., Professor of Medicine, Cardiology, University Hospital, 3010 Bern, Switzerland

MILLER, V.M., Ph.D., Department of Surgery and Physiology, 9 Guggenheim Building, Mayo Clinic and Foundation, Rochester, MN 55905, USA

NEWBY, A.C., Ph.D., Reader Cardiovascular Biochemistry, Department of Cardiology, College of Medicine, University of Wales, Health Park, Cardiff CF4 4XN, UK

OEMAR, B.S., M.D., PD Dr., Department of Research, University Hospital, 4031 Basel, Switzerland

PFISTERER, M., MD, FESC, FACC, Professor of Cardiology, University Hospital Basel, 4031 Basel, Switzerland

SAWADA, S.G., M.D., University of Michigan Medical Center, 1500 E. Medical Center Dr., UH B1G505, Ann Arbor, MI 48109-0028, USA

SCHWAIGER, M., Prof. Dr., Nuklearmedizidische Klinik und Poliklinik, Technische Universität München, Klinikum rechts der Isar, Ismaningerstr. 22, 81657 München, Germany

VON SEGESSER, L.K., PD Dr., Department of Cardiovascular Surgery, University Hospital Zurich, 8091 Zurich, Switzerland

SEIDEL, D., PD. Dr., Direktor des Institutes für Klinische Chemie, Klinikum Grosshadern, Ludwig-Maximilians-Universität München, Marchioninistrasse 15, 81366 München, Germany

SERGEANT, P., M.D., Cardiac Surgery Department, Gasthuisberg, University Hospital, Herestraat, 3000 Leuven, Belgium

SUMA, H., M.D., Department of Cardiovascular Surgery, Mitsui Memorial Hospital, 1, Kanda Izumi-cho, Chiyoda-ku, Tokyo 101, Japan

THOMTON, J.C., M.D., Associate Professor of Surgery, Case Western Reserve University, Cleveland, OH 44104, USA

TURINA, M., M.D., Professor of Surgery, Chairman, Dept. of Cardiovascular Surgery, University Hospital Zurich, 8091 Zurich, Switzerland

URBAN, P., M.D., Professor of Medicine, Centre de Cardiologie, Hôpital Cantonal Universitaire, 24, rue Micheli-du-Crest, 1211 Genève, Suisse

WACKERS, F.J.T., M.D., Yale University School of Medicine, Department of Diagnostic Radiology and Medicine, 333 Cedar Street, TE-2, New Haven, CT 06510, USA

YACOUB, M., SIR, Professor of Surgery, National Heart & Lung Institute, Academic Department of Cardiothoracic Surgery, Dovehouse Street, London SW3 6LY, UK

YANG, Z., M.D., Cardiovascular Research, Cardiology, University Hospital, 3010 Bern, Switzerland

The Problem

The Natural History of Saphenous Vein Grafts

C.M. Grondin and J.C. Thornton

The saphenous vein (SV) was used as a bypass conduit first in the peripheral circulation for the relief of claudication by Kunlin in 1949 [1] and later in cardiac surgery for the correction of anomalous origin of the left coronary artery by Garrett and associates in 1966 [2]. Today, it remains the graft material of choice in peripheral vascular surgery and the conduit most often used in coronary artery surgery [3]. Detailed knowledge of the fate of the SV has come from serial angiographic studies conducted in patients subjected to coronary bypass grafting although a good deal of information had appeared in earlier reports on femoropopliteal bypass grafts. These indicated, on the one hand, that early occlusions of the SV are the result of faulty technique or poor arterial run-off and suggested, on the other, that graft atherosclerosis is a major factor in late occlusions [4, 5].

The response of SV appears to vary little whether it is used peripherally or centrally, although in certain areas specific characteristics may be observed with greater frequency, for instance, aneurysmal dilatation in aortorenal grafts [6]. This chapter reviews the natural history of the SV as used in the coronary arterial circuit. As angiographic findings and clinical results cannot be easily separated from one another or from morphological findings, a brief review of posttransplantation histological changes is first appropriate.

Histological Changes in Aortocoronary Vein Grafts

Early Changes

Although the normal SV may show localized fibrous thickening, it is not believed that phlebosclerosis predisposes the vein to late graft atherosclerosis. Indeed, phlebosclerosis increases with age [7] whereas graft disease does not. Graft disease may in fact may affect younger patients, who are expected to have better veins to a greater extent [3], probably because the disease both in their native arteries and in their grafts is a more active process.

In grafts recovered early after operation a variety of changes are noted which, for the most part, involve the intimal layer [8]. These acute changes include endothelial denudation or sloughing, edema and deposition of fibrin, leukocytes and platelets. Muscle necrosis is also noted in the media. Denudation of the endothelium probably triggers the whole reaction by attracting blood elements – platelets and monocytes – which in turn, through secretion of various factors, promote further platelet aggregation, hyperplasia, and migration of medial cells to the intimal layer [9–11]. After a few weeks the endothelium returns to cover a much thicker intima [8]. Fibrointimal hyperplasia, a term used to describe the more chronic phase of the process after 1 month [12–15], represents regeneration of the intimal layer which, at that point, consists of a thick layer of fibroblasts, smooth muscle cells, and occasional foam cells, all in a matrix rich in mucopolysaccharides [15]. There is also loss of smooth muscle cells in the media and ultimately some fibrosis [12]. All this renders the vein more rigid and at angiography reduces the lumen of the graft. The latter as a consequence does not recoil with myocardial shortening as the coronary arteries do on the surface of the heart. The graft also shortens so that in the 1-year study it appears to tug on the distal anastomosis and causes tenting. It is estimated that the SV length shrinks by 10% during the first year.

These early changes in the histology of the transplanted vein are ubiquitous but vary in degree. In some grafts the thickening is limited and may not translate to a reduced lumen at angiography. During the first postoperative year, 25% of grafts show no appreciable angiographic change in diameter. On the other hand, all grafts recovered at operation or postmortem show some fibrous intimal hyperplasia, and the intimal thickening usually reduces the graft lumen by 30% [16]. Intimal hyperplasia is a reparative process, a reaction to the trauma and stress which result from transplantation of the vein into the arterial circuit. This does not appear to occur in transplanted arteries, probably because the arteries, although still subject to transplantation ischemia and loss of their vasa vasorum, are already prepared for the dynamics of arterial pressure and oxygen content [9] and harbor a more resistant endothelium which clears lipids and fibrin or secretes prostacyclin and other protective substances at a more favorable rate than the vein endothelium [17–20].

Late Changes

Beyond the first year and until the third or fouth year very little change occurs. The vein wall – both intima and media – may become more fibrous, i.e., it shows greater matrix and fewer nuclei, but on the whole the lumen to wall thickness ratio stabilizes. On the other hand, an increase in lipid contents and number of foam cells may be noted [14]. Several authors believe that both the foam cells and the intimal thickening are early signs or precursors of atherosclerosis [13, 14, 21]. Intimal thickening, for one, precedes atherosclerosis in human aortas [22] and coronary arteries [23]. In certain arteries, such as the internal mammary, intimal thickening is seen only in the fifth or sixth decade [24] whereas it usually appears during the first decade in the coronary arteries [23]; this may account for the difference in the degree of disease noted in these two arterial systems.

Although discrete atherosclerosis may be seen as early as 3 months postoperatively histologically [13] and at 1 year at angiography [25], most features of graft disease manifest themselves beyond the third year. The disease as it affects the transplanted vein is histologically indistinguishable from arterial atherosclerosis [13, 15]. Grossly, it is somewhat diffuse, often friable [26], rarely calcified, and on occasion leads to aneurysmal dilatation [27] (perivenous fibrous reaction probably limits dilatation in the aortocoronary position). In the early phase only a yellow fibrous plaque may be seen, but rupture of plaques is frequent – as high as 40% in surgical specimens [28]. In all, atherosclerosis in coronary vein grafts appears to be a more active disease with more fragile, unstable features than its arterial counterpart, which takes decades to develop [29]. It is also more unpredictable, leading in some instances to sudden events either in the natural setting or upon manipulation of the graft [30, 31].

Angiographic Changes in Aortocoronary Vein Grafts

Early Patency Rate and Angiographic Findings

In the peripheral vascular circuit as well as in the heart, the SV remains open in 85%–90% of cases at 1 month and in 75%–85% at 1 year, which means that cumulatively the attrition rate during the first year approximates 20%–25% [32, 33] (Table 1). Factors responsible for occlusion include the quality of runoff, the technique, which is often dependent on the experience of the surgical team, and perhaps the graft itself which develops fibrointimal hyperplasia and other changes described above.

The quality of the recipient bed is assessed visually at operation and by measuring graft flow as well as its response to injection of a vasodilator such

Table 1. Patency rate of vein grafts in consecutive series of patients, first 3 postoperative years (from [16])

	No. of patients	No. of grafts	Occlusions	
			n	%
1 month	98	141	16	11.3
1 year	79	108	22	20.4
3 years	65	86	4	5.1

Table 2. Influence of surgical experience on fate of aortocoronary vein grafts (from [35])

	Early experience[a] (%)	Longer experience[b] (%)	*p* value
Early patency (1 month)	86.3	91.8	NS
Late patency (1 year)	67	87.5	0.0005
Patency			
Graft Q > 50 ml	90	90	NS
Graft Q < 50 ml	28	73	0.0005
Graft narrowing			
Localized (>40%)	16.5	6	0.025
Diffuse (>40%)	31	12	0.001

NS, Not significant.
[a] Less than 2 years; 105 patients; 154 grafts.
[b] More than 2 years; 67 patients; 152 grafts.

as papaverine. Basal flow and response to vasodilatation predict with considerable accuracy patency of the graft, both at 1 month and at 1 year. Thus, in a series of 70 patients, all grafts with flow greater than 50 ml/min remained open; those with a flow of 20 ml/min or less or which failed to respond to papaverine were occluded [34]. At 1 year 90% of grafts with flow greater than 50 ml/min remained open, compared to 72% of grafts with more limited flow (<50 ml/min) [35]. Experience of the surgical team, like the quality of the distal bed, may influence results during the first 12 months but not beyond. Table 2 shows a marked difference in cumulative patency rate at 1 year in the same study when the surgical team had a 2-year experience with the procedure compared to an earlier period.

The mechanism responsible for fibrointimal hyperplasia (FIH) as a cause of graft closure is, on the other hand, a more debated point. Indeed, although FIH (which accounts for diffuse reduction in the radiological diameter of grafts over time) occurs in 75% of grafts [16], it may in the same subject affect one graft and not the other, which suggests that the process does not represent normal adaptation of the vein to arterial surroundings. Some vein segments, perhaps from different areas or from the other leg, handled differently or subjected to somewhat different dynamics, may either not lose as much endothelial function or respond less to mitogenic factors and remain relatively intact. It must be pointed, however, that, as seen in our study in patients whose grafts showed FIH, most if not all grafts with mild to moderate diffuse reduction in caliber showed the same degree of reduction. Patients whose grafts showed severe diffuse reduction were the exception, i.e., they might have other grafts showing no reduction. Severe diffuse reduction usually occurs in grafts with poor runoff, and ultimately, 1–2 years later, these grafts show total occlusion. Grafts with mild reduction

Table 3. Changes in vein graft diameter at 1 year (between studies at 1 and 12 months) and outcome at 3 years (65 patients; from [16])

Type of reduction (year)	No. of grafts	No. occluded (3 years)
Diffuse		
Nove (<20%)	21	0
Mild (20%–40%)	41	0
Moderate (40%–60%)	22	1
Severe (>70%)	2	1
Segmental		
Mild (25%)	11	0
Moderate (<50%)	13	0
Severe (>70%)	2	2

of luminal diameter (20%–40%) or moderate reduction (<60%) do not suffer such a fate [16] (Table 3). On the whole, in grafts with mild to moderate reduction the larger the initial diameter on the early study the greater is the reduction, which suggests some adaptation on the part of the graft to the size of the recipient artery.

Although FIH is considered by most to be a precursor to atherosclerosis [13, 14], it does not appear to progress beyond the first year or to influence graft patency beyond the first or the third year [16]. Blood flow has little to do with FIH [16]. Agents known to inhibit platelet function, such as aspirin, improve patency but only that of grafts with limited flow [36]. As low flow does not appear to equal FIH, it must be assumed that better patency by platelet inhibitors is not achieved through prevention/retardation of FIH. Indeed, FIH is not altered by these agents, whose effect on patency may not continue beyond the first year.

Grafts may remain open but due to technical error perfuse only the proximal or the distal limb of the anastomosis (Fig. 1). Occlusion at a later date often follows the former situation but not the latter [16]. With greater experience these technical faults become less frequent, and the rate of graft loss drops [35]. Localized stenoses are also seen in the body of the graft during the first year and are believed secondary to local factors such as placement of an occlusive clamp or forceps at the time of operation, an incomplete twist of the graft, or the presence of venous valves. These may cause occlusion later. With experience the incidence of early localized narrowing also decreases (Table 2). Sometimes there is no apparent cause for graft occlusion during the first 3 years.

Although early angiographic changes suggestive of atherosclerosis have been reported in vein grafts 1 year after operation, most authors agree that such changes become more evident between the fifth and the tenth post-operative year [37, 38].

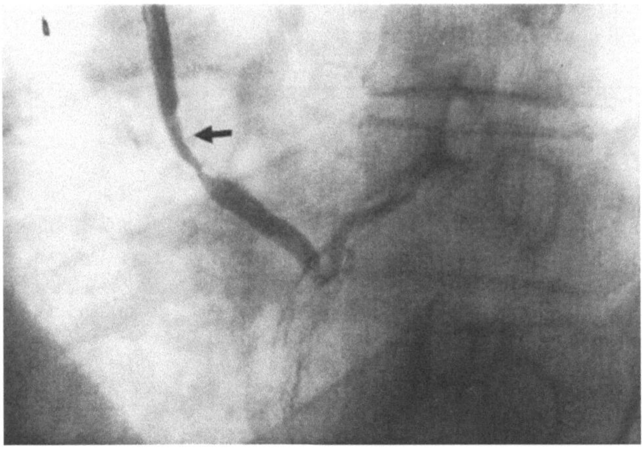

Fig. 1. Saphenous vein graft to left anterior descending artery (LAD) 10 years postimplantation, showing long irregular stenosis in midportion of graft (*arrow*). Previous angiogram 3 years earlier had shown normal graft. Note occlusion of LAD distal to graft also present on previous study

Late Patency Rate and Angiographic Changes

Although it is now believed that late graft occlusion (>5 years after operation) is due to progression of atherosclerosis, one must distinguish between histological and radiological evidence of atherosclerosis. Histological evidence of the process may be found as early as 3–6 months [13, 14] after the operation in the form of fibrous plaque and foam cells, but less subtle changes such as ulcerated, hemorrhagic, and calcified plaques are visible much later. For instance, in our 3-year angiographic study [16], no such changes were detected although, in retrospect, some irregular walls (more evident at 5–6 years) probably represented such a process. FitzGibbons and coworkers, on the other hand, using more rigid criteria, described so-called B lesions (decrease in the graft lumen by at least 50%) as probable evidence of atherosclerosis based on the fact that at 5 years there was a higher incidence of occlusion or increase in the severity of the narrowing [25]. This, however, may be equivalent to our own localized narrowing – not ascribed to atherosclerosis – which worsened but was not considered necessarily to be secondary to atherosclerosis. On the other hand, all agree that at 5–6 years unmistakable angiographic evidence of the process exists, often confirmed histologically – in 14% of grafts in our study [37] and in 38% in that of FitzGibbons and associates [25].

The occlusion rate of grafts, which between the first and fifth years decreases considerably (2%–2.5% per year), accelerates anew and doubles to 5% per year between the fifth and tenth postoperative years [39] (Table 4). At angiography the lesions are no longer discrete, and several grafts

Table 4. Attrition rate (AR) and cumulative occlusion rate (COR) of aortocoronary vein grafts (consecutive series) as determined at 1 month, 1 year, and 10 years after surgery

	1 month (%)	1 year (%)		10 years (%)	
	AR	AR	COR	AR	COR
FitzGibbons et al. [38]	8	7	15	30	45
Grondin et al. [43]	10.9	8	18.9	31	49.9

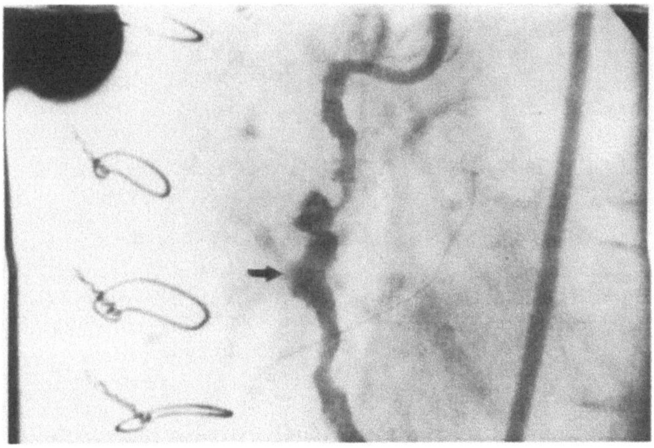

Fig. 2. Saphenous vein graft to right coronary artery 12 years after operation, displaying all features of graft disease including stenosis, ulceration, aneurysmal dilatation (*arrow*), elongation, and tortuosity. Risk of embolization spontaneously or at time of manipulation is indisputable in such grafts

show multiple signs of advanced disease such as irregular lining, ulcers, elevated irregular plaques, dilatation, spurs, conventional stenoses, clefts, and thrombi [37–39] (Fig. 2). In fact, more than 50% of the patent grafts show these changes, so that only 20%–25% of vein grafts appear intact, i.e., patent with smooth lining (Fig. 3). The atheroma is friable and may embolize. The incidence of embolic events is probably underestimated. Many patients present with unstable angina which may represent microscopic emboli from diseased grafts [30]. Embolization may also occur during manipulation at the time of operation or catheterization [40, 41].

Various surgical steps have been devised to avoid intraoperative manipulation of grafts [31]. In essence, the current emphasis is on minimal dissection prior to cardiopulmonary bypass, the use of retrograde cardioplegia, transection of the diseased grafts before manipulation, and completion of the distal anastomosis and the performance of the proximal anastomosis under aortic clamping (to avoid ischemia in the area dependent

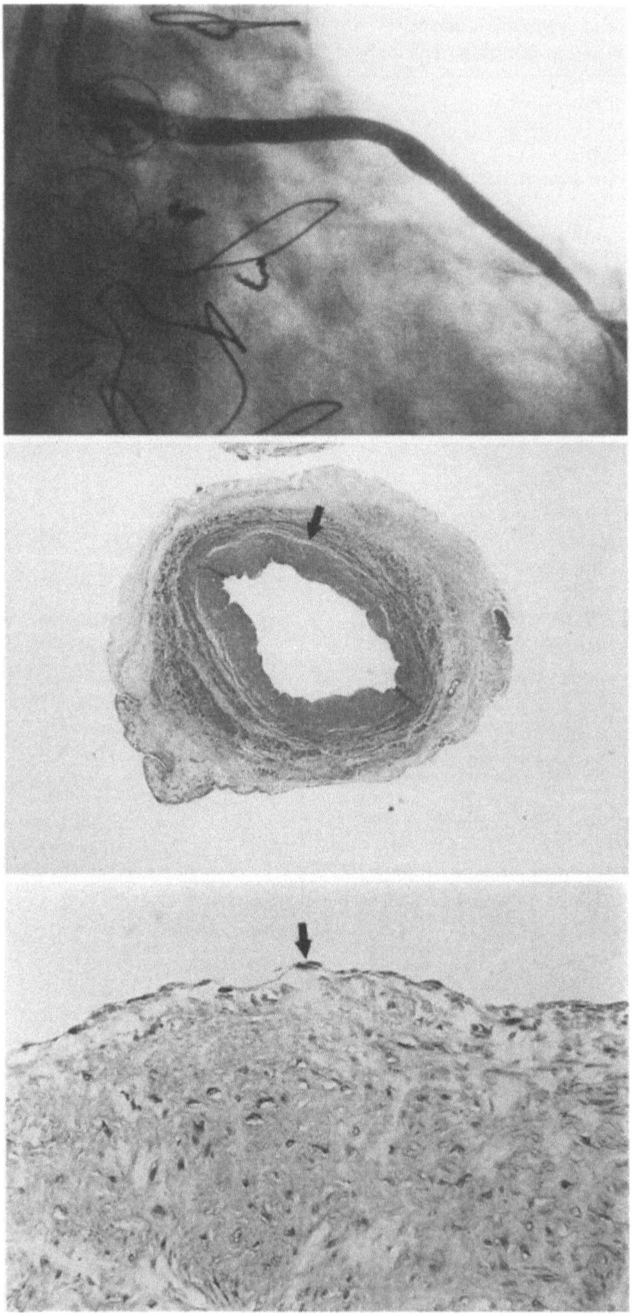

a

b

c

Fig. 3. **a** Graft to left anteriory descending artery (LAD) 10 years after operation in a patient who needed replacement of biological aortic valve prosthesis. Note perfect contours. Graft was removed prophylactically and replaced with LIMA. **b** Histology of LAD graft (same patient) showing mild intimal fibrous hyperplasia (*arrow* limits intima). Graft was grossly normal: soft, thin-walled with shiny intimal surface. **c** High-power view of intima showing absence of foam cells and other signs of atherosclerosis. Note endothelial cell (*arrow*) on old transected grafts). Mortality and morbidity are thus diminished significantly [29]. Angioplasty of these grafts (or grafts older than 5–6 years) is also fraught with danger [41].

In summary, several reports on late patency of SV grafts indicate that at 10 years nearly 50% of grafts have become occluded, i.e., between the first and tenth years 30–40 grafts of 100 become occluded, in addition to the 15–20 which occlude during the first year [38, 42, 43].

Factors Responsible for Late Graft Occlusion

Graft flow, runoff, and technique have little effect on late (10-year) graft patency [42]. On the other hand, the relationship with lipid profile is strong. Plasma levels of low-density lipoprotein are higher, and high-density lipoprotein (HDL) is lower in patients with graft disease and progression of disease in nongrafted vessels [44]. Smoking has also been linked to graft disease and decreased postoperative survival [45, 46].

Although occlusion at 10 years is believed to be the result of progression of graft disease that took root in the preceding 5 years, absolute proof of this sequence of events is not available in a significant number of patients. Indeed, grafts which appear normal at 5 years may become occluded at 10 years without angiographic demonstration of graft disease in the intervening years [38]. However, since at 5 years 15%–35% of patent grafts display signs of atherosclerosis [25, 37], it is logical to hold this process responsible for late occlusion. Indeed, in one series 60% of grafts displaying atherosclerosis at 5 years showed progression (more diffuse disease, more severe narrowing) of the disease at 10 years, and an additional 30% became occluded [38]. Occlusion, on the other hand, may be sudden secondary to thrombosis or to hemorrhage into a ruptured plaque with formation of an occluding flap. All this can occur in a graft that might have shown little or no disease on a recent earlier study. Further, about one-third of the 25% of grafts harbor significant disease or occlusion within 3 years in our study [47], and in a more recent report only 70 (25%) of an original group of 278 grafts found free of disease at 5 years remained so 5 years later [38]. Thus, freedom from disease at 5 or at 10 years constitutes no guarantee of trouble-free years ahead.

On the other hand, many surgeons, cardiologists, and angiographers can recall patients with perfectly normally appearing grafts at angiography 10–12 years after operation who developed occlusive disease in nongrafted arteries or in the left main coronary artery and required operation, only to be found to have pristine (as suggested at angiography) vein grafts, i.e., soft and thin throughout their length at operation, and for whom the wise decision was ultimately not to tamper. There are too few such examples to draw meaningful conclusions on these patients' habits (e.g., eating or exercise), their lipid profile, or the precise technique, if different, that lead to such fortunate and rare outcomes.

Future of Saphenous Vein Grafting

From this review, one could conclude that with time and notable exception all vein grafts used in the aortocoronary circuit will fail and few will exceed 20 years. On the other hand, sufficient progress has been made in risk factor management and surgical technique for hope to persist. A large trial is underway in multiple North American centers (grouping several of the original CASS centers and sponsored by NHLBI) which looks at the effect of lowering serum cholesterol, low dose anticoagulation, and other risk containment. Angiographic and clinical results should become available in 1996. Further, the use of arterial grafts is spreading. In addition to the internal mammary artery, whose excellent long-term patency and freedom from disease has been documented [48], other arterial grafts such as the gastroepiploic [49], the inferior epigastric [50], and the radial artery [51] are currently being used and studied. On our own service, in 1991, 32% of patients receiving multiple grafts had at least two arteries bypassed with arterial conduits. This percentage may be higher in other centers. Excellent early patency rates have been reported with the right gastroepiploic (no late results available at this writing) and the inferior epigastric artery [52] (patency rate of the latter at 1 year appears equal to that of free internal mammary artery grafts, i.e., $\geqslant$80%). On the other hand, the SV will continue to be utilized since arterial grafts are not likely to become the sole conduits in all patients. It remains to be seen whether technical advances such as those advocated by Mills and his group [53] (removal of all venous valves) and Angelini and coworkers [54] (performance of proximal anastomosis first, said to preserve endothelial function), and Boncek [55] (abstention from mechanical distension of the vein) will prevent or delay occlusion/disease of vein grafts. Experimental evidence of these refinements awaits clinical confirmation in man. Efficacy of cholesterol lowering agents as suggested in recent reports [56, 57] also await further confirmation.

References

1. Kunlin J (1949) Le traitement de l'arterite obliterante par la greffe veineuse (1949). Arch Mal Coeur 42:371–379
2. Garrett HE, Dennis EW, DeBakey ME (1973) Aorto coronary bypass with saphenous vein: a 7 year angiographic follow-up. JAMA 223:792–796
3. Grondin CM, Campeau L, Thornton JC, Engle JC, Cross FS, Schreiber H (1989) Coronary artery bypass grafting with the saphenous vein. Circulation 79(I):24–29

4. LiCalzi LK, Stansel HC (1982) Failure of autogenous reversed saphenous vein femoropopliteal grafting. Pathophysiology and Prevention. Surgery 91:352–359
5. Szilagyi DE, Elliott JP, Hageman JH, Smith RF, Dall'olmo CA (1973) Biologic fate of autogenous vein implants as arterial substitute. Ann Surg 178:232–240
6. Stanley JC, Ernest CB, Fry WJ (1973) Fate of 100 aortorenal vein grafts. Characteristics of late graft expansion, aneurysmal dilatation and stenosis. Surgery 74:937–946
7. Milroy CM, Scott JA, Beard JD, Horrocks M, Bradfield JW (1989) Histological appearance of the long saphenous vein. J Pathol 159:311–316
8. Fuchs JCA, Mitchener JS, Hagen P (1978) Postoperative changes in autologous vein grafts. Ann Surg 188:1–15
9. Brody WR, Kosek JC, Angell WW (1972) Changes in vein grafts following aorto-coronary bypass induced by pressure and ischemia. J Thor Cardiovasc Surg 64:847–854
10. Groves HM, Kinlough-Rathbone RL, Richardson M, Moore S, Mustard JF (1979) Platelet interactions with damaged rabbit aorta. Lab Invest 40:194–200
11. Packham MA, Mustard JF (1986) The role of platelets in the development and complications of atherosclerosis. Semin Hematol 23:8–26
12. Barboriak JJ, Pintar K, Korns ME (1974) Atherosclerosis in aorto coronary vein grafts. Lancet 2:621–624
13. Bulkley BH, Hutchins GM (1977) Accelerated atherosclerosis: a morphological study in 97 saphenous vein grafts. Circulation 55:163–169
14. Kalan JM, Roberts WC (1990) Morphological findings in saphenous veins used as coronary arterial bypass conduits for longer than one year: necropsy analysis of 53 patients, 123 saphenous veins. Am Heart J 119:1164–1184
15. Unni KK, Kottke BA, Titus JL, Frye RL, Wallace RB, Brown AL (1974) Pathologic changes in aortocoronary saphenous vein grafts. Am J Cardiol 34:526–532
16. Grondin CM, Lesperance J, Bourassa MG, Pasternac A, Campeau L, Grondin P (1974) Serial angiographic evaluation in 60 consecutive patients with aorto-coronary artery vein grafts 2 weeks, 1 year and 3 years after operation. J Thorac Cardiovasc Surg 67:1–6
17. Malone JM, Kischer CW, Moore WS (1981) Changes in venous endothelial fibrinolytic activity and histology with in vitro venous distension and arterial implantation. Am J Surg 142:178–186
18. DeMey JG, Vanhoutte PM (1982) Heterogenous behavior of the canine arterial and venous wall. Importance of the endothelium. Circ Res 51:439–446
19. Henderson VJ, Cohen RG, Mitchell RS, Kosek JC, Miller DC (1986) Biochemical (functional) adaptation of "arterialized" vein grafts. Ann Surg 203:339–345
20. Shafi S, Palinski W, Born GVR (1987) Comparison of uptake and degredation of low density lipoproteins by arteries and veins of rabbits. Atherosclerosis 66:131–138
21. Vlodaver Z, Edwards JE (1972) Pathologic analysis in fatal cases following saphenous vein coronary arterial bypass. Chest 64:555–563
22. Movat HZ, More RH, Haust MD (1958) The diffuse intimal thickening of the human aorta with aging. Am J Pathol 34:1023–1030
23. Velican C, Velican D (1976) Intimal thickening in developing coronary arteries and its relevance to atherosclerotic involvement. Atherosclerosis 23:345–355
24. Sims FH (1983) A comparison of coronary and internal mammary arteries and implications of the results in the etiology of arteriosclerosis. Am Heart J 105:560–566
25. Fitzgibbon GM, Leach AJ, Keon WJ, Burton JR, Kafka HP (1986) Coronary bypass graft fate: angiographic study of 1179 vein grafts early, one year and five years after operation. J Thorac Cardiovasc Surg 91:773–778
26. Ratliff NB, Myles JL (1989) Rapidly progressive atherosclerosis in aorto coronary saphenous vein grafts. Arch Pathol Lab Med 113:772–780
27. Teja K, Dillingham R, Mentzer RM (1987) Saphenous vein aneurysm after aorto coronary bypass grafting: postoperative interval and hyperlipidemia as determining factors. Am Heart J 113:1527–1529

28. Walts AE, Fishbein MC, Matloff JM (1987) Thrombosed, ruptured atheromatous plaques in saphenous vein coronary artery bypass grafts: ten year's experience. AM Heart J 114:718–723
29. Grondin CM (1986) Graft disease in patients with coronary bypass grafting. Why does it start? Where do we stop? J Thorac Cardiovasc Surg 92:323–329
30. Lytle BW, Loop FD, Taylor PC, Simpfendorfer C, Kramer Jr, Ratliff NB, Goormastic M, Cosgrove DM (1992) Vein graft disease: the clinical impact of stenosis in saphenous vein bypass grafts to coronary arteries. J Thorac Cardiovasc Surg 103:831–840
31. Grondin CM, Pomar JL, Hebert Y, Bosch Y, Santos JM, Enjalbert M, Campean L (1984) Reoperation in patients with patent atherosclerotic coronary vein grafts, a different approach to a different disease. J Thorac Cardiovasc Surg 87:379–385
32. Walker JA, Friedberg HD, Flemma RJ, Johnson WD (1972) Determinants of angiographic patency of aortocoronary vein bypass grafts. Circulation 45(I):86–92
33. Grondin CM, Castonguay YR, Lesperance J, Bourassa MG, Campeau L, Grondin P (1972) Attrition rate of aortocoronary vein grafts after one year. Ann Thorac Surg 14: 223–231
34. Grondin CM, Lepage G, Castonguay YR, Meere C, Grondin P (1971) Aortocoronary bypass graft. Initial blood flow through the graft and early postoperative patency. Circulation 44:815–819
35. Campeau L, Crochet D, Lesperance J, Bourassa MG, Grondin CM (1975) Postoperative changes in aortocoronary saphenous vein grafts revised. Angiographic studies at 2 weeks and at 1 year in two consecutive series of patients. Circulation 52:369–377
36. Fuster V, Cheseboro JH (1985) Aortocoronary artery vein-graft disease. Experimental and clinical approach for the understanding of the role of platelets and platelet inhibitors. Circulation 72(II):65–70
37. Grondin CM, Campeau L, Lesperance J, Solymos BC, Vouhe P, Castonguay YR, Meere C, Bourassa MG (1979) Atherosclerotic changes in coronary vein grafts six years after operation. J Thorac Cardiovasc Surg 77:24–31
38. FitzGibbons GM, Leach AJ, Kafka HP, Keon WJ (1991) Coronary bypass graft fate: long-term angiographic study. J Am Coll Cardiol 17:1075–1080
39. Campeau L, Enjalbert M, Lesperance J, Vaislic C, Grondin CM, Bourassa MG (1983) Atherosclerosis and late closure of aortocoronary saphenous vein grafts: sequential angiographic studies 2 weeks, 1 year, 5 to 7 years, and 10 to 12 years after surgery. Circulation 68(II):1–9
40. Keon WJ, Heggvetit HA, Leduc J (1982) Perioperative myocardial infarction caused by atheroembolism. J Thorac Cardiovasc Surg 84:849–855
41. Platko WP, Hollman J, Whitlow PL, Franco I (1989) Percutaneous transluminal angioplasty of saphenous vein graft stenosis: long term follow-up. J Am Coll Cardiol 14:1645–1650
42. Grondin CM, Campeau L, Lesperance J, Enjalbert M, Bourassa MG (1984) Comparison of late changes in internal mammary artery and saphenous vein grafts in two consecutive series of patients 10 years after operation. Circulation 70(I):208–212
43. Lytle BW, Loop FD, Cosgrove DM, Easley K, Taylor PC (1983) Long-term sequential studies of internal mammary artery and saphenous vein coronary bypass grafts. Circulation 68(III):114–120
44. Campeau L, Enjalbert M, Lesperance J, Bourassa MG, Kwiterovich P, Wacholder S, Sniderman A (1984) The relationship of risk factors to the development of atherosclerosis is saphenous vein bypass grafts and the progression of disease in the native circulation. A study 10 years after surgery. N Engl J Med 311:1329–1332
45. FitzGibbons GM, Leach AJ, Kafka HP (1987) Atherosclerosis of coronary artery bypass grafts and smoking. Can Med Assoc J 136:45–47
46. Cavender JB, Rogers WJ, Fisher LD, Gersh BJ, Coggin CJ, Myers WO (1992) Effect of smoking on survival and morbidity in patients randomized to medical or surgical therapy in the Coronary Artery Surgery Study (CASS): a 10 year follow-up. J Am Coll Cardiol 20:287–294

47. Grondin CM (1986) The removal of still functioning albeit old grafts: not in our genes? Ann Thorac Surg 42:122–123
48. Grondin CM (1984) Late results of coronary artery grafting: is there a flag on the field? J Thorac Cardiovasc Surg 87:161–166
49. Pym J, Brown PM, Charette EP, Parker JO, West RO (1987) Gastroepiploic – coronary anastomosis. J Thorac Cardiovasc Surg 94:256–259
50. Puig LB, Ciongolli W, Cividanes GV, Dontos A, Kopell, Bittencourt D, Assis V, Jatene A (1990) Inferior epigastric artery as a free graft for myocardial revascularization. J Thorac Cardiovasc Surg 99:251–255
51. Acar C, Jebara VA, Portoghese M, Dervanian P, DeSouza M, Chachques C, Fabiani JN, Deloche A, Carpentier A (1992) The radial artery for coronary bypass operations: revival of an old conduit. Ann Thorac Surg 54 (in press)
52. Buche M, Schoevaerdts JC, Louagie Y, Schroeder E, Marchandise B, Chenn P, Dion R, Verhelst R, Delos M, Gonzales E, Chalant CH (1992) Use of the inferior epigastric artery for coronary bypass. J Thorac Cardiovasc Surg 103:665–670
53. Mills NL, Ochsner JL (1976) Valvulotomy of valves in the saphenous vein graft before coronary artery bypass. J Thorac Cardiovasc Surg 71:878–879
54. Angelini GD, Breckenridge IM, Williams HM, Newby AC (1987) A surgical preparative technique for coronary bypass grafts of human saphenous vein which preserves medial and endothelial functional integrity. J Thorac Cardiovasc Surg 94:393–398
55. Bonchek LI (1980) Prevention of endothelial damage during preparation of saphenous vein for bypass grafting. J Thorac Cardiovasc Surg 79:911–915
56. Blankenhorn DH, Nessini SA, Johnson RL, Sanmarco ME, Azen SP, Cashin-Hemphill L (1987) Beneficial effects of combined colestipol-niacin therapy on coronary atherosclerosis and coronary venous bypass grafts. JAMA 257:3233–3240
57. Brown G, Alberts JJ, Fisher LD, Schaefer BA, Lin JT, Kaplan C, Zhao X-Q, Bisson BD, Fitzpatrick VF, Dodge HT (1990) Regression of coronary artery disease as a result of intensive lipid-lowering therapy in men with high levels of apolipoprotein B. N Engl J Med 323:1289–1298

Risks and Prediction of Adverse Events After Coronary Bypass Grafting Based on a Single Center Experience

P. Sergeant

Introduction

This chapter discusses four clinical cardiac events after coronary bypass surgery. Their prevalence over time is presented, and, where possible, events are related to graft failure using the incremental risk factors active in the different phases of activity of these events.

Every patient is situated within his own multivariate environment, and, in particular, he is subjected to external influences such as pharmacological regimens and dietary and smoking habits. Internal influences such as lipid metabolism, insulin-dependent diabetes, and hypertension are also important components of this multivariate environment. An additional problem is that these influences and their interactions are not constant but changing over time. It therefore becomes essential that events after a certain treatment for coronary pathology be studied in a time-related manner and using multivariate methods. The immediate limitations in studying these events are evident and most frequently due to the absence of variables identifying these internal and external influences and the difficulty of interpretating this information. It is possible that the resumption of smoking after surgery enhances the progression of graft disease and failure; this then represents a time-related covariant. It is easy to determine whether or not the patient resumed smoking, but if he has, it is unlikely that he does so at a constant level. More likely, he stopped for a certain number of months after surgery then resumed smoking gradually, then stopped again, resumed at a different level, and stopped again, etc. The quantification and interpretation of this information is virtually impossible. This chapter presents only pre- and perioperative information as incremental risk factors in an attempt to explain postoperative events, although most of this postoperative information is available in the Katholieke Universiteit of Leuven Coronary Surgery Database [1, 2].

The primary analyses [3, 4], including that of the multivariate risk factors, were carried out parametrically in a time-related manner [5]. In the figures a solid line represents the solution of the independently determined parametric equation for freedom from the event, with thinner lines enclosing the 70% confidence limits. In the identification of incremental risk factors a *p* value of less than 0.05 was required for inclusion of a variable in the final multivariate models. The analyses identified patient, surgical procedure, and graft-related risk factors. Appendix A lists the variables selected for entering into the analyses, but many more were tested in extensive univariate and multivariate explorations since various transformations of ordinal or continuous variables (logarithmic, exponential, power, inverse) were used to represent the shape of the relationship of the variable to the distribution of events, and extensive interactions among the variables were explored. Since the data set is representative [6] of surgical practice from 1971–1987, this study permitted evaluation of variables unavailable in most databases because of patient exclusion criteria. The nature of the models used in the analysis was such that probability and hazard function estimates can be obtained for exploration of the shape and strength of the risk factors and for making patient-specific predictions.

The Studied Events

Four events were studied and their possible relationship to the grafts used or to the method of use of these grafts: death by any mode, freedom from any ischemic symptom, freedom from first reoperation, and freedom from first reintervention. Angina after surgery for coronary artery bypass graft (CABG) was the return of new, even minimal, angina pectoris, without an infarct or death the same day. Myocardial infarction included only the first fatal or nonfatal post-CABG infarction, excluding perioperative infarcts (those occuring during the hospital stay that could reasonably be attributed to cardiac surgery). Sudden death was unexpected sudden death in a patient in generally good health who might previously have had return of angina or even a post-CABG infarct. The first ischemic event was defined as the earliest occurrence of any of these three ischemic events. Reoperation was defined as repeat coronary surgery, mitral value surgery for ischemic disease, or cardiac transplantation. Reintervention was either percutaneous transluminal coronary angioplasty (PTCA) or reoperation sometime during follow-up. For the nonfatal events, surviving patients not experiencing the event by the end of their follow-up, were evaluated at the date of last follow-up or death.

Death by Any Mode

The study population was a consecutive series of 5880 patients operated on for isolated primary CABG surgery at the Katholieke Universiteit of Leuven in Belgium from 1971 to 1987. Repeat procedures were excluded for statistical reasons, but the first operation was included if it had been performed

Table 1. Results of CABG surgery using IMA and venous graft material

	Bilateral IMA grafts ± veins	Single IMA grafts ± veins	Only venous grafts	Total
Alive at follow-up				
Number	259	2444	2634	5337
Percentage	4	42	45	91
Row percentage	5	46	49	–
Column percentage	94	95	87	–
Death				
Number	17	129	397	543
Percentage	0.3	2	7	9
Row percentage	3	24	73	–
Column percentage	6	5	13	–
Total				
Number	276	2573	3031	5880
Percentage	5	44	52	100

at our institution. A cross-sectional follow-up study was made of all patients in November 1987.

Table 1 describes the results of surgery using the internal mammary artery (IMA). Only 9% of the patients died between surgery and the end of follow-up. Differentiation by the grafts used demonstrates that only 6% of the bilateral-IMA patients died and 5.0% of the single IMA patients but 13% of the venous grafts only patients. The chi-square statistic, likelihood ratio chi-square, and Mantel-Haenszel chi-square all have values below 0.0001. The elation that one might feel over the success of using single and bilateral IMAs is dampened by the fact that this analysis is univariate and not time related and is therefore totally inappropriate. This method of analysis does not consider how long each patient had been at risk of death when he died, or how these differed from the surviving patients. A univariate actuarial survival analysis (Fig. 1) of the populations with and without an IMA graft in addition to venous material suggests the relationship of death to time and the possible benefit of using of the IMA. Furthermore, although this analysis is time related, the data may be biased by the multivariate climate of the patient and his environment. It could very well be that only young patients with good ventricular function received IMA bypasses, and that the elderly with bad ventricular function were grafted using venous material.

A time-related multivariate analysis is therefore necessary. In a first step death after CABG surgery was analyzed over time. The 1-, 5-, 10-, and 15-year parametric survival rates of the study population were 97%, 93%, 81%, and 57%, respectively (Fig. 2). These data are interesting as basic information for quality control purposes but are scientifically irrelevant because they depend on the study population and the presence of risk

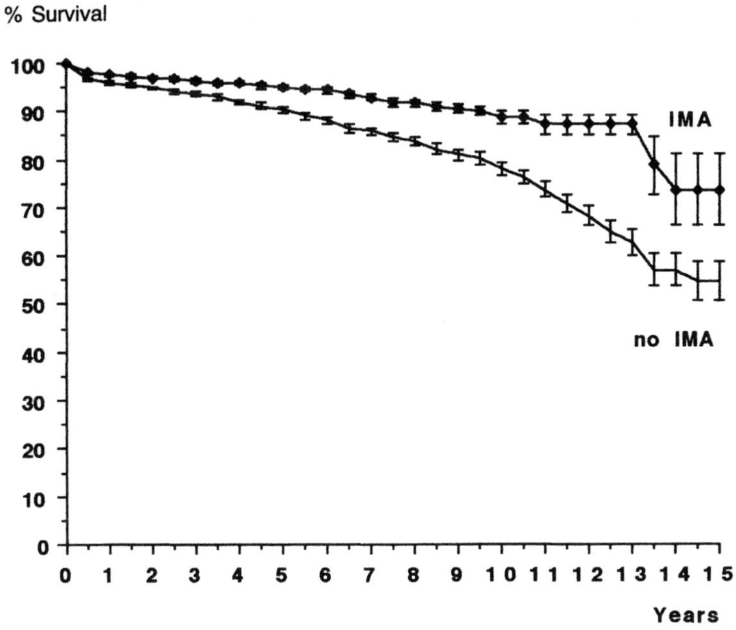

Fig. 1. Total survival after CABG surgery: univariate analysis by use of IMA regardless of other graft material used

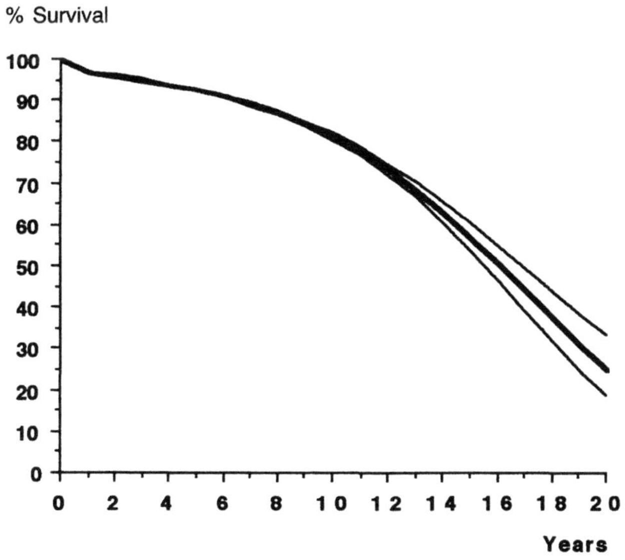

Fig. 2. Parametric survival of the total study population (n = 5880). *Solid line*, the solution of the independently determined parametric equation for freedom from the event; *thinner lines*, 70% confidence limits

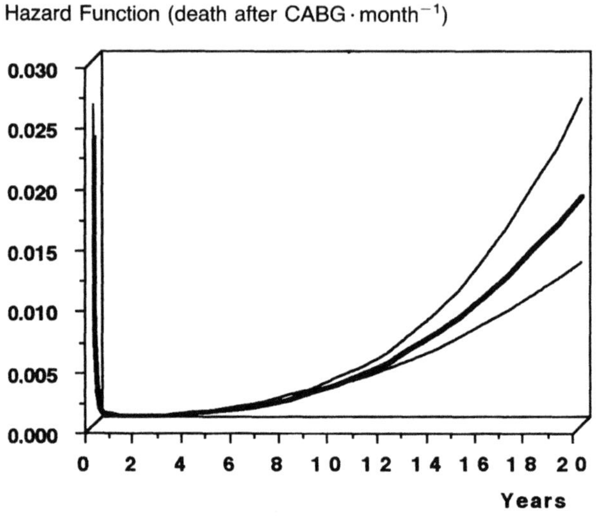

Fig. 3. Hazard function for death after CAGB surgery, representing the immediate risk of dying by any means, on the condition that the patient survives

factors in this population. More information is provided by the hazard function for death (Fig. 3). In this Figure only the form of the curve is interesting, not the values on the vertical axis, since these values are, again, influenced by the presence or absence of risk factors in the study population. Figure 3 demonstrates that the instantaneous risk of dying over 20 years after coronary surgery is not constant but changes over time. The analysis identifies three phases, which are sometimes present simultaneously: (a) an early phase from the start of anaesthesia but declining in effect to 1.25 years after surgery when it ceases to be present; (b) a constant phase from the start of anaesthesia and present with similar strength to the end of the study interval; and (c) a late phase starting a minimal influence at around 3 years after surgery and increasing in influence to the end of the study period. The second most important feature from this information is that the analysis can now identify risk factors present in each phase (Table 2, "Appendix B").

The interpretation of this information requires information about the selection process of risk factors in multivariate analyses. The absence of a risk factor may be due to three reasons: the variable can have no influence, the information residual in the variable is better expressed in a variable that is already selected, or there are no patients with this variable at risk in a certain phase. These different possibilities are discussed further in the analysis of the influence of the use and method of use of graft material on total survival.

The use and method of graft material can reduce but also increase risk; therefore, in addition to the presence of this information, data on the influence of variables identifying the graft material are important.

Table 2. The incremental risk factors active in each phase for death by any means at any time after CABG surgery

	Early hazard	Constant hazard	Late hazard
Age			
Higher	*		*
Lower			*
Coexisting condition			
Worse pulmonary function	*		*
Elevated lipid values (HDL triglycerides)		*	*
Presence of insulin-treated diabetes	*		*
Coronary disease and distribution			
Presence of left main stenosis >90%	*		
Extension of vessel disease			*
Presence of smaller coronary vessels	*		*
Left ventricular function			
Lower ejection fraction	*	*	*
Worse hemodynamic instability	*		
Presence of left ventricular hypertrophy	*		
Presence of mitral insufficiency		*	
Preoperative angina			
Higher anginal class	*	*	
Atherosclerotic disease			
Presence of peripheral vascular disease	*	*	*
Surgical factors			
High-risk surgeon	*		
Earlier date of surgery	*		
Presence of coronary endarterectomy	*		
Higher ratio of distal to proximal anastomoses	*		
Presence of incomplete revascularization		*	
Nonuse of IMA			*

The use and method of the IMA covers a 16-year period down to 1971 and is not at all representative of current practice at the our institution. At least one IMA, excluding the free grafts, was used after 1972 and in 2849 patients from this study material. The left IMA was used in 2837 patients and the right in 289. The IMA revascularized the left anterior descending (LAD) system in 2469 patients and another system in 341 patients. The ages of the patients with or without an IMA bypass were almost identical (albeit statistically different with IMA 55 ± 8 years, without IMA 56 ± 8 years, $p = 0.0001$), but the age range was similar (25–82 years with IMA and 23–79 without). There was no difference in sex distribution. There has been a tendency to limit the use of IMAs in patients with restricted pulmonary function. The following data demonstrate that this is not a correct decision, and that pulmonary dysfunction is no contraindication for IMA surgery. The vital capacity percentage pulmonary function and 1-s percentage values of the patients with or without an IMA differed (with

IMA, vital capacity 94% ± 13%, 1-s 96% ± 15%; without IMA vital capacity 90% ± 13%. 1-s 90% ± 15%, $p = 0.0001$), but the ranges were, again, similar. The distribution by ventricular function also differed ($p < 0.01$). An IMA graft was constructed, respectively, in 47%, 52%, 47%, and 40% of the patients with a normal, slightly reduced, moderately reduced, and very bad ventricular function. Although the mean values and ranges are very similar, it is clear that the populations with or without an IMA graft were different.

The multivariate parametric model (Table 2, Figs. 2, 3) selected the nonuse of IMA as incremental risk factor for the late phase, without the specification right or left or of the area reperfused by the graft. The benefit from a single IMA is seen only after a few months and differs for each patient because it depends on the presence of the risk factors which are active in the early and constant phase, i.e. before a possible benefit of the IMA. It is therefore impossible to depict this benefit for a whole population; however, the parametric methodology allows a patient-specific prediction using the patient's own values for the incremental risk factors. This also helps us later to understand the possible benefit of multiple IMA grafting.

A first patient-specific prediction (Fig. 4a) confirms the benefit of a single IMA graft, whatever graft material is used for the other distal anastomoses, in a given patient A with minimal risk factors. Patient A is defined as aged 65 years, no diabetes, stable angina before surgery, no peripheral vascular surgery, triple-vessel disease, minimal ventricular dysfunction due to a single preoperative infarct, no left ventricular hypertrophy, and no coronary endarterectomy. The 5-, 10-, and 15-year survival rates are 94%, 67%, and 24%, and 97%, 87%, and 66%, respectively, without and with an IMA graft. The differences are very impressive. Since virtually no risk factors are active in the early or the constant phase, the even minimal early benefit of IMA grafting is very apparent.

A second patient-specific prediction (Fig. 4b) validates the benefit of a single IMA graft, whatever graft material is used for the other distal anastomoses, in a given patient B with similar risk factors as patient A but inaccurate ventricular dysfunction. Patient B is defined as aged 66 years, no diabetes, stable angina before surgery, no peripheral vascular surgery, triple-vessel disease, ejection fraction (EF) of 45%, no left ventricular hypertrophy (LVH), and no coronary endarterectomy. The 5-, 10-, and 15-year survival results are 89%, 53%, and 9%, and 93%, 77%, and 45%, respectively, without and with an IMA graft. The survival results have deteriorated here considerably, but the benefit of the IMA grafting is still present. Due to the diminished ventricular function, present in all phases (also in the late phase), the minimal early benefit of IMA grafting is not evident.

A third patient-specific prediction (Fig. 4c) confirms the benefit of a single IMA graft, whatever other graft material is used for the other distal anastomoses, in a given patient C with similar risk factors as patient B but much older. Patient C is defined as aged 75 years, no diabetes, stable angina

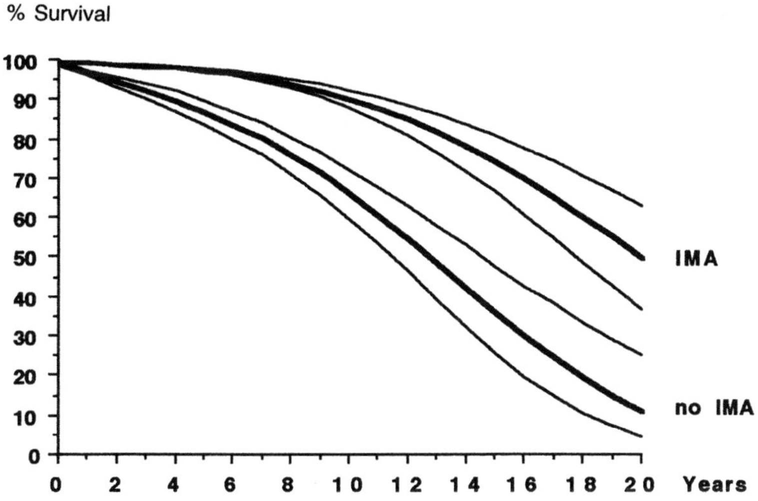

a

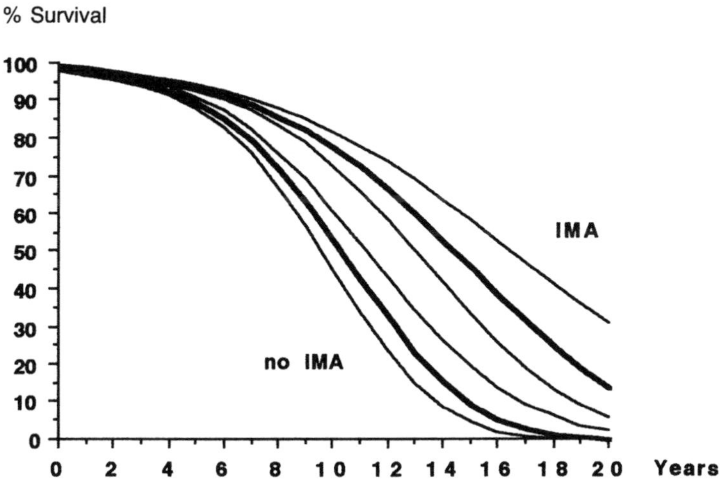

b

Fig. 4a–c. Patient-specific total post-CABG survival of patients A (**a**), B (**b**), and C (**c**) with and without an IMA graft. **a** Patient A = 65 years, no diabetes, stable angina, no peripheral vascular surgery, triple vessel disease, slight ventricular dysfunction due to infarct, no LVH, no endarterectomy. **b** Patient B = 66 years, no diabetes, stable angina, no peripheral vascular surgery, triple vessel disease, EF 45%, no LVH, no endarterectomy

before surgery, no peripheral vascular surgery, triple-vessel disease, ejection fraction of 45%, no left ventricular hypertrophy, and no coronary endarterectomy. The 5-, 10-, and 15-year survival results are 84%, 24%, and 0%, and 91%, 61%, and 17%, respectively, without and with an IMA graft. The

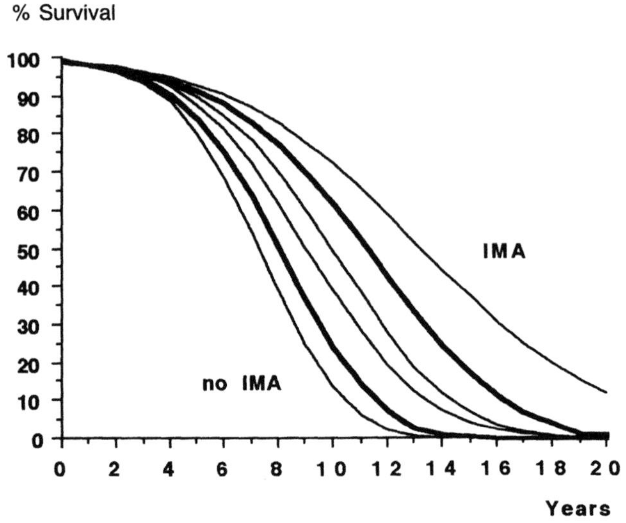

c

Fig. 4. c. Patient C = 75 years, no diabetes, stable angina before surgery, no peripheral vascular surgery, triple vessel disease, EF 45%, no LVH, no endarterectomy

increased benefit of IMA grafting against patients A and B indicates that, even with expected unfavorable survival in this 75-year-old hypothetical patient, an IMA anastomosis remains an essential element in his surgical treatment.

Table 2 also indicates that no deleterious effect, early or late, is found in the use of a single IMA since the variable did not enter the model with a risk-increasing effect in the early or late phase. Adding to the analysis interaction variables combining the effect of bad ventricular function and IMA grafting does not change the model.

Sequential IMA grafting [7] was started in 1978. A total of 439 patients (7.5% of the study population) had a double or triple IMA graft (excluding the free grafts). The following sequences of side-to-side and end-to-side anastomoses were used: LAD-LAD, Diag-Diag, Diag-LAD, Diag-Diag-LAD, Diag-Diag-Diag-LAD, Obt Marg-Diag, CX-CX, CX-CX-CX, and LAD-Diag. The range of the ages of the patients was 31–78 years. The distribution by ventricular function differed ($p < 0.01$) with, respectively, 9% and 1%, 12% and 1%, 10% and 1%, and 8% and 1% of the patients with a normal, slightly reduced, moderately reduced, or very bad ventricular function with two and three IMA anastomoses. Sequential IMA grafting was not retained in the model with a total mortality increasing effect. No additional benefit was found in addition to that from a single IMA graft. Is there then no possible benefit from sequential IMA grafting? All patients with sequential IMA grafting were at risk of a risk-increasing effect in the early phase, but the maximum available follow-up was only 9 years, and only the few patients operated on in 1979 and 1980 with this technique really had a benefit. It is therefore possible that the patient population was underpowered to demonstrate a possible benefit. Another possible explanation is that, as seen in patient A with his predicted 10-year survival of 87% using one IMA graft, there is very little room for possible additional benefit during the first 10 years in a patient with acceptable ventricular function.

Total mortality is divided in to equal proportions with cardiac and noncardiac mortality. Thus only 7% of patients with a profile similar to that of patient A die the first 10 years from cardiac causes. A single venous graft, even in the presence of one or more IMA grafts, that occludes may cause an infarct and death, as can a rhythm disturbance. In the patients with reduced ventricular function more benefit is possible, but probably not enough patients had the combination of impaired ventricular function, sequential IMA grafting, and enough follow-up in this database (underpowered number of patients). A new concept must be added in this search for possible benefits of multiple IMA anastomoses. Nearly all sequential IMA grafts are single-area, multiple IMA distals. It is very rare that multiple areas can be revascularized with a single in situ IMA graft. It is therefore more difficult to find an additional benefit for this surgical procedure.

Bilateral in situ IMA grafting was used in 276 patients in this database. The first bilateral IMA grafts were implanted in 1973, but this was only occasional, and a more routine use began in 1978. The surgical strategy until 1983–1985 was to graft the right IMA, in the 60% of the patients in whom it was used, to the LAD system, most frequently to a diagonal artery. The left IMA was grafted to the LAD system in 91% of the patients in whom it was used, most frequently to the LAD. Most of these patients therefore received single-area, bilateral IMA grafts. Since 1986 the right IMA has been used preferentially to the LAD and the left IMA to the circumflex system in a single or sequential mode. Bilateral IMA grafting was not retained in the model with a total mortality increasing effect, and no additional benefit was found in addition to that from a single IMA graft. This is probably due to a combination of factors. One is an insufficient (i.e. statistically underpowered) number of patients at risk in the periods during which an additional benefit could be present. As for sequential IMA grafting, there is very little room for improvement of the survival in the first 10 years after surgery in most patients with good ventricular function. A more appropriate use of both IMA grafts similar to our current strategy would probably increase the chances of bilateral IMA benefit in late survival in the 10–20 years after surgery.

Complete arterial (in situ) revascularization was achieved in 324 patients, but probably for similar reasons as for sequential and IMA grafting the variables identifying this information were not selected for the model of total survival.

Saphenous grafts were used in all patients in whom incomplete arterial revascularization was achieved. It is intriguing that a higher ratio of distal to proximal anastomoses was identified as increasing the early risk. In 1978–1984 it was routine to construct a single venous multiple jump graft revascularizing three or four lateral branches of the circumflex artery and ending on the posterior descending artery. Early occlusion of some of these grafts supplying a very large area at risk may explain negative early results. No late benefit of this extreme in sequential grafting was observed. High preoperative values of high-density lipoprotein levels reduce the constant risk of dying; low preoperative values of triglyceride levels reduce the late hazard of dying. Both of these lipid disorders (analyzed as absolute values of cholesterol and triglycerides) are probably responsible for progression of the atherosclerotic disease on the native grafted and non-grafted coronary vessels, but they are doubtless also present in the venous grafts. Medication treating one of these two lipid disorders can therefore have effect only on the constant or late phases after coronary surgery (see chapter by H. Drexel and F. Amman). An interesting element of the hazard function is the nearly exponential rise after 12–15 years. A similar effect is seen for most events after CABG surgery. It seems clear that this cannot be due only to progression, but that the attrition rate for graft failure increases rapidly during this period. This information forced us to replace, whereever possible with arterial reconstructions, all old venous grafts in repeat procedures.

Prosthetic grafts and cephalic veins have, as in most centers, been used only in exceptional circumstances, to the worst vessels. Nearly all of these grafts were occluded when these patients had early or late repeat angiograms, but this information is not very relevant.

Regardless of the graft material used, the method, the clinical, angiographical, and hemodynamic status of the patient, the experience or the routine of the center or the surgeon, a statistical difference was found between different surgeons. This difference was found only in the early hazard phase, and this is distressing and reassuring as well for the patient. The difference can be quantified by noting that the negative effect of a high-risk surgeon on death in the early phase is similar to that of the presence of insulin-treated diabetes in the operated patient.

Figure 3 indicates that improvement of surgical technique, whether for myocardial protection, choice and method of graft, or any other element of the operation, can still improve the results. Under ideal circumstances the early hazard phase should disappear. The late hazard phase could certainly be reduced in size and be lowered if a stricter lipid-intervention and anti-smoking protocol were followed by the patients (see chapters by H. Drexel and F. Amman and D. Seidel, this volume).

Freedom from First Ischemic Symptom Anytime After CABG Surgery

The 1-, 5-, 10-, and 15-year parametric freedom from first ischemic event for the total study population was 93%, 79%, 54%, and 21%, respect-

Table 3. The components of first post-CABG ischemic event

Type of event	*n*
Angina return	1053
Only	905[a]
Before post-CABG infarct	124[a]
Before sudden death	21[a]
Before post-CABM infarct and later sudden death	2[a]
After post-CABG infarct	1[a]
Post-CABG infarct	322
Only	192[a]
After angina return	124
After angina return, before sudden death	2
Before sudden death	3[a]
Before angina return	1[a]
Sudden death	78
Only	52[a]
After angina return	21
After post-CABG infarct	3
After angina return and post-CABG infarct	2

[a] These categories constitute the 1300 patients suffering a first ischemic event.

ively. Table 3 presents the components of the event first ischemic event (1453 events in 1300 patients). Figure 5 presents the parametric freedom from this event for the 5880 patients of the study population. Similarly as for total survival, this information is totally irrelevant for a particular patient with his specific risk factors. More information is found in the hazard function for this event of the study population (Fig. 6). Here only the form of the curve is interesting, not the values on the vertical axis, since these values are again influenced by the presence or absence of risk factors in the study population.

The analysis identifies three phases in the hazard function for this event: (a) an early phase starts in the 1st week after surgery, is at its peak effect 2 months after surgery, and returns to the level of the constant phase at 18 months; a constant phase is present from the 1st h and remains present with similar strength until the end of the study period; and (c) a late phase begins with a minimal effect around 3–4 years after surgery and increases in effect to the end of the study period. These phases are present simultaneously in some time periods. The immediate hazard for this event, on the condition that the patient stays alive, 15 years after surgery is nearly tenfold the hazard 1 year after surgery. As for death after CABG surgery, the analysis identifies risk factors periods in each phase (Table 4, "Appendix C").

A fourth patient-specific prediction quantifies the benefit of a single IMA graft to the LAD, whatever graft material is used for the other distal anastomoses, in patient D with minimal risk factors. Patient D was defined as aged 62 years, male, no diabetes, stable but fairly severe angina before

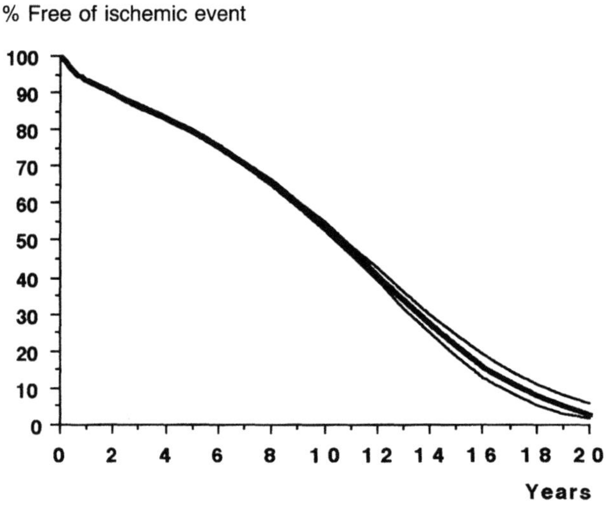

Fig. 5. Parametric freedom from first ischemic event for the total study population. *Solid line*, the solution of the independently determined parametric equation for freedom from the event; *thinner lines*, the 70% confidence limits

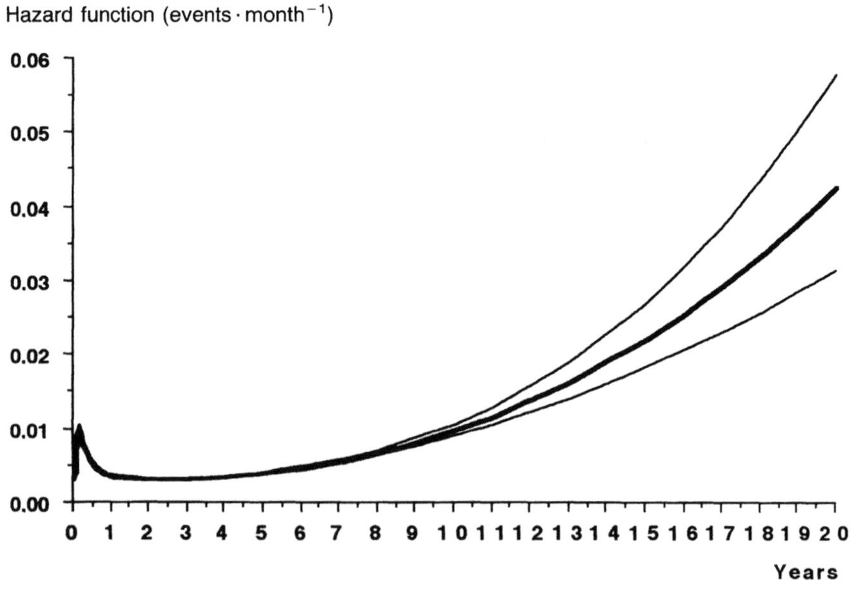

Fig. 6. Hazard function for return of ischemic events after CABG surgery, representing the immediate risk of return of clinical ischemia, on the condition that the patient survives

Table 4. Incremental risk factors for return of ischemic symptoms after CABG surgery

	Early hazard	Constant hazard	Late hazard
Younger age	*		
Female sex		*	
Coexisting condition			
Elevated lipid values (triglycerides)			*
Degree of diabetes			*
Presence of hypertension		*	
Coronary disease and distribution			
Absence of left main stenosis >50%		*	
Presence of smaller coronary vessels			*
Left ventricular function			
Higher left ventricular end-diastolic pressure		*	
Higher number of preoperative infarcts		*	
Worse hemodynamic instability	*		
Preoperative angina			
Higher anginal class	*	*	
Longer anginal history		*	*
Atherosclerotic disease			
Presence of peripheral vascular disease	*		
Presence of diseased aorta		*	
Presence of diffusely diseased vessels		*	
Surgical factors			
Higher-risk surgeon	*		
Higher ratio of distal to proximal anastomoses			*
Presence of incomplete revascularization	*		
Nonuse of IMA	*		

surgery, no peripheral vascular surgery, no hypertension, preoperative triglyceride level of 154 mg/dl, left ventricular end-diastolic pressure of 11 mmHg, and a low-risk surgeon. The 1-, 2-, and 3-year parametric freedom from first ischemic event were 97%, 95%, and 92%, and 98%, 95%, and 93%, respectively, without and with an IMA graft to the LAD. The 5-, 10-, and 15-year parametric freedom from first ischemic event was 86%, 60%, and 23%, and 87%, 60%, and 23%, respectively, without and with an IMA graft to the LAD (Fig. 7). It is clear that, with the techniques of surgery and postoperative dietary and medical regimens used in this database, all patients will have developed clinical signs of ischemia 20 years after surgery, if they stay alive. The differences with and without IMA, left or right, to the LAD are statistically significant but might appear very small. A more profound analysis of these differences is necessary before conclusions can be reached, however. Early graft failure and its time course becomes more apparent it presented as in Fig. 6. This early graft failure phase ends 1 year after surgery, and its level of hazard is only twice that in the constant phase. Therefore one can expect that the magnitude of the influence of a risk factor

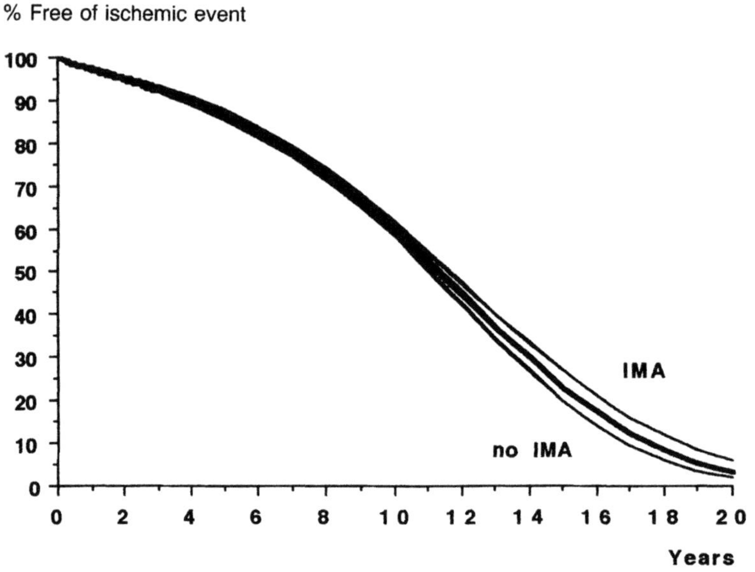

Fig. 7. The 1- to 20-year patient-specific freedom from post-CABG first ischemic event for patient D with and without an IMA graft to the LAD. Patient D = 62 years, male, no diabetes, severe angina, no peripheral vascular surgery, no hypertension, tryglicerides 145 mg/dl, LVEDP 11 mmHg, low risk surgeon

present in this phase to be only minimal, even if the effect is statistically very significant. In addition, most of the patients had nearly four distal anastomoses, consisting of a single IMA graft and further venous grafts. It is sufficient that one of these venous grafts should occlude for the patient to suffer a first ischemic symptom.

Bilateral single- or double-area IMA grafting and sequential mammary artery grafting were not selected as risk-reducing variables in this analysis, but we can anticipate where their influence should be seen. Multiple IMA grafting techniques will not affect progression of the disease, so their influence should not be expected in a late phase. A closer look at the early and constant phase is therefore needed. In the early phase they might enter the models, but their effect increase gradually as a function of the growing ratio of IMA anastomoses against venous anastomoses. Mathematically it can be expected that a patient with one IMA anastomosis in the presence of another single venous anastomosis would behave similarly in the early hazard phase for first ischemic return as a patient with two IMA anastomoses in the presence of two venous anastomoses. In patients with a complete arterial reconstruction and complete revascularization it is expected that the early phase should be absent, but the data do not confirm this. The constant phase, which is pronounced with this event, contains an element progression

Table 5. Results of post-CABG reintervention and reoperation using IMA

	Bilateral IMA grafts ± veins	Single IMA grafts ± veins	Only venous grafts	Total
PTCA				
Number	2	10	29	41
Percentage	1	5	15	21
Row percentage	5	24	71	
Column percentage	50	19	21	
PTCA + reoperation				
Number	0	3	3	6
Percentage	0	1.5	1.5	3
Row percentage	0	50	50	
Column percentage	0	5	2	
Reoperation				
Number	2	42	103	147
Percentage	1	22	53	76
Row percentage	1	29	70	
Column percentage	50	76	76	
Total				
Number	4	55	135	194
Percentage	2	28	70	100

and an attrition rate of graft failure. For this reason an influence of extensive IMA grafting should be seen in this phase.

Freedom from Reintervention and Reoperation After CABG Surgery

Reoperation as an event combines the coronary repeat procedures, mitral valve reconstructions or replacements for ischemic disease, and cardiac transplantations. The event reintervention combines PTCA and reoperations after CABG surgery. Table 5 presents the distribution of the type of reintervention by the use of IMA. The chi-square of the data is 0.4690 and the likelihood ratio chi-square 0.524. Since 55% of the cells had expected counts less than 5, the chi-square may not be a valid test. The limitations of univariate non-time-related analysis are, once more, undeniable and will be solved by using new multivariate time-related methodologies.

The 1-, 5-, 10-, and 15-year parametric freedom from first post-CABG reoperation for the total population was 99%, 98%, 93%, and 74%, respectively. Figure 8 presents the parametric freedom from this event for the 5880 patients of the study population. The hazard function for this event is more informative (Fig. 9). In this depiction only the form of the curve is interesting, not the values on the vertical axis, since these values are again influenced by the presence or absence of risk factors in the study population. Figure 9 demonstrates again that the immediate risk of return of ischemic

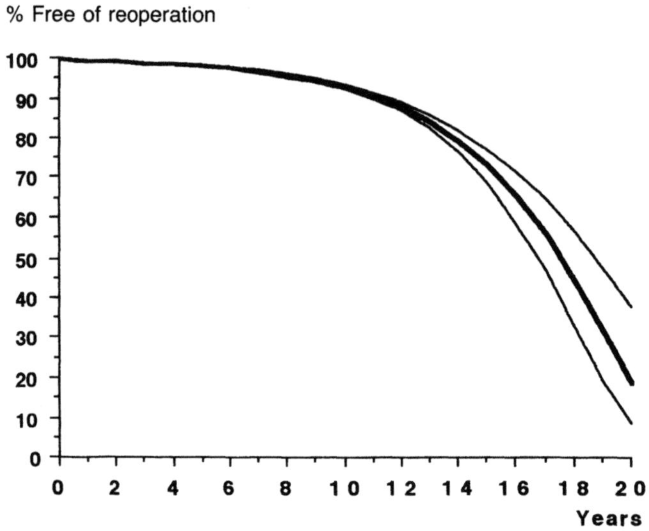

Fig. 8. Parametric freedom from first post-CABG reoperation. *Solid line*, the solution of the independently determined parametric equation for freedom from the event; *thinner lines*, 70% confidence limits

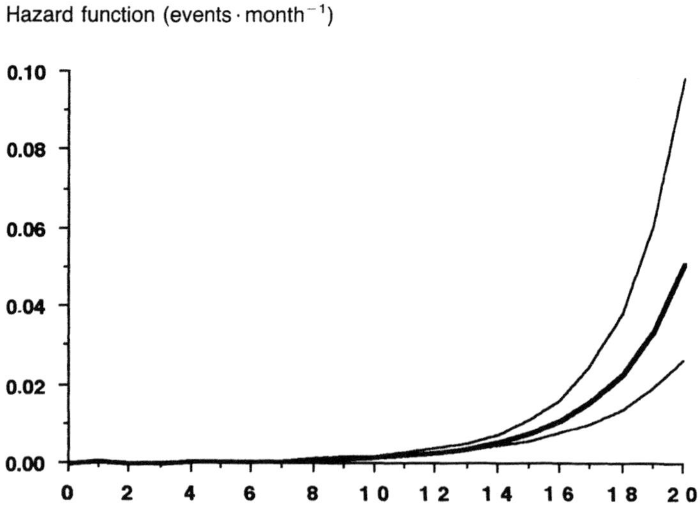

Fig. 9. Hazard function for first post-CABG reoperation, representing the immediate risk of reoperation, on the condition that the patient survives

Table 6. Incremental risk factors for first reoperation after CABG surgery

	Early hazard	Late hazard
Younger age	*	*
Coexisting condition		
Presence of hypertension		*
Higher triglyceride level		*
Lower triglyceride level	*	
Coronary disease and distribution		
Greater number of vessels diseased		*
Presence of smaller coronary vessels		*
Less diffusely diseased vessels		*
Left ventricular function		
Higher ejection fraction		*
Preoperative angina		
Higher anginal class	*	
Presence of unstable angina	*	*
Presence of nonexertional angina	*	
Surgical factors		
Nonuse of IMA	*	

symptoms after CABG surgery changes over time. The analysis detects two phases. An early phase starts in the 1st week after surgery, is at its peak effect 8 months after surgery, and returns to the level of the constant phase at 18 months; a late phase starts with minimal effect around 24 months after surgery and increases in effect to the end of the study period. These phases are present simultaneously. The hazard 15 years after surgery is nearly 200 times that 1 year after surgery. The analysis also identifies, as for death after CABG surgery, risk factors present in each phase (Table 6).

The 1-, 5-, 10-, and 15-year parametric freedom from first post-CABG reintervention for the total population was 99%, 98%, 91%, and 67%, respectively (Fig. 10). The immediate risk (Fig. 11) of return of ischemic symptoms after coronary surgery changes over time and rises almost exponentially 15 years after surgery.

The analysis detects two phases (although they are not apparent due to overlap of a flat curve with an increasing curve). An early phase starts in the 1st week after surgery, is at its peak effect 7 months after surgery and returns to the level of the constant phase at 18 months; a late phase starts with minimal effect around 28 months after surgery and increases in effect until the end of the study period. These phases are present simultaneously. The hazard 15 years after surgery is nearly 200 times that at 1 year after surgery. Table 7 identifies the incremental risk factors for first reintervention.

Tables 6 and 7 include the nonuse of IMA as a risk-increasing factor for reoperation and reintervention. Patient-specific predictions quantify this

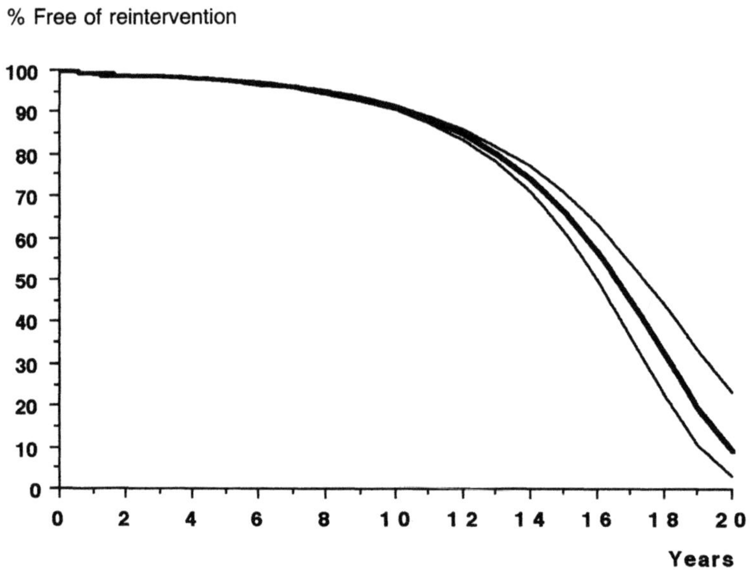

Fig. 10. Parametric freedom from first post-CABG reintervention. *Solid line*, the solution of the independently determined parametric equation for freedom from the event; *thinner lines*, the 70% confidence limits

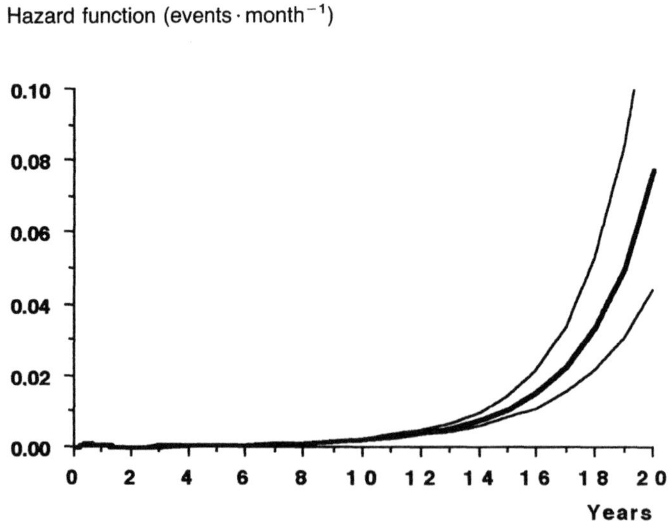

Fig. 11. Hazard function for first post-CABG reintervention, representing the immediate risk of reoperation on the condition that the patient survives

Table 7. Incremental risk factors for first reintervention after CABG surgery

	Early hazard	Late hazard
Younger age	*	*
Coexisting condition		
Presence of hypertension		*
Higher triglyceride level		*
Lower triglyceride level	*	
Coronary disease and distribution		
Greater number of vessels diseased		*
Presence of smaller coronary vessels		*
Less diffusely diseased vessels		*
Left ventricular function		
Higher ejection fraction	*	*
Atherosclerotic disease		
Presence of peripheral vascular disease	*	
Preoperative angina		
Higher anginal class	*	
Presence of unstable angina	*	*
Presence of nonexertional angina	*	
Surgical factors		
Nonuse of IMA	*	
More use of sequential grafting		*

benefit as very minor (0.4%) at peak effect in both models, but the total group suffering the event after 10 years is only 7% for reoperation and 9% for reintervention. It can be expected that extensive bilateral and sequential grafting will enter the model at least in the early phase and probably also in the late phase. The reason probably differs for each phase. The attenuating effect on early return of ischemia provoked by less early graft failure should preclude the effect on an early hazard phase. Technical reasons probably influence the late hazard phase. It is very unlikely that surgeons are anxious to reoperate on patients with patent bilateral IMA grafts and perhaps a patent gastroepiploic artery merely to construct a venous graft to a smaller coronary vessel. A new surgical technique warning emerges in the analysis against extensive sequential grafting, appearing as a risk factor in the late phase of post-CABG reintervention.

Conclusion

More substantial knowledge can be obtained about certain events the more cautious one is in drawing conclusions. At least one IMA should be used in each primary or repeat CABG procedure. Neither limited pulmonary function, older age, nor impaired ventricle function is a contraindication to this technique. It is possible that the patient is in profound shock or cardiac massage by the time he is put onto the operating table. In these circumstances the IMA can be dissected once the patient has been placed on extracorporeal circulation.

Mathematical models have never confirmed a benefit for extensive IMA grafting, but they have shown that no increased risk for an event is associated with this technique. Extensive IMA grafting should therefore be used for nearly all patients, with very few limitations due to the patient's status. Bilateral IMA grafting has been excluded for most insulin-dependent diabetics because of an apparently increased sternal infection rate. In our experience a stepwise logistic model for sternal infection has not indicated the relationship between insulin-treated diabetes, bilateral IMA grafting, and sternal wound infections.

Certain surgical teams have postponed the use of a single or bilateral IMA to the repeat procedure, at least during the time period of this analysis. There are no medical or statistical bases for this decision. Patients develop myocardial infarcts or even die during follow-up because of venous graft failure. This should be avoided by all means since these events are irreversible. Bilateral IMA grafting, if performed, should preferably go to two myocardial areas, and sequential IMA grafting expands the possible, but as of yet unconfirmed, benefit of this technique.

Other in situ or free arterial grafts can be useful. By 1 October 1992 more than 105 patients, 25% of them reoperations, had undergone coronary revascularization using a right or left gastroepiploic artery. The 1-month early patency was 98% and only one patient, after a third reoperation, died. This information is casuistic, but the effort is made to demonstrate that an extension of arterial grafting to non-IMAs does not increases the operative risk. It can be expected that at least a decade will be needed to confirm a possible benefit.

A new data set was completed 1 January 1992 including 10000 patients undergoing isolated primary or repeat coronary surgery. Several thousand patients have received extensive sequential and bilateral IMA grafting. It is hoped that some of the much needed answers will emerge from this data set.

Appendix A

The Variables Entered in the Analysis

Demographic: age (years), female sex, obesity, history of smoking

Distribution of coronary artery disease: coronary score, left main stenosis (%), left main stenosis >50%, left main stenosis >90%

Left ventricular function: presence of aneurysm, left ventricular end diastolic pressure (mmHg), ejection fraction, left ventricular hypertrophy, NYHA class, mitral insufficiency

Angina: anginal class (0 = no angina, 1 = mild symptoms, 2 = moderate to severe symptoms, 3 = nonexertional angina, 4 = unstable angina), no anginal symptoms, stable angina, nonexertional angina, unstable angina, anginal history, urgency grade (0 = nonurgent, 1 = unstable symptoms, 2 = unstable ST segment responding to intravenous medication, 3 = fixed ST segment nonresponding to intravenous medication), no ST changes, unstable ST segment, grade of instability of the ST segment

Pre-CABG myocardial infarction: anterior infarct, apical infarct, septal infarct, posterior infarct, number of infarcted areas, number of preoperative infarcts, infarct same day, infarct in the last 30 days

Hemodynamic status: cardiogenic shock, congestive heart failure, unstable hemodynamics

Peripheral vascular disease: vascular pathology, ascending aortic disease (0 = normal, 1 = calcified, 2 = extremely thin and fragile, 3 = caseous)

Carotid artery disease: carotid disease, operated carotid artery, occluded carotid artery, occluded other cerebral centripetal artery

Small coronary arteries, vessel quality: mean size of the vessels (mm), mean quality of the distal vessels (0 = normal, 1 = nonstenotic diffuse disease, 2 = stenotic diffuse disease, 3 = endarterectomy needed), the size of the vessels, number of vessels $\leq$1 mm in size

Coexisting conditions: diabetes (0 = normal, 1 = pathological glucose tolerance test, 2 = peroral antidiabetic medication, 3 = insulin treated diabetes), insulin-treated diabetes, dialysis, family history of coronary pathology, hypertension, malignancy, pulmonary vital capacity (% of normal), pulmonary one second value (% of normal), neurological symptoms

Coagulation abnormalities: intracoronary thrombolysis history

Hyperlipidemia: cholesterol, HDL, triglyceride value

Surgical environment: surgeon, year of surgery, serial number of procedure, serial number of procedure performed by a particular surgeon

Management of myocardium: cardioplegia, lidoflazine, clamptime, cooling, clamptime, using cardioplegia, clamptime using lidoflazine, other myocardial protection

Bypassing conduit: bilateral IMA, IMA, IMA on the LAD, only IMA, IMA and saphenous bypasses, left IMA, left IMA to circumflex, left IMA to LAD, IMA jumpgraft, one IMA distal, two IMA distals, IMA triple jumpgraft, number of IMA distals, number of IMA grafts, right IMA, right IMA to circumflex, right IMA to LAD, right IMA to right coronary artery, presence of saphenous bypasses, only saphenous grafts, single IMA

Other operative details: number of distals, number of endarterectomies, number of conduits, pump time, ratio of distals anastomoses to conduits, any concomitant surgery, carotid endarterectomy, abdominal aorta aneurysm resection as combined procedure, other combined surgical procedure.

Completeness of revascularization: incomplete revascularization (a vessel of size 1.5 mm or greater with a stenosis of more than 70% left unrevascularized)

Appendix B

Multivariable Risk Factor Equation for Death by Any Mode After the Coronary Bypass Operation (modified from [3])

For the three hazard phases, parameter estimates and incremental risk factors, their coefficients, standard deviations, and p values were:

Early: $\delta = 0$, $\rho = 0.1113$, $\nu = 1.443$, $m = 0$, intercept $= -5.901$, age (years) $= 0.05760 \pm 0.0138$ ($p < 0.0001$), left main disease ($0 =$ no, $\geqslant 90\%$ stenosis $= 1$) 0.6730 ± 0.31 ($p = 0.03$), ejection fraction $= -2.082 \pm 0.77$ ($p = 0.007$), left ventricular hypertrophy ($0 =$ no, $1 =$ yes) $= 0.8049 \pm 0.29$ ($p = 0.006$), severity of angina ($0 =$ none, $1 =$ mild stable angina, $2 =$ moderate or severe stable angina, $3 =$ severe nonexertional angina, $4 =$ unstable angina) $= 0.6126 \pm 0.111$ ($p < 0.0001$), hemodynamic instability ($0 =$ none, $1 =$ instability without shock, $4 =$ cardiogenic shock) $= 0.4533 \pm 0.125$ ($p = 0.003$), peripheral vascular disease ($0 =$ no, $1 =$ yes) $= 0.6345 \pm 0.22$ ($p = 0.004$), small coronary arteries (ratio of number of 1 mm or smaller distal coronary anastomoses to number of distal anastomoses) $= 1.396 \pm 0.43$ ($p = 0.001$), insulin-treated diabetes ($0 =$ no, $1 =$ yes) $= 0.8807 \pm 0.35$ ($p = 0.01$), 1-s expiratory rate (% of normal) $= -0.02125 \pm 0.0056$ ($p = 0.0001$) date of operation (years since Jan. 1971) $= -0.08312 \pm 0.032$ ($p = 0.01$), surgeon B ($0 =$ no, $1 =$ yes) $= 0.5546 \pm 0.22$ ($p = 0.01$), number of endarterectomies $= 0.6609 \pm 0.24$ ($p = 0.007$), sequential grafting (ratio of number of distal anastomoses to number of conduits) $= 0.3538 \pm 0.122$ ($p = 0.004$).

Constant: intercept $= -4.709$, ejection fraction $= -3.806 \pm 0.77$ ($p < 0.0001$), ischemic mitral incompetence ($0 =$ no, $1 =$ yes) $= 0.7834 \pm 0.26$ ($p = 0.002$), no anginal symptoms ($0 =$ no, $1 =$ yes) $= 0.6196 \pm 0.23$ ($p = 0.007$), unstable angina ($0 =$ no, $1 =$ yes) $= 0.7944 \pm 0.20$ ($p < 0.0001$), peripheral vascular disease $= 0.6226 \pm 0.23$ ($p = 0.007$), high-density lipoprotein level (mg/dl) $= -0.01820 \pm 0.0092$ ($p = 0.05$), incomplete revascularization ($0 =$ no, $1 = \geqslant 70\%$ stenosis remaining unbypassed) $= 0.8025 \pm 0.190$ ($p < 0.0001$).

Late (rising): $\tau = 1'$, $\gamma = 1$, $\alpha = 1$, $\eta = 3.526$, intercept $= 9.827$, age $= 0.2620 \pm 0.080$ ($p = 0.001$), age (natural logarithm transformation) $=$

-11.18 ± 4.1 ($p = 0.006$), number of diseased vessels (1–3, ≥70% stenosis) = 0.3219 ± 0.140 ($p = 0.02$), ejection fraction = -2.287 ± 1.10 ($p = 0.04$), peripheral vascular disease = 0.6530 ± 0.23 ($p = 0.005$), small coronary arteries = 1.229 ± 0.40 ($p = 0.002$), insulin-treated diabetes = 1.756 ± 0.41 ($p < 0.0001$), 1-s expiratory rate = -0.01493 ± 0.0056 ($p = 0.008$), trigliceride level (mg/dl, natural logarithm transformation) = 0.4884 ± 0.169 ($p = 0.004$), nonuse of internal mammary (thoracic) artery as a conduit (0 = no, 1 = yes) = 1.234 ± 0.29 ($p < 0.0001$).

Appendix C

Multivariable Risk Factor Equation for Return of First Ischemic Symptom After the Coronary Bypass Operation (from [4])

For the three hazard phases, parameter estimates and incremental risk factors, their coefficients, standard deviations, and p values were:

Early: $\delta = 0$, $\rho = 2.561$, $\nu = -0.564$, $m = 3.1419$, E2 = 2.10272 ± 1.93844 ($p = 0.278$), E3 = -0.571133 ± 0.4218735 ($p = 0.1758$), E4 = 1.14483 ± 2.535476 ($p = 0.6516$), intercept = -1.59949 ± 0.8332003 ($p = 0.0549$), age (years) = $-0.0405148 \pm 0.01016712$ ($p < 0.0001$), angina at rest = 0.6038821 ± 0.2537803 ($p = 0.0173$), level of support of unstable angina = 0.5559621 ± 0.1845576 ($p = 0.0026$), peripheral vascular disease (vascular pathology) 1.075684 ± 0.1847098 ($p < 0.0001$), nonuse of IMA to LAD = 0.5837915 ± 0.227054 ($p = 0.0101$), surgeon X = 0.3931646 ± 0.2268607 ($p = 0.0831$), surgeon Y (surgeon Y) = -0.686987 ± 0.3015056 ($p = 0.0227$), incomplete revascularization (complete revascularization = 0, incomplete = 1) = 0.9141202 ± 0.2005738 ($p < 0.0001$).

Constant: intercept = -7.74272 ± 0.6439814 ($p < 0.0001$), female patient = 0.709169 ± 0.1712434 ($p < 0.0001$), left main >50% (left main stenosis greater than 50%) = -0.627524 ± 0.3484979 ($p = 0.0718$), logarithm of the end-diastolic pressure = 0.2600223 ± 0.1530931 ($p = 0.0894$), enrinfar (natural logarithm transformation of the number of infarcts) = $0.02901628 \pm 0.01305821$ ($p = 0.0263$), anginal history = $0.004456822 \pm 0.001159014$ ($p = 0.0001$), severity of angina (0 = none, 1 = mild stable angina, 2 = moderate or severe stable angina, 3 = severe non-exertional angina, 4 = unstable angina) = 0.1285804 ± 0.04992487 ($p = 0.01$), aortscor (quality of the aorta ascendens different from normal 0 = normal, 1 = calcified, extremely thin or caseous) = 0.6993435 ± 0.4045241 ($p < 0.0838$), mean quality of the grafted vessels = 0.3159076 ± 0.07495202 ($p < 0.0001$), small coronary arteries (ratio of number of 1 mm or smaller distal coronary anastomoses to number of distal anastomoses) = 0.9785607 ± 0.2887966 (p = 0.0007), hypertension (syst. bp > 160 or dist. bp > 100) = 0.3930363 ± 0.1397823 (p = 0.0049).

Late: $\tau = 1$, $\gamma = 3.326$, $a = 1$, $\eta = 1$, L2 = 1.201893 ± 0.09452374 ($p <$ 0.0001), intercept = −20.5282 ± 2.088272 ($p < 0.0001$), anginal history (duration in months of the anginal history) = 0.003759441 ± 0.002492586 (p = 0.1315), diabetes (no diabetes = 0, abnormal glucose tolerance test = 1, peroral antidiabetic medication = 2, insulin treated diabetes = 3) = 0.2879517 ± 0.1384528 (p = 0.0375), logarithm of the preoperative triglyceride level = 0.5351755 ± 0.1547362 (p = 0.0005), sequential grafting (logarithm of the ratio of number of distal anastomoses to number of conduits + 0.5) = 1.054712 ± 0.3889804 (p = 0.0067).

Appendix D

Multivariable Risk Factor Equation for Reoperation for Ischemic Disease After the Coronary Bypass Operation (unpublished material)

For the two hazard phases, parameter estimates and incremental risk factors, their coefficients, standard deviations, and p values were:

Early: E2 = 2.010144 ± 0.1068594 ($p < 0.001$), E3 = −1.27255 ± 0.2109373 ($p < 0.0001$), E0 = 0.6086181 ± 2.351275 (p = 0.7950), age (years) = −0.067354 ± 0.0219104 (p = 0.0021), angina grade = 0.4208089 ± 0.1739434 (p = 0.0137), log(preoperative triglyceride level) = −0.84776 ± 0.4090836 (p = 0.0502), nonuse of IMA to LAD = 1.478115 ± 0.6034320 (p = 0.0143).

Late: L1 = 4.879965 ± 0.1249261 ($p < 0.0001$), L0 = −7.63 . . . 85 ± 1.507538 ($p < 0.0001$), log(preoperative triglyceride level) = 0.5970178 ± 0.1915692 (p = 0.0018), square of years of age = −4.8120 ± 1.275479 (p = 0.0002), ejection fraction (%) = 2.496803 ± 1.235366 (p = 0.0433), vessel disease = 0.402486 ± 0.1419770 (p = 0.0046), unstable angina without IMA = 0.5682132 ± 0.2278622 (p = 0.0126), number of anastomosed vessels with a size of 1 mm = 1.470499 ± 0.4770453 (p = 0.0021), mean quality vessel = −0.353805 ± 0.1666890 (p = 0.0338), hypertension (systolic BP > 160 or diastolic BP > 100) = 0.5447042 ± 0.1906559 (p = 0.0043).

Appendix E

Multivariable Risk Factor Equation for Reintervention for Ischemic Disease After the Coronary Bypass Operation (unpublished material)

For the two hazard phases, parameter estimates and incremental risk factors, their coefficients, standard deviations, and p values were:

Early: E2 = 2.061046 ± 0.1057478 ($p < 0.0001$), E3 = −1.1473 ± 0.1740811 ($p < 0.0001$), E0 = −1.53271 ± 2.520013 ($p = 0.5430$), age (years) = −0.0541722 ± 0.01966909 ($p = 0.0059$), ejection fraction (%) = 3.834577 ± 1.932274 ($p = 0.0472$), angina grade = 0.3086074 ± 0.15425 ($p = 0.0454$), peripheral vascular pathology = 1.174435 ± 0.3789576 ($p = 0.0018$), log(preoperative triglyceride level) = −0.980436 ± 0.3505755 ($p = 0.0063$), nonuse of IMA to LAD = 1.306090 ± 0.4738752 ($p = 0.0058$).

Late: L1 = 4.024555 ± 0.0988910 ($p < 0.0001$), L0 = −7.78792 ± 1.370853 ($p < 0.001$), ejection fraction (%) = 2.56465 ± 1.114209 ($p = 0.0213$), log(preoperative triglyceride level) = 0.6032546 ± 0.1736234 ($p = 0.0005$), square of years of age = −4.46977 ± 1.133766 ($p < 0.0001$), vessel disease = 0.2693849 ± 0.1268673 ($p = 0.0337$), unstable angina without IMA = 0.6814102 ± 0.1960351 ($p = 0.0005$), number of anastomosed vessels with a size of 1 mm 1.275200 ± 0.4524433 ($p = 0.0048$), mean quality vessel = −0.589405 ± 0.1555188 ($p = 0.0123$), hypertension (syst. BP > 160 or diast. BP > 100) = 0.3891457 ± 0.1726070 ($p = 0.0242$), LRTEDIGR (logarithmic transformation of the ratio between the number of distals against the number of grafts) = 0.8062774 ± 0.3681095 ($p = 0.0285$).

References

1. Sergeant P (1989) Methodology of the K.U. Leuven Coronary Surgery Database. Medicina Informatica 6(2):127–135
2. Sergeant P, Lesaffre E (1991) The K.U. Leuven Coronary Surgery Database: a clinical research database. In: Meester GT, Pinciroli F (eds) Databases for cardiology. Kluwer Academic, Amsterdam, pp 223–237
3. Sergeant P, Lesaffre E, Flameng W, Suy R (1990) Internal mammary artery: methods of use and their effect on survival after coronary bypass surgery. Eur J Cardiothorac Surg 4:72–8
4. Sergeant P, Lesaffre E, Flameng W, Suy R, Blackstone E (1991) The return of clinically evident ischemia after coronary artery bypass grafting. Eur J Cardiothorac Surg 5:447–457
5. Blackstone E, Naftel D, Turner M Jr (1986) The decomposition of time-varying hazard into phases, each incorporating a separate stream of concomitant information. J Am Stat Assoc 81:615–624
6. Sergeant P. Hazard analysis in coronary bypass surgery. PhD thesis, Katholieke Universiteit Leuven Belgium, Acco Leuven
7. Sergeant P, Flameng W, Suy R (1988) The sequential internal mammary artery graft. J Cardiovasc Surg 29(5):596–600

Mechanisms of Plaque Formation and Occlusion in Venous Coronary Bypass Grafts

I.K. Jang and V. Fuster

The progression of venous coronary bypass graft disease can be divided into three phases [12]: (a) acute thrombotic phase, (b) intimal hyperplasia, and (c) atherosclerosis (Fig. 1). Acute thrombotic occlusion occurs within the first month after operation and is mediated mainly by platelets. Between 1 and 12 months after operation smooth muscle cells begin to proliferate, and connective tissue synthesis increases. After 3 years atherosclerotic lesions progress further, and the natural history of venous bypass grafts becomes similar to that of native coronary arteries with advanced atherosclerosis.

In this chapter we discuss the pathogenesis of venous graft disease in relation to risk factors. The changes at each phase are discussed separately.

Acute Thrombotic Phase

Endothelial injury may be caused by handling of the vein during harvest, ischemia due to disruption of vasa vasorum and time delay before anastomosis, the type of preservation solution used during operation, and rheologic factors after restoration of blood flow [25, 36]. The injury leads to exposure of collagen in the subendothelium which in combination with thrombin generated by the extrinsic and intrinsic coagulation pathways and adenosine diphosphate from red blood cells activates platelets. Acivated platelets expose membrane receptors such as glycoprotein Ia, Ib, and IIb/IIIa [42] (Fig. 2). Glycoprotein Ia binds to exposed collagen. Glycoprotein Ib is important in platelet adhesion to subendothelium through von Willebrand factor, especially at high shear rate such as in the venous bypass graft connected to the arterial system [2, 3, 47, 53, 57]. Von Willebrand factor plays a crucial role not only in platelet-subendothelium interaction but also in platelet-platelet interaction through glycoprotein IIb/IIIa.

When subendothelium is exposed to circulation, the coagulation system is also activated by collagen and tissue factor (Fig. 2). Tissue factor activates not only the intrinsic pathway but also the extrinsic pathway by stimulating factor IX in the presence of calcium. The final product, thrombin, catalyzes fibrinogen to fibrin, activates factor XIII to promote cross-linking of fibrin, and produces new thrombin by stimulating factors V and VIII. At the same

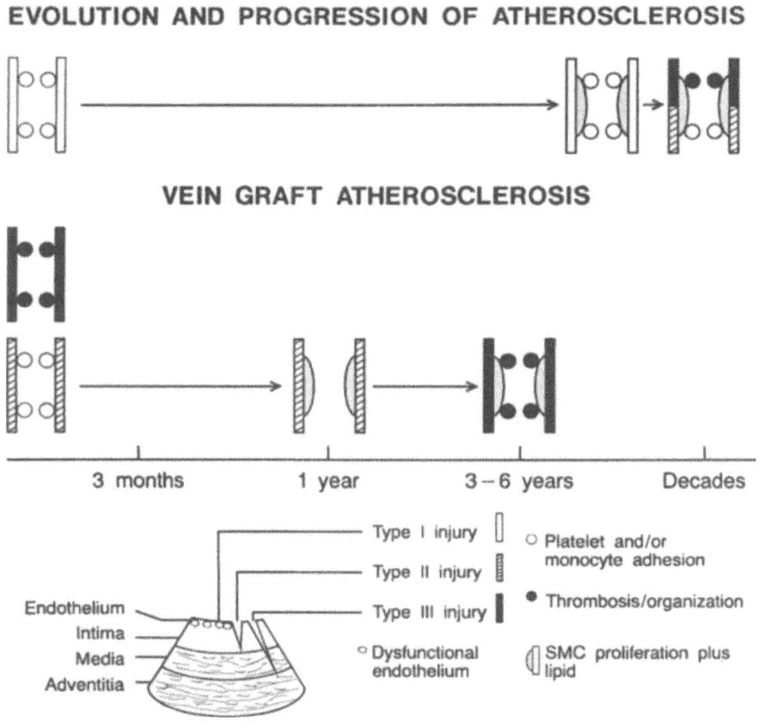

Fig. 1. Pathogenesis of plaque formation and occlusion of venous bypass graft compared with that of native vessel. Endothelial injury (type III) during operation causes platelet deposition, resulting in thrombus formation and subsequent release of growth factors. Connective tissue synthesis from smooth muscle cells (*SMC*) and fibroblasts is the main mechanism of luminal narrowing between 1 and 12 months. Incorporation of lipid into the lesions, which is accelerated by hyperlipidemia and smoking, develops atheromatous plaques, which can rupture and cause acute thrombotic occlusion of the graft

time, thrombin is a strong agonist for platelet aggregation [30, 33, 35], and activated platelets increase prothrombinase activity, resulting in further thrombin production from prothrombin. Under a high shear condition as in the arterial system, the venous graft undergoes an adaptive process, so-called "arterialization," thereby decreasing the synthesis of prostacyclin and increasing the thrombotic potential.

Indeed, in pathologic studies platelet deposition on the surface and formation of mural thrombus were evident in 75% of vein grafts obtained within 24 h after operation [6, 26, 36]. Although careful handling of the venous graft and improved surgical skill without vein distension before anastomosis can reduce this endothelial damage to a certain extent [39], there are other factors that cannot be completely avoided. Chesebro et al. [13] identified two important risk factors for early bypass graft occlusion: low vein-graft blood flow (less than 40 ml/min) and small luminal size of the

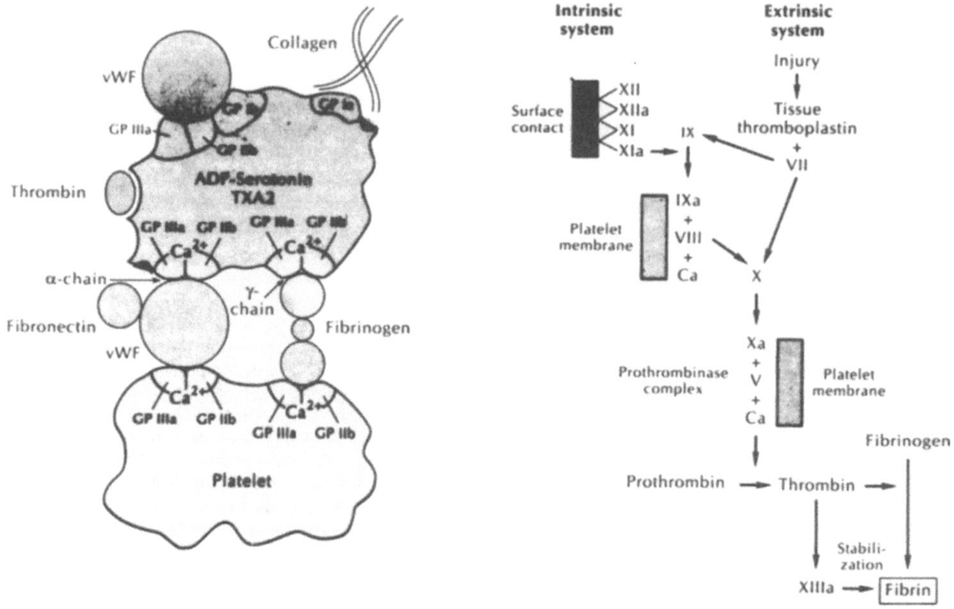

Fig. 2. *Left*, platelet membrane receptors and adhesive molecules; *Right*, intrinsic and extrinsic coagulation pathways. Factor VII activates both intrinsic and extrinsic pathways and thereby playing a key role in vivo coagulation. (From [27])

grafted artery (less than 1.5 mm). Other risk factors are endarterectomy, bypass to the circumflex or right coronary artery, local atheromas at the arteriotomy site or extension of the arteriotomy into a branch vessel, postoperative elevated serum lipids, and smoking [8, 13]. Further, angioscopic study has shown mechanical narrowing at the distal anastomosis which may result in low blood flow and thrombotic occlusion in up to 20% of grafts [29].

Intimal Hyperplasia

Within 1 month after bypass operation smooth muscle cells begin to proliferate, and this becomes a main cause of occlusion between 1 and 12 months after operation [37, 41, 54]. This smooth muscle cell proliferation can be divided into three phases [12]. In phase I smooth muscle cells in the media show hyperplastic changes, which peak at 48 h. In phase II, which starts at 4 days and lasts up to 14 days, smooth muscle cells migrate from the media to the intima and proliferate within the intima [15, 40]. Phase III, or late smooth muscle cell proliferation, starts after 2 weeks, when intimal hypertrophy and extracellular matrix production become evident [15, 52].

The hyperplastic changes of smooth muscle cells in the media in phase I is probably caused by vessel injury during operation and at the site of anastomosis (the so-called "response to injury" hypothesis) and appear to be related to the release of growth factors from platelets, monocytes, endothelial cells, and smooth muscle cells as well as elimination of the suppressive effect of endothelium [38]. The strong correlation between the amount of platelet deposition and the degree of smooth muscle cell proliferation [15], together with a lesser degree of intimal hyperplasia in the rabbit with severe thrombocytopenia [24] and the suppression of intimal hyperplasia by antiplatelet therapy [31], supports the notion that platelets play a key role in the development of smooth muscle cell proliferation and subsequent migration.

Activated platelets release platelet-derived growth factor (PDGF) from alpha granule [46]. PDGF is a basic protein, consisting of two polypeptide chains (A and B). PDGF can be synthesized by cells other than platelets, such as endothelial cells, macrophages, and smooth muscle cells. This explains why smooth muscle cells continue to proliferate even after the completion of reendothelialization. Walker et al. [56] showed that smooth muscle cells from the intima 2 weeks after a balloon injury produce PDGF-like substance in an amount ten times higher than cells from the non-injured area. Multiple growth factors as well as various neurotransmitters and hormones are implicated in vascular smooth muscle cell proliferation (interleukin-1, alpha- and beta-fibroblast growth factors, serotonin and thrombospondin, catecholamines, and angiotension II).

Vascular smooth muscle cells have different phenotypes: synthetic and contractile. During the developmental period synthetic phenotype smooth muscle cells actively proliferate and produce large amounts of collagen, elastin, and proteoglycans. Once development ceases, contractile phenotype smooth muscle cells become predominant and regulate vessel wall tension. However, when the vessel is stimulated, smooth muscle cells in the media turn into the synthetic phenotype and increase the production of a synthetic matrix, thereby developing intimal hyperplasia. In cell culture these phenotypic changes in vascular smooth muscle cells were inhibited by endothelial cells, demonstrating the suppressive effect of endothelium [7, 11, 49]. There is evidence that the changes in phase I may be enhanced by thrombin [4].

The mechanism of migration of smooth muscle cells from the media to the intima in phase II has not been fully explored. Among different growth factors, only PDGF has been shown to induce directed migration in cell culture [28]. There is some evidence that platelet factor 4 and interleukins may also play a role in the migration of the cells [43, 50]. It is in this phase that platelets, PDGF, and other growth factors play a key role [21, 40].

Proliferation of smooth muscle cells in phases II and III plays the most important part in the pathogenesis of atherosclerosis of the venous bypass graft. Analysis of smooth muscle cells using titrated thymidine shows that about half of the cells which migrate from the media into the intima never divide further and comprise only 10% of intimal cells [14]. This means that proliferation of smooth muscle cells within the intima is the main cause of intimal hyperplasia rather than migration of cells from the media. The proliferative ability of the smooth muscle cells varies from cell to cell. There are some cells that do not seem to proliferate [9, 32]. Whether the ratio of cells that proliferate and those that do not is important for the degree of intimal hyperplasia is not known. However, there seems to be a correlation between the amount of platelet deposition on the vessel wall and the degree of intimal thickening [15, 36, 41, 52]. Once the surface is covered with new endothelium, smooth muscle cells in the intima appear to cease their proliferation, probably by endothelium-synthesized inhibitors [10, 22, 45]. Several studies have shown the inverse relationship between the rate of reendothelialization and the degree of smooth muscle cell proliferation [22, 44, 55]. The mechanism of suppression of smooth muscle cell proliferation by endothelium is not clear. Changes in the type of glycoaminoglycan may also be responsible for determining the degree of smooth muscle cell proliferation [1, 10, 34, 45, 59]. In cell culture, endothelial cells produce a heparinlike substance that suppresses smooth muscle cell proliferation [10]. In the another study [45], heparan sulfate containing glycosaminoglycan, which has been shown to suppress smooth muscle cell proliferation, accumulated in higher concentration in the area with regenerated endothelium compared to the area without endothelium.

Extracellular fibrous tissue within the vessel wall in phase III is an important component of luminal narrowing, and this predisposes the vessel to atherosclerotic changes. Four important elements of fibrous tissue are collagen, elastin, glycosaminoglycan, and glycoprotein. Collagen, synthesized by smooth muscle cells stimulated by various growth factors, is a main component of atherosclerotic plaque. Although the concentration of elastin in atherosclerotic plaque is relatively low, abnormal elastin in the atherosclerotic arterial wall may enhance lipid uptake and contibute to calcification of plaques [59]. Dermatan sulfate, one of the glycosaminoglycans, as well as glycoprotein is synthesized by smooth muscle cells, when stimulated by growth factors [46, 58, 59]. Dermatan sulfate also seems to contribute to lipid uptake of the vessel wall. Although these biochemical changes have been studied mainly in arteries, the same changes are expected to occur in venous bypass grafts and constitute the transitional phase to atherosclerosis.

Atherosclerosis

Atherosclerosis becomes evident after 3 years, and the pathogenesis of plaque formation in this stage is similar to that of the native vessel. Recent pathologic studies have shown that there is continuous damage of the intima in varying degrees [18, 19]. The damaged area is sealed with thrombus consisting of platelets and fibrin, and this healing process seems to play an important role in the progression of atherosclerosis. Indeed, Bini et al. [5] demonstrated that atherosclerotic lesions contain fibrin and related products. These products were also found in early lesions and in normal arteries. Platelets and thrombin in the thrombus not only promote smooth muscle cell proliferation but also enhance the lipid uptake of macrophages, thereby accelerating the foam cell formation and the progression of atherosclerosis [16, 49, 51]. Smooth muscle cells and fibroblasts also synthesize connective tissue and incorporate lipid into the cells. Consequently, risk factors such as hyperlipidemia and smoking accelerate this process and lead to vascular occlusion.

Rupture of atheromatous plaque with superimposed thrombus results in acute coronary syndromes such as acute myocardial infarction, unstable angina pectoris, and sudden ischemic death. The rupture is caused by a tear of the thin fibrous "cap" covering a soft atheromatous plaque and separating it from the arterial lumen. The exact mechanism of plaque rupture is unkown. It may include ulceration by shear forces engendered by hypertension, changes in coronary arterial tone or turbulent flow at the site of stenosis, or disruption of ingrown vasa vasorum causing intraplaque hemorrhage and plaque expansion [17]. It may be simply an incidental event in the evolution and growth of the atheromatous plaque, which occurs when the cap has become thinned to the extent that normal hemodynamic stresses may tear it [20]. It has also been suggested that macrophages release enzymes which digest collagen and elastin and thereby weaken the cap. Then, several events may occur: (a) the contents of the atheromatous plaque may discharge into the lumen and embolize distally, (b) blood from the lumen may enter into the plaque and cause intraplaque hemorrhage, (c) platelet aggregation may occur at the site of the rupture leading to peripheral embolization of platelet clumps or progression towards luminal occlusion, and (d) the occlusive thrombus may propagate both proximally and distally [17, 20, 23]. The composition of the thrombus at the site of the rupture consists mainly of platelets, with some red cells and fibrin. Once the initial thrombus grows and occludes the lumen, the proximal and distal parts are filled with stasis-type red cell-rich thrombus, thereby forming "head" and "tail" parts of an occlusive thrombus. Since the venous bypass graft does not have side branches, thrombus propagates rapidly and fills the proximal and sometimes distal parts of the vessel to the anastomosis sites. This may explain the poor reponse of venous graft occlusion to thrombolytic therapy.

References

1. Ausprunk DH, Boudreau CL, Nelson DA (1981) Proteoglycans in the microvasculature. I. Histochemical localization in microvessels of the rabbit. Am J Pathol 103:353–366
2. Badimon L, Badimon JJ, Turitto VT, Fuster V (1987) Platelet deposition in von Willebrand factor deficient vessel wall. J Lab Clin Med 110:634–647
3. Badimon L, Badimon JJ, Turitto VT, Vallabhajosuia S, Fuster V (1988) Platelet thrombus formation on collagen type I. Influence of blood rheology, von Willebrand factor and blood coagulation. Circulation 78:1431–1442
4. Berk BC, Taubman MB, Gragoe EJ, Fenton FW, Griendling KK (1990) Thrombin signal transduction mechanism in rat vascular smooth muscle cells. Calcium and protein kinase C-dependent and-independent pathways. J Biol Chem 265:17334–17440
5. Bini A, Fenoglio JJ, Mes-Tejada R, Kerdryk B, Kaplan KL (1989) Identification and distribution of fibrinogen, fibrin and fibrin (ogen) degradation products in atherosclerosis: use of monoclonal antibodies. Atherosclerosis 1:109–121
6. Bulkley BH, Hutchins GM (1978) Pathology of coronary artery bypass graft surgery. Arch Pathol Lab Med 102:273–280
7. Campbell GR, Campbell JH (1985) Smooth muscle phenotypic changes in arterial wall homeostasis: implication for the pathogenesis of atherosclerosis. Exp Mol Pathol 42: 139–162
8. Campeau L, Enjalbert M, Lesperance J, Bourassa MG, Kwiterovich P, Wacholder S, Sniderman A (1984) The relation of risk factors to the development of atherosclerosis in saphenous-vein bypass grafts and the progression of disease in the native circulation. N Engl J Med 311:1329–1332
9. Caplan AI, Fizman MC, Eppenbeiger HM (1983) Molecular and cell isoforms during development. Science 221:921–927
10. Castellot JJ, Addonizio ML, Rosenberg R, Karnovsky MJ (1981) Cultured endothelial cells produce a heparin-like inhibitor of smooth muscle cell growth. J Cell Biol 90:372–377
11. Chamley-Campbell JH, Campbell GR, Ross R (1979) The smooth muscle cell in culture. Physiol Rev 59:1–61
12. Chesebro JH, Goldman S (1992) Coronary artery bypass surgery: antithrombotic therapy. In: Fuster V, Verstraete M (eds) Thrombosis in cardiovascular disorders. Saunders, Philadelphia, pp 375–388
13. Chesebro JH, Clements IP, Fuster V, Elveback LR, Smith HC, Bardsley WT, Frye RL, Homes DR, Vlietstra RE, Pluth JR, Wallace RB, Puga FJ, Orszulak TA, Piehler JM, Schaff HV, Danielson GK (1982) A platelet-inhibitor-drug trial in coronary-artery bypass operations: benefit of perioperative dipyridamole and aspirin therapy on early postoperative vein-graft patency. N Engl J Med 307:73–78
14. Clowes AW, Schwartz SM (1985) Significance of quiescent smooth muscle migration in the injured rat carotid artery. Circ Res 56:139–145
15. Clowes AW, Reidy MA, Clowes NM (1983) Kinetics of cellular proliferation after arterial injury. I. Smooth muscle growth in the absence of endothelium. Lab Invest 49: 327–333
16. Cunningham DD, Farrell DH (1986) Thrombin interaction with cultured fibroblasts: relationship to mitogenic stimulation. Ann NY Acad Sci 485:240–248
17. Davies MJ, Thomas AC (1985) Plaque fissuring: the cause of acute myocardial infarction, sudden ischemic death, and crescendo angina. Br Heart J 53:363–373
18. Davies MJ, Woolf N, Rowles PM, Pepper J (1988) Morphology of the endothelium over atherosclerotic plaques in human coronary arteries. Br Heart J 60:459–464
19. Davies MJ, Bland MJ, Hartgartner WR, angelini A, Thomas AC (1989) Factors influencing the presence or absence of acute coronary thrombi in sudden ischemic death. Eur Heart J 10:203–208

20. Falk E (1983) Plaque rupture with severe pre-existing stenosis precipitating coronary thrombosis: characteristics of coronary atherosclerotic plaques underlying fatal occlusive thrombi. Br Heart J 50:127–134
21. Fingerle J, Au WPT, Clowes AW, Reidy MA (1990) Intimal lesion formation in rat carotid arteries after endothelial denudation in absence of medial injury. Arteriosclerosis 10: 1082–1087
22. Fishman JA, Ryan GB, Kamorsky MI (1977) Endothelial regeneration in the rat carotid artery and the significance of endothelial denudation in the pathogenesis of myointimal thickening. Lab Invest 32:339–351
23. Friedman M, van den Bovenkamp GJ (1966) The pathogenesis of a coronary thrombus. Am J Pathol 48:19–44
24. Friedman RJ, Stemerman MB, Wenz B, Moore S, Gauldie J, Gent M, Tiell ML, Spaet TH (1977) The effect of thrombocytopenia on experimental arteriolsclerotic lesion formation in rabbit. J Clin Invest 60:1191–1201
25. Fuster V, Chesebro JH (1986) Role of platelets and platelet inhibtors in aortocoronary artery vein-graft disease. Circulation 73:227–232
26. Fuster V, Dewanjee MK, Kaye MP, Josa M, Metke MP, Chesebro JH (1979) Noninvasive radioisotopic technique for deterioration of platelet deposition in coronary artery bypass grafts in dogs and its reduction with platelet inhibitors. Circulation 60:1508–1512
27. Fuster V, Badimon L, Cohen M, Ambrose JA, Badimon JJ, Chesebro JH (1988) Insight into the pathogenesis of acute ischemic syndromes. Circulation 77:1213–1220
28. Gortendorst G (1984) Alteration of the chemotactic response of NIH/3T3 cells to PDGF by growth factors, transformation and tumor promotors. Cell 36:279–285
29. Grundfest WS, Litvack F, Sherman T, Carroll R, Lee M, Chaux A, Kass R, Matloff J, Berci G, Swan HJC, Morgenstern L, Forrester J (1985) Delineation of peripheral and coronary detail by intraoperative angioscopy. Ann Surg 202:394–400
30. Hanson SR, Harker LA (1988) Interruption of acute platelet-dependent thrombosis by the synthetic antithrombin D-phenylalanyl-L-prolyl-L-arginyl chloromethyl ketone. Proc Natl Acad Sci USA 85:3184–3188
31. Harker LA, Harlan JM, Ross R (1983) Effect of sulfinpyrazone on homocystein-induced endothelial injury and arteriosclerosis. Circ Res 53:731–739
32. Haudenschild CC, Grunwald J (1985) Proliferative heterogeneity of vascular smooth muscle cells and its alteration by injury. Exp Cell Res 157:364–370
33. Heras M, Chesbro JH, Penny WJ, Bailey KR, Badimon L, Fuster V (1989) Effects of thrombin inhibition on the development of acute platelet-thrombus deposit during angioplasty in pigs. Heparin vs. hirudin, a specific thrombin inhibitor. Circulation 79:657–665
34. Hollman J, Schmidt A, von Bassewitz DB, Buddecke E (1989) Relationship of sulfated glycosaminoglycans and cholestrol content in normal and atherosclerotic human aorta. Arteriosclerosis 9:154–158
35. Jang IK, Gold HK, Ziskind AA, Leinbach CR, Fallon JT, Collen D (1990) Prevention of platelet-rich arterial thrombosis by selective thrombin inhibition. Circulation 81:219–225
36. Josa M, Lie JT, Bianco RL, Kaye MP (1981) Reduction of thrombosis in canine coronary bypass graft vein grafts with dipyridamole and aspirin Am J Cardiol 47:1248–1254
37. Lie LT, Lawrie GM, Morris GC (1977) Aortocoronary bypass saphenous vein graft atherosclerosis. Am J Cardiol 40:906–914
38. Lindner V, Lappi DA, Baird A, Majack RA, Reidy MA (1991) Role of basic fibroblast growth factor in lesion formation. Circ Res 68:106–113
39. LoGerfo FQ, Haudenschild CC, Quist WC (1984) A clinical technique for prevention of spasm and preservation of endothelium in saphenous vein grafts. Arch Surg 119:1212–1214
40. Majesky MW, Reidy MA, Bowen-Pope DF, Hart CE, Wilcox JN, Schwartz SM (1990) PDGF ligand and receptor gene expression during repair of arterial injury. J Cell Biol 111:2149–2158

41. Metke MP, Lie JT, Fuster V, Josa M, Kaye MP (1979) Reduction of intimal thickening in canine coronary bypass vein grafts with dipyridamole and aspirin. Am J Cardiol 43: 1144–1148
42. Peerschke EIB (1985) The platelet fibrinogen receptor. Semin Hematol 22:241–259
43. Raines EW, Dower SK, Ross R (1989) Interleukin-I mitogenic activity for fibroblasts and smooth muscle cells is due to PDGF-AA. Science 243:393–396
44. Reidy MA, Clowes AW, Schwartz SM (1983) Endothelial regeneration. V. Inhibition of endothelial regrowth in arteries of rat and rabbit. Lab Invest 49:569–575
45. Richardson M, Ihnatowycz I, Moore S (1980) Glycosaminoglycan distribution in rabbit aortic wall following balloon catheter deendothelialization: an ultrastructural study. Lab Invest 43:509–516
46. Ross R, Raines EW, Bowen-Pope DF (1986) The platelet derived growth factor. Cell 46:155–169
47. Sakariassen KS, Nievelstein FF, Coller BS, Sixma JJ (1986) The role of platelet membrane glycoprotein Ib and IIb/IIIa is platelet adherence to human artery subendothelium. Br J Haematol 63:681–191
48. Schwartz SM, Reidy MA (1987) Common mechanism of proliferation of smooth muscle in atherosclerosis and hypertension. Hum Pathol 18:240–247
49. Schwartz CJ, Valente AJ, Kelly JL, Sprague EA, Edwards EH (1988) Thrombosis and the development of atherosclerosis: Rokitansky revisited. Semin Thromb Hemost 14:189–194
50. Senior RM, Griffin GL, San Huang J, Walz AA, Deuel TF (1983) Chemotactic activity of platelet alpha granule proteins for fibroblast. J Cell Biol 96:382–385
51. Shuman MA (1986) Thrombin-cellular interactions. Ann NY Acad Sci 485:288–239
52. Snow AD, Bolender RP, Wright TN, Clowes AW (1990) Heparin modulates the composition of the extracellular matrix domain surrounding arterial smooth muscle cells. Am J Pathol 137:313–330
53. Turitto VT, Weiss JH, Baumgartner HR (1984) Platelet interaction with rabbit subendothelium in von Willebrand's disease: altered thrombus formation distinct from defective platelet adhesion. J Clin Invest 74:1730–1741
54. Uni KK, Kottke BA, Titus JL, Frye RL, Wallace RB, Brown AL (1974) Pathologic changes in aortocoronary saphenous vein grafts. Am J Cardiol 34:526–532
55. Walker LN, Ramsey MM, Bowyer DE (1983) Endothelial healing following defined injury to rabbit aorta: depth of injury and mode of repair. Atherosclerosis 47:123–130
56. Walker LN, Bowen-Pope DF, Ross R, Reidy MA (1986) Production of platelet-derived growth factor-like molecule by cultured arterial smooth muscle cells accompanied proliferation after arterial injury. Proc Natl Acad Sci USA 83:7311–7315
57. Weiss HJ, Turitto VT, Baumgartner HR (1978) Effect of shear rate on platelet interaction with subendothelium in citrated and native blood. I. Shear rate-dependent decrease of adhesion in von Willebrand's disease and the Bernard-Soulier syndrome. J Lab Clin Med 92:750–754
58. Wight LN (1989) Cell biology of arterial proteoglycans. Arteriosclerosis 9:1–20
59. Yea-Herttuala S, Sumuvuori H, Karkola K, Mottonen M, Nikkari P (1986) Glycosaminoglycans in normal and atherosclerotic human coronary arteries. Lab Invest 54:402–408

Surgical Aspects

Arterial and Venous Coronary Bypass Grafts: Surgical Techniques and Outcome

F.D. Loop

Introduction

The choice of conduits in coronary artery surgery is restricted to lower extremity superficial veins and a variety of small arteries. Currently no synthetic material smaller than 6 mm is used in humans, although research is ongoing. Significantly lower graft patency is reported for cephalic veins, radial and splenic arteries, cryopreserved homografts, and synthetic conduits. This chapter deals with selection of the proper conduit, grafting techniques, complications, and outcome adjusted for the type of conduit.

Long-term serial studies [9, 28] confirm the durability of the internal thoracic artery compared with saphenous vein bypass grafts. This information coupled with clear and consistent survival benefit at 10 years, which is reported in more detail below, made the left internal thoracic artery the graft of choice to revascularize the anterior descending coronary artery. Since the anterior descending is prognostically the most important of the major vessels, left main coronary artery excepted [20], revascularization of this vessel with a durable conduit significantly improves long-term survival. Technical experience with the internal thoracic artery has led to its greater use as bilateral, free, and sequential anastomoses, and has stimulated development of other arterial conduits, namely the gastroepiploic and inferior epigastric arteries. The preliminary results of these newer arterial grafts are discussed in another chapter.

The prevalence of internal thoracic artery grafting continues to increase around the world as surgeons become more facile with small vessel anastomoses. In a personal series of 1000 consecutive patients, the author used an internal thoracic artery graft in 95% of patients who received bypass grafts. Whether the internal thoracic artery is used at the first operation is the single greatest determinant of the incidence of coronary artery reoperation.

The relative freedom from atherosclerosis in the internal thoracic arterial conduit is attributed to yet undefined vasoactive properties of the arterial wall. The thoracic artery releases endothelium-derived relaxing factor [27], now identified as nitrous oxide derived from arginine in the cell, and prostacyclin [11] significantly more so than the saphenous vein graft. In a comprehensive report of intimal ultrastructure of the internal thoracic artery [37], a more uniform elastic lamina was found compared with other small arteries. While the role of endothelial factors is not elucidated, the internal thoracic artery has an adaptability which enables it to increase flow in response to changes in coronary peripheral vascular resistance.

The saphenous vein should not be discounted, however, because it is plentiful, versatile, and provides a greater initial flow than the internal thoracic artery. The vein graft is still the most widely used conduit in coronary bypass surgery. However, problems frequently occur after the fifth postoperative year when the vein develops atheroma, which tends to be progressive and results in graft closure. The patency at 10 years ranges from 50% to 60% in many studies and approximately half of the vein grafts still open at 10 years have visible signs of lumen narrowing, presumably from atherosclerosis [9, 28].

Selection Factors

The principal factors that influence conduit selection are age, gender, comorbidity, clinical status at the time of operation, and the type of operation intended. Most experienced coronary artery surgeons tend to use the left internal thoracic artery for anterior descending coronary artery obstruction irrespective of the patient's age. The following recommendations are substantiated in the outcome section. In general, the younger the patient, the more emphasis is placed on an all-arterial graft operation. The problem is in determining who is old. Being over 65 is not necessarily elderly, especially for purposes of conduit selection. Physiologic age, activity, employment, and mental condition all weigh in the assessment of the patient. If life expectancy is longer than 5 or 10 years beyond the operation, it is better to plan for the future and provide the most durable conduit.

Older men and women are similarly afflicted with coronary atherosclerosis. The number of women as surgical candidates is increasing, particularly as the population ages. Women tend to present with a greater prevalence of diabetes, hypertension, hypercholesterolemia, and left ventricular hypertrophy, which may contribute to a poorer clinical outcome early after treatment. Generally the *risk* of coronary artery surgery has been slightly higher in women than men. The hospital mortality has been about twice as high in women as in men. Including emergencies, the surgical mortality for women is still higher than that for men. The New York State registry for coronary bypass surgery recorded risk-adjusted mortality rates of 3.3% for men and 4.5% for women in 1989 [18]. Therefore, gender is a factor in selection as a whole but should not appreciably affect the decision for use of the internal thoracic artery. Arterial grafts are excellent conduits in women because their diameter closely corresponds to the diameter of their generally smaller recipient arteries.

The comorbidity exhibited by the patient preoperatively may affect risk and subsequent hospital course, but with few exceptions comorbidity does not affect selection of the conduit. One such exception is extensive peripheral vascular disease that involves the brachiocephalic and specifically the subclavian arteries. This finding may preclude use of one or both thoracic arteries as in situ grafts. Another exception is diabetes, which may influence the use of both thoracic arteries since it has been shown that there is a higher wound infection rate in diabetic patients in whom both thoracic arteries have been used [23].

The stability of the patient at the time of surgery dictates some decisions regarding conduits and expediency. Patients in extremis rescued from a cardiac catheterization laboratory are unlikely to receive internal thoracic arteries, the flow of which may be affected by shock and vasopressor support. Similarly, patients with poor left ventricular function may benefit more from vein grafts because of flow considerations. Vein grafts are less dependent on normal blood pressure compared with internal thoracic artery grafts. The reoperation candidate often presents a dilemma because of diffuse coronary atherosclerosis and worse left ventricular function than their primary counterparts. Diffuse disease is often a reason to use internal thoracic arteries rather than the larger vein grafts.

Recently, risk of surgery has been predicted more accurately by a statistical assessment of preoperative characteristics. Using variables such as emergency status, serum creatinine level, patient's age and body surface area, presence of heart failure, peripheral vascular disease, or left main coronary atherosclerosis, and severity of angina, one is able to stratify risk. The clinical risk index so constructed is based on weights or scores assigned to each preoperative variable determined by logistic regression. Clinical risk score is the sum of all risk factor weights for that individual [19]. The point is that patients who lie in the highest risk echelons may be candidates for vein grafts because of flow considerations. Conversely, small coronary arteries, irrespective of risk score, may better be grafted using the smaller arterial conduits.

There are relative contraindications for internal thoracic arteries and vein grafts. As mentioned earlier, brachiocephalic disease may affect in situ use of internal thoracic arteries, but free thoracic artery grafts may still be a viable alternative. In our experience, patients who have had extensive chest wall irradiation, usually for breast cancer or Hodgkin's disease, often have unsuitable internal thoracic arteries. Furthermore, if one is contemplating an endarterectomy, the internal thoracic artery is usually not a good choice because its small size does not lend itself to use as a long onlay patch to cover the extended arteriotomy. Rarely, a patient with poor ventricular function may be cause for concern about use of an arterial conduit that is affected by pressure and vasopressor support.

The saphenous vein is generally a satisfactory conduit. Rarely are there size changes or evidence of phlebosclerosis. Even under these circumstances a vein can usually be procured from the greater saphenous systems high or low in the leg, and the necessary length is usually found. A greater problem is the patient with absent saphenous veins. Some of these patients may have a short saphenous system that has not been stripped, but occasionally the saphenous system has been removed surgically in all areas. When this finding is appreciated on the preoperative examination, selective arteriography of each internal thoracic artery may be indicated, particularly if the patient is undergoing a reoperation. Otherwise, we do not advocate catheterization of the internal thoracic arteries routinely.

Technique

Conduit Preparation

The internal thoracic artery must be detached from its chest wall. This preparation requires skill and a respect for the principles of fine dissection. The artery itself must not be touched with forceps or in any way handled roughly. The fragile arterial wall is prone to endothelial disruption and even dissection of the arterial layers. The conduit is removed as a pedicle with the venae comitantes. Generally the pedicle is less than 2 cm wide and should be removed with low cautery and little thermal damage of the surrounding chest wall. We spray 3:1 saline/papaverine through a fine needle onto the artery but do not inject papaverine into the vessel itself for fear of endothelial disruption.

Proper saphenous vein procurement is also important to the success of the bypass operation. The lower extremity vein may be tougher than the internal thoracic artery, but it too may be damaged by overexpansion and external injury. Any endothelial trauma may result in platelet adhesion, fibrin deposition, smooth muscle cell proliferation, vasospasm, and reduced fibrinolytic activity [1]. The vein is best procured atraumatically after heparinization. The vein specimen may be irrigated gently with a balanced electrolyte solution and dilute papaverine, but storage should be brief [33]. In other words, whenever the vein is procured from the leg and prepared, it should be used as soon as possible. Pretreatment with papaverine may reduce vein graft endothelial loss, which occurs because of contraction (Fig. 1).

Myocardial Protection

The evolution of myocardial protection has advanced to the nearly routine use of cold chemical cardioplegia. These cardioplegic solutions cause a potassium arrest. Numerous experiments have indicated that blood cardioplegia is

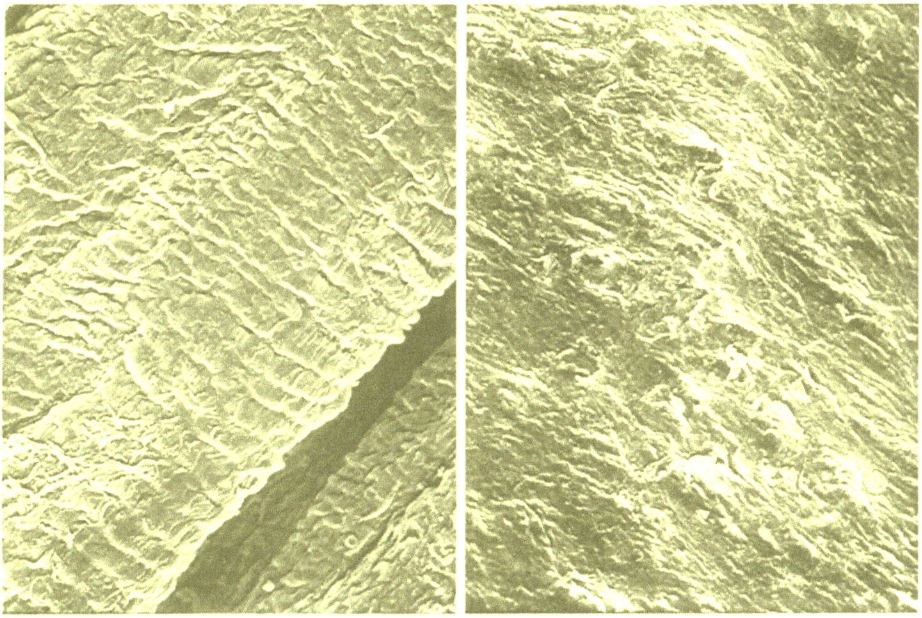

a b

Fig. 1. **a** Smooth muscle cell extensions push up underneath or between cells in the endothelial layer. This herniation causes subsequent sloughing of the endothelial cells. **b** Note the smooth endothelium resulting from a lack of spasm in the procured vein segment

advantageous over other cardioplegic solutions because it provides oxygen for aerobic metabolism during cardiac arrest and reduces perfusion injury [6]. Blood is allegedly a better oncotic medium and buffer than crystalloid solution. Clinical experience appears to confirm these experimental findings [25]. We have used a blood cardioplegia protocol, antegrade and retrograde delivery, and a terminal warm reperfusate since 1986.

The single cross-clamp method, rather than multiple episodes of aortic cross-clamping, results in less aortic manipulation. Ascending aortic atheroembolism is one of the leading causes of stroke and myocardial complications [31]. Aortic disease may be suspected in patients with brachiocephalic atherosclerosis, extensive peripheral vascular disease, or left main coronary narrowing. Aortic atheroemboli appear to occur more frequently in patients undergoing coronary artery surgery than other cardiac procedures [3]. Signs of extensive atherosclerosis may be further evaluated by transesophageal echocardiography and mobile atheromatous disease may contraindicate aortic cross-clamping [35, 42].

Grafting Techniques

The following conditions affect graft patency: (a) the degree of narrowing of the proximal coronary arterial obstruction, (b) overall condition of the

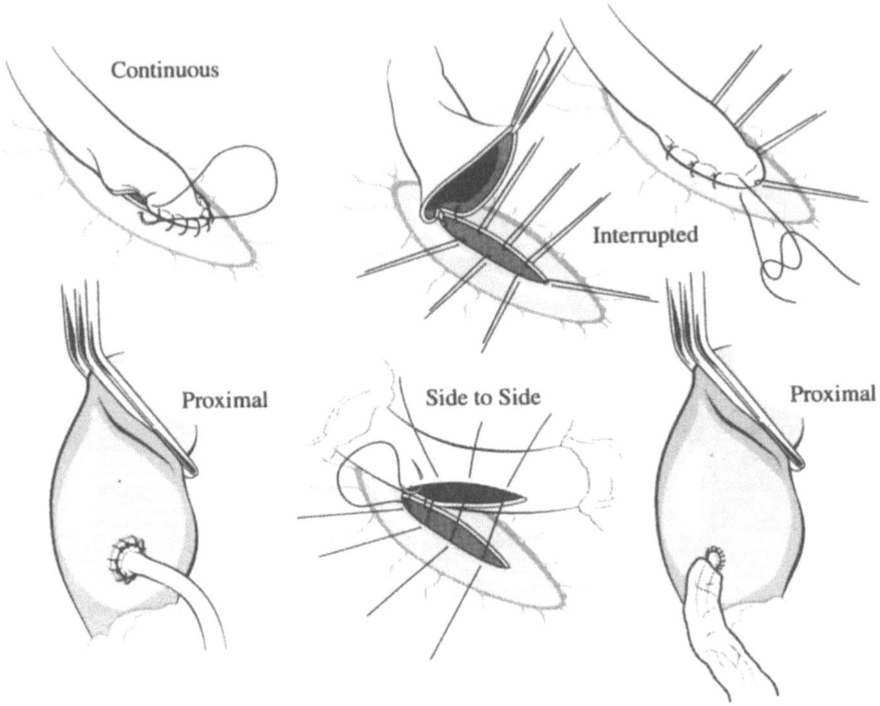

Fig. 2. The various techniques of constructing distal and proximal anastomoses. The continuous technique is usually achieved with 6-0 or 7-0 polypropylene distally and 5-0 polypropylene for proximal anastomoses. We have used the interrupted suture technique with siliconized 7-0 silk for nearly 25 years. Approximately ten sutures are used to effect the anastomosis. Free internal thoracic artery graft proximal anastomoses (*lower righthand panel*) may be performed with continuous 6-0 polypropylene

recipient coronary artery and the characteristics of its distal arterial runoff, (c) extent of wall motion of the segment perfused by the recipient coronary artery, (d) patient's lipid profile, (e) skillfulness of surgical technique, and (f) the type of conduit used.

The actual technique of performing the anastomosis is standardized and consists of a continuous monofilament plastic suture or an interrupted siliconized silk technique. Figure 2 shows a collage of arterial and vein grafting techniques for end-to-side, distal, side-to-side, and proximal anastomoses. In vein grafting, our preference is to perform the distal anastomosis first and construct the proximal anastomosis under full aortic cross-clamping. When vein grafts are combined with one or two arterial grafts, the vein grafts are best performed first and the arterial grafts last to lessen the potential for disruption of the anastomosis by retraction.

Complications

Major morbidity after arterial or vein bypass surgery includes bleeding requiring reoperation, myocardial infarction, stroke, respiratory distress, wound infection, and renal failure. Other complications are rare. Infections at saphenous vein procurement sites are highly unusual and almost always occur in diabetic patients. In our experience, wound infections are more likely to occur in diabetic patients, but the sternal blood supply is not reduced in diabetic compared with nondiabetic patients [10]. Bilateral internal thoracic artery usage leads to a higher sternal wound complication rate but only in insulin-dependent patients [23]. Other factors implicated in higher wound complication rates are longer operation times, obesity, and higher number of units of blood transfused. We have found that bilateral internal thoracic artery grafting in nondiabetic patients poses no greater risk of mediastinitis than in patients with vein grafts or those with one internal thoracic artery graft. Today we believe that bilateral internal thoracic artery grafting may be used safely in diabetic patients. We underscore the need for strict aseptic technique, meticulous procurement of this conduit, an expeditious procedure, and meticulous, layered, interrupted suture closure. We recommend polypropylene wound closure with sutures remaining in place for 2 weeks. This technique has resulted in an exceedingly low infection rate, even in diabetic patients.

Other major complications mentioned above are not related to the type of conduit, but more to the cardiac status and comorbidity of the patient at the outset of the procedure.

Graft Patency

The internal thoracic artery graft enjoys a patency in the 90th percentile over time, up to 10–15 years after the bypass operation. The vein graft is subject to deterioration; however, the early patency is quite satisfactory. One of the earliest and most comprehensive studies on vein graft results reported an 89% patency in 1400 consecutive vein grafts prior to hospital discharge and 81% patency at 1 year [16]. Several groups have reported higher patency of sequential vein grafts. Late thrombosis of saphenous vein coronary bypass grafts is related to several factors, the most important of which is cigarette smoking [39].

Aspirin is widely used for ischemic heart disease. Numerous studies of aspirin use have shown a decrease in the incidence of new myocardial infarction in men and women [43], even in those without clinically apparent ischemic heart disease, especially for those who are over 50 years old and have some cardiovascular risk factors. There have been trials in which the stroke incidence is increased but not to significant levels. Whether to use aspirin after a myocardial infarction is conjectural.

In the original Mayo Clinic studies, aspirin and dipyridamole were prescribed according to a protocol with the reasoning that two platelet-inhibitors affecting different platelet metabolic pathways might be more effective than use of one antiplatelet drug [12]. The effect of antiplatelet drugs was less striking at 1 year compared with early after the operation (14% occlusion in placebo versus 9% in treated group late). Investigators concluded that the effect of these drugs is not related to prevention of primary occlusive proliferative disease but rather to the prevention of complicating thrombosis superimposed on intimal hyperplasia. Subsequently, other investigators have shown that aspirin alone [17] and even low-dose aspirin [26] improve graft patency compared with placebo. There did not seem to be additional benefit when dipyridamole was added to aspirin, and aspirin once a day is as effective as aspirin three times a day. Anticoagulant therapy to enhance graft patency is generally not practiced and has several disadvantages: (a) it does not decrease platelet deposition, (b) it must be started a few days after the operation; and (c) it necessitates laboratory monitoring.

The deterioration of the vein graft accelerates after the fifth year. Montreal investigators found that late luminal changes occur with twice the frequency between 7 and 12 years compared with between the first and the seventh years. In these time frames the mean yearly attrition rate changed from 2% per year to 5.3% per year, and 10–12 years after surgery the graft patency was 63% [8].

It is theorized that atherosclerosis in a vein graft represents a continuum from platelet deposition to smooth muscle proliferation. When one sees intimal hyperplasia and foam cells in contact with blood, these cells are considered a precursor of atherosclerosis. Vein graft atherosclerosis in its complicated form is frequently concentric in distribution, as opposed to the eccentricity of native vessel atherosclerosis, and more often diffuse than localized. These lesions are fragile and may have a poorly defined fibrous cap. Numerous foam cells and inflammatory cells are present, including multinucleate giant cells. Instability of these lesions, which are composed of soft debris, are conducive to atheroembolism to the distal coronary circulation. This atheroembolism may result from manipulation of the vein during reoperation or through coronary balloon angioplasty. Vein graft atherosclerosis may be more related to the patient's lipid profile than originally thought.

Figure 3 shows preliminary correlation of four preoperative serum cholesterol levels as they relate to vein graft stenosis [40]. There is a correlation, which reaches statistical significance at times, between a higher incidence of graft stenosis and the highest cholesterol values. A similar relationship may be drawn between serum triglyceride levels and the frequency of vein graft narrowing. Blankenhorn and colleagues [2] believe that since 60% of the weight of these atheroma is composed of cholesterol esters

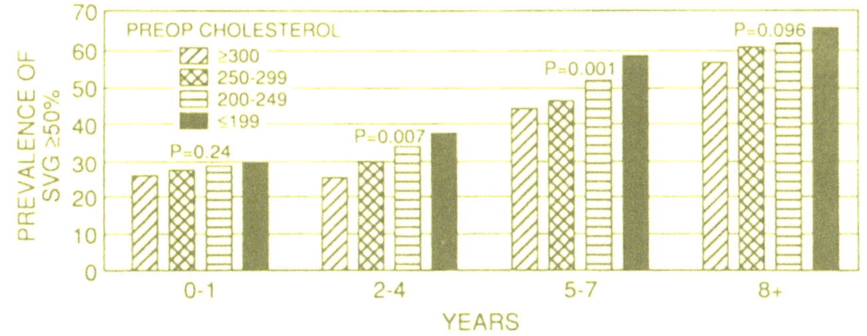

Fig. 3. The prevalence of vein graft stenosis over time related to the preoperative cholesterol level. Note that the highest cholesterol values are a result in the highest percentage of vein grafts stenosed. The level of statistical significance is shown at the top of the bar. (Adapted from Stewart et al. [40])

and phospholipids, a reduction of plaque cholesterol may occur when plasma cholesterol levels are reduced.

Late vein graft failure is not always caused by atherosclerosis. Thrombosis associated with intimal hyperplasia may occur even after 5 years postoperatively [28]. This finding may be a reason to continue antiplatelet drugs beyond 1 year.

Progression of Atherosclerosis

The effect of conduits on native vessel atherosclerosis is interesting. Initially, Montreal Heart Institute investigators found that the rate of progression in the native circulation is higher in grafted arteries, irrespective of whether the grafts are open or closed [4]. In the first year after surgery, half of the grafted arteries demonstrated progressive change at the site of the original lesion compared with about 10% progression in ungrafted vessels. Progression appears to depend on time and the amount of narrowing at the proximal obstruction [5]. Five years after surgery, the progression rates in the ungrafted vessels essentially caught up with the grafted vessels. Interestingly, the effect of internal thoracic artery grafting on the proximal native vessel occlusion is much less prominent [14]. Those studying these findings reason that accelerated proximal closure may indeed occur because the graft flow dominates and reduces or eliminates the flow across the proximal lesion. Anastomotic stenosis may also decrease flow between the proximal lesion and the distal anastomosis. The internal thoracic artery with a lower flow appears to have less effect on native vessel progression.

Survival

Studies have shown that the use of an internal thoracic artery grafted to the anterior descending coronary artery performed alone or combined with vein grafts to other coronary vessels improves 10-year survival compared with vein grafting only [22]. Furthermore, it reduces the incidence of important cardiac events, especially myocardial infarction, rehospitalization for cardiac causes, and reoperation (Fig. 4). The difference in 10-year survival for those who had one internal thoracic artery graft to the anterior descending coronary artery as treatment for one-vessel disease compared with vein grafting was 93.4% and 88%, respectively; for two-vessel disease, the difference in favor of arterial grafting was 90% and 79.5%, and for three-vessel disease the spread was 82.6% and 71%. These differences were highly significant and were irrespective of gender or ventricular performance.

More recently, Cameron and colleagues [7] completed a 20-year follow-up showing that the 20-year actuarial survival for vein graft patients was 38%, whereas it was 50% for patients with one internal thoracic artery graft, and at 19 years, 63.5% with two internal thoracic artery grafts. Other than these long-term studies, there is scant evidence that two internal thoracic artery grafts offer substantially more benefit. This year, Cleveland Clinic investigators found an incremental benefit of two internal thoracic artery grafts in patients under the age of 60 at the time of their revascularization [15]. At 8 years postoperatively, for those less than 60 years old at time of operation, the survival with two internal thoracic artery grafts was 93% versus 88% for one internal thoracic artery and 77% for vein grafts only. A similar and significant difference was found in cardiac event-free survival and reoperation-free survival. At age 60 or above, the benefit was less striking: 8-year survival, 75% with two internal thoracic artery grafts, 77% with one arterial graft, and 68% for vein grafts only (NS). The difference in cardiac event-free survival and no statistical difference in reoperation-free survival was barely significant.

Diabetes is a strong predictor of outcome in some series [32]. In fact, it may be as strong as failure to use an internal thoracic artery graft. While use of internal thoracic artery grafts improves survival over vein grafts only in both nondiabetic and diabetic patients, diabetes is such an important risk factor for late cardiac mortality that use of the thoracic artery does not negate the adverse effect of diabetes on survival. Indeed, in the Duke University experience, vascular disease and diabetes were associated with late death [38]. However, the single greatest determinant of mortality in medical and surgical series is extent of left ventricular damage.

The Veterans' Affairs Cooperative Study involved 686 patients with chronic stable angina. The survivors were followed a median of 16.8 years, and the actuarial 18-year survival rates of 33% for medicine and 30% for surgery are representative of that era of bypass surgery and of the vein graft operation. Their findings showed that in some subsets surgery was advan-

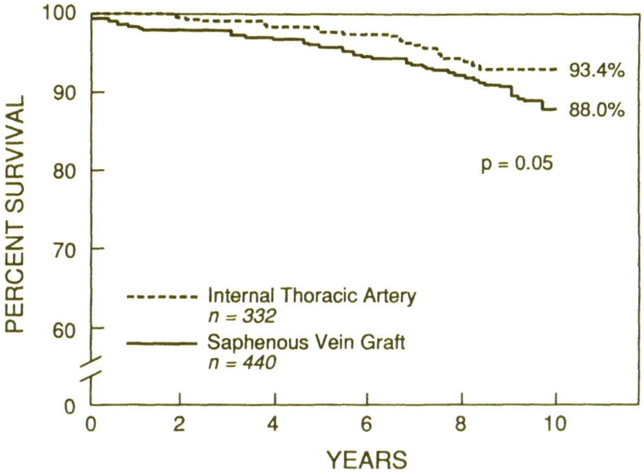

a

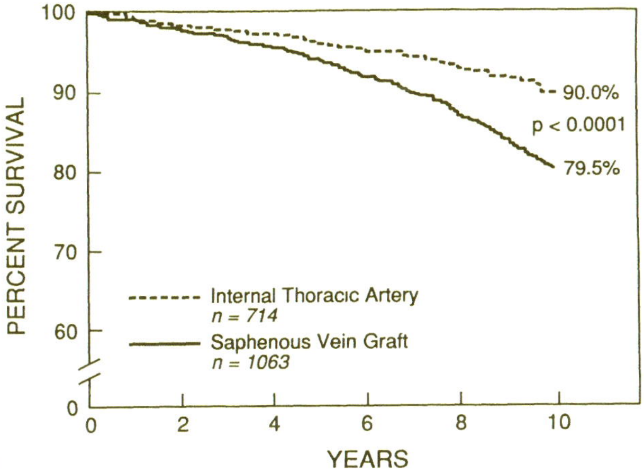

b

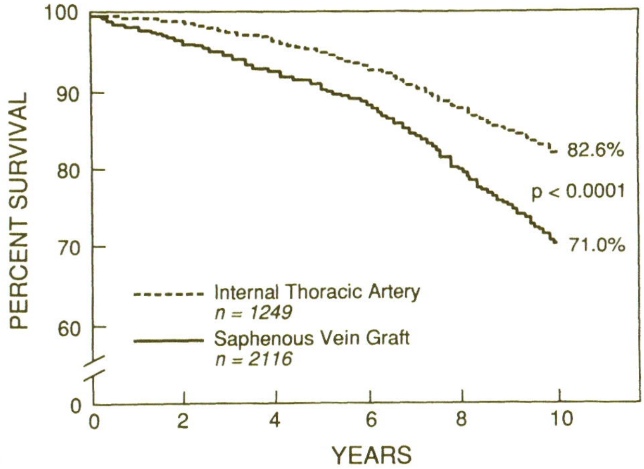

c

Fig. 4a–c. The comparative cohorts of patients who received a left internal thoracic artery graft to the anterior descending coronary artery alone or combined with vein grafts, compared with patients who had vein grafts only are compared for 10-year survival according to the extent of coronary artery disease. The difference in favor of the arterial graft group is significant univariately in one- (**a**), two- (**b**), and three-vessel (**c**) disease subsets. (Reprinted with permistageous up to 11 years, but after that point the medical and surgical results were virtually the same, as was the fatal and nonfatal myocardial infarction rates. The principal reason for the diminution in clinical benefit was graft closure [41].

Between 1968 and 1975, approximately 1700 patients underwent coronary bypass surgery by one surgeon and were followed up to 20 years [21]. All patients received vein grafts only. The overall survival was about 30%, for one-vessel disease 40%, two-vessel 26%, three-vessel 20%, and left main coronary artery disease 25%. The vein graft patency was 81% up to 5 years, 68% 6–10 years, 60% 11–15 years, and 46% 16–20 years. Of the surviving patients, 76% had one or more patent grafts at 15–20 years postoperatively.

In contrast, the experience of the St. Vincent Hospital in Portland, Oregon [34] found a 15- to 20-year survival after bypass surgery in an era similar to that of the Veterans Administration study (1969–1973) and compared approximately 500 patients operated on in that earlier time with approximately 7000 patients operated on from 1974 through 1988. The earlier group was younger and had less coronary disease but incurred a higher operative mortality and a 15- to 20-year survival of 47% compared with 33% for the later group. Patients in the later series showed a 15-year survival of 55%, which was significantly higher than the first series. Men had a significantly higher 15-year survival of 56% versus 52% for women.

Angina. Recent studies [36] have shown that only about half of the patients originally angina-free at year 5 remain so at years 10–12. No studies have shown a relationship between the type of conduit used and late angina relief. Late angina does relate to hyperlipidemia and hypertension. Sudden death relates more to the status of the left ventricle preoperatively.

Reoperation

Vein graft atherosclerosis has become the leading angiographic reason for reoperation, more so than progressive coronary atherosclerosis. As use of arterial conduits increases, the rate of reoperation may decline. Other factors that may lessen the reoperation rate include use of antiplatelet agents, cessation of cigarette smoking, and reduction of serum lipids. Factors associated with a favorable 10-year survival after coronary artery reoperation include age younger than 65 years at the time of reoperation, no major comorbidity and mild angina preoperatively, absence of left main coronary disease, good left ventricular performance, and use of an internal thoracic artery graft. One or more arterial grafts used either at the first operation or the reoperation yielded a significantly higher 10-year survival [24]. The internal thoracic artery tends to preserve left ventricular contractility when used at the first operation [13]. Approximately a third of patients lose

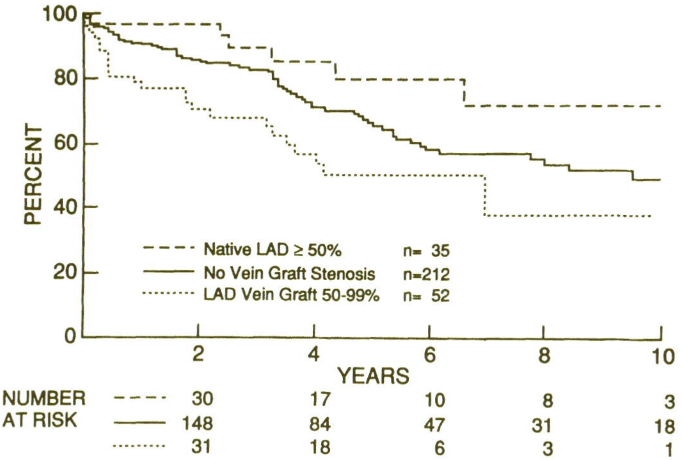

Fig. 5. The zero point in time is the point at which the postoperative catheterization was performed (approximately 5 years after reoperation). The three curves depict the survival for patients with an anterior descending coronary artery narrowing of 50% or greater (---), no vein graft stenosis (—), and narrowing of 50%–99% in a vein graft to the anterior descending coronary artery (----). Note that the latter group exhibits a significantly worse survival than either of the other two categories ($p = 0.002$). (Reprinted with permission from [29])

previously normal left ventricular function in the interval between operations. Patients who have an open internal thoracic artery graft constructed initially have better left ventricular function at the time of reoperation than patients who have received vein grafts only.

Vein graft disease affects prognosis, particularly when atherosclerosis affects a vein graft to the anterior descending coronary artery. Lytle and colleagues [29] have reported that stenosis of the vein graft to the left anterior descending coronary artery is a strong predictor of decreased survival, decreased reoperation-free survival, and decreased event-free survival (Fig. 5). Patients more than 5 years postoperative with an estimated 50% or greater narrowing in a vein graft to the anterior descending had a survival rate of 70% and 50% 2 and 5 years after the second catheterization, the first of which was performed about 5 years postoperatively. These figures compare with 97% and 80% for those with an estimated 50% or greater stenosis of the native left anterior descending coronary artery. The major findings here are that late vein graft stenoses are more dangerous than native coronary stenoses, and that the anterior descending graft lesions have great predictability in determining death and cardiac events.

The question of whether a reoperation should be advocated for late stenoses in vein grafts has also been addressed by Cleveland Clinic investigators [30]. Given that the prognosis for late stenosis in vein grafts to the anterior descending coronary artery is worse than late stenosis in vein grafts to other coronary arteries, it appeared reasonable to compare those subjected

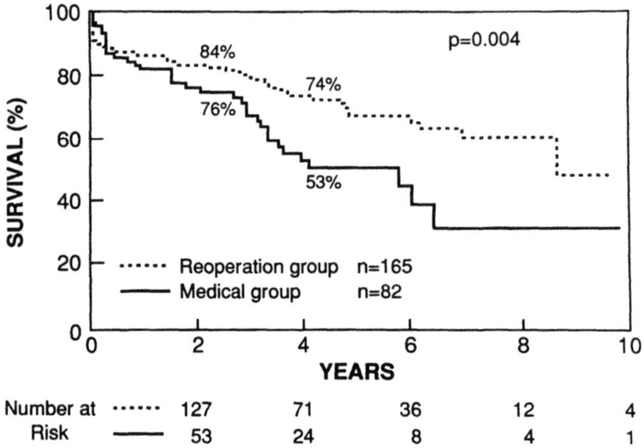

Fig. 6. Two 10-year actuarial survival curves are shown for patients who had late stenosis of vein grafts to the anterior descending coronary artery. The reoperation patients had significantly better 10-year survival compared with their medical counterparts. (Reprinted with permission from [30])

to reoperation with those who were managed conservatively. If the vein graft stenosis appeared *early* and was not likely an atheroma, the overall survival was relatively good, and the patients were treated conservatively because they did not appear to be at high risk of death. However, patients with *late* vein graft stenoses treated surgically fared significantly better than their counterparts treated medically (Fig. 6). Patients who underwent reoperation for vein graft atherosclerosis experienced a 3% hospital mortality. The mortality rose to 8.5% when the atherosclerotic lesion occurred in a vein graft to the anterior descending coronary artery; however, those patients who had a patent internal thoracic artery graft to the anterior descending or an occluded vein graft to the anterior descending had no in-hospital mortality with reoperations, which were performed between 1972 and 1989.

One may conclude from these two studies of Lytle and colleagues on vein graft atherosclerosis that late stenosis in a vein graft to the anterior descending is a strong indication for reoperation, even if the patient is not severely symptomatic. Prolonged life expectancy occurs with reoperation in this subset.

Summary

The internal thoracic artery is the graft of choice. In both arterial and vein grafting, one must follow the principles of graft procurement precisely. Long-term aspirin therapy appears practical for vein graft patients in view of the risk of recurring coronary thrombotic events and the possibility of early and late vein graft thrombosis. Risk factor modification should be pursued explicitly, including absolute cessation of cigarette smoking, which is implicated in vein graft thrombosis. All patients who receive coronary bypass surgery should have their lipid characteristics analyzed and a treatment regimen prescribed if lipids are abnormal.

References

1. Baumann FG, Catinella FP, Cunningham JN Jr, Spencer FC (1981) Vein contraction and smooth muscle cell extensions as causes of endothelial damage during graft preparation. Ann Surg 194:199–211
2. Blankenhorn DH, Nessim SA, Johnson RL, Sanmarco ME, Azen SP, Cashin-Hemphill L (1987) Beneficial effects of combined colestipol-niacin therapy on coronary atherosclerosis and coronary venous bypass grafts. JAMA 257:3233–3240
3. Blauth CI, Cosgrove DM, Webb BW, Ratliff NB, Boylan M, Piedmonte MR, Lytle BW, Loop FD (1992) Atheroembolism from the ascending aorta: an emerging problem in cardiac surgery. J Thorac Cardiovasc Surg 103:1104–1112
4. Bourassa MG, Lesperance J, Corbara F, Saltiel J, Campeau L (1978) Progression of obstructive coronary artery disease 5 to 7 years after aortocoronary bypass surgery. Circulation 58 [Suppl I]:100–106
5. Bruschke AVG, Kramer JR Jr, Bal ET, Haque IU, Detrano RC, Goormastic M (1989) The dynamics of progression of coronary atherosclerosis studied in 168 medically treated patients who underwent coronary arteriography three times. Am Heart J 117:296–305
6. Buckberg GD (1986) Studies of controlled reperfusion after ischemia: a series of experimental and clinical observations from the Division of Thoracic Surgery, UCLA School of Medicine. J Thorac Cardiovasc Surg 92:483–648
7. Cameron A, Brogno DA, Green GE (1991) Internal thoracic artery grafts, twenty years clinical follow-up. Circulation 84 [Suppl II]:II-463
8. Campeau L, Enjalbert M, Lesperance J, Vaislic C, Grondin CM, Bourassa MG (1983) Atherosclerosis and late closure of aortocoronary saphenous vein grafts: sequential angiographic studies at 2 weeks, 1 year, 5 to 7 years, and 10 to 12 years after surgery. Circulation 68 [Suppl II]:1–7
9. Campeau L, Enjalbert M, Lesperance J, Bourrassa MG, Kwiterovich P Jr, Wacholder S, Sniderman A (1984) The relation of risk factors to the development of atherosclerosis in saphenous-vein bypass grafts and the progression of disease in the native circulation. A study 10 years after aortocoronary bypass surgery. N Engl J Med 311:1329–1332
10. Carrier M, Gregoire J, Tronc F, Cartier R, Leclerc Y, Pelletier LC (1992) Effect of internal mammary artery dissection on sternal vascularization. Ann Thorac Surg 53:115–119
11. Chaikhouni A, Crawford FA, Kochel PJ, Olanoff LS, Halushka PV (1986) Human internal mammary artery produces more prostacyclin than saphenous vein. J Thorac Cardiovasc Surg 92:88–91
12. Chesebro JH, Fuster V, Elveback LR, Clements IP, Smith HC, Holmes DR Jr, Bardsley WT, Pluth JR, Wallace RB, Puga FJ, Orszulak TA, Piehler JM, Danielson GK, Schaff HV, Frye RL (1984) Effect of dipyridamole and aspirin on late vein-graft patency after coronary bypass operations. N Engl J Med 310:209–214
13. Coltharp WH, Decker MD, Lea JW IV, Petracek MR, Glassford DM Jr, Thomas CS Jr, Burrus GR, Alford WC, Stoney WS (1991) Internal mammary artery graft at reoperation: risks, benefits, and methods of preservation. Ann Thorac Surg 52:225–229

14. Cosgrove DM, Loop FD, Saunders CR, Lytle BW, Kramer JR (1981) Should coronary arteries with less than fifty percent stenosis be bypassed? J Thorac Cardiovasc Surg 82: 520–530
15. Cosgrove DM, Lytle BW, Hill AC, Taylor PC, Stewart RW, Novoa R, McCarthy PM, Golding LR, Goormastic M, Loop FD (1992) Are two internal thoracic arteries better than one? J Thorac Cardiovasc Surg (in press)
16. FitzGibbon GM, Burton JR, Leach AJ (1978) Coronary bypass graft fate: angiographic grading of 1400 consecutive grafts early after operation and of 1132 after one year. Circulation 57:1070–1074
17. Goldman S, Copeland J, Moritz T, Henderson W, Zadina K, Ovitt T, Doherty J, Read R, Chesler E, Sako Y, Lancaster L, Emery R, Sharma GVRK, Josa M, Pacold I, Montoya A, Parikh D, Sethi G, Holt J, Kirklin J, Shabetai R, Moores W, Aldridge J, Masud Z, DeMots H, Floten S, Haakenson C, Harker LA (1988) Improvement in early saphenous vein graft patency after coronary artery bypass surgery with antiplatelet therapy: results of a Veterans Administration Cooperative Study. Circulation 77:1324–1332
18. Hannan EL, Bernard HR, Kilburn HC Jr, O'Donnell JF (1992) Gender Differences in mortality rates for coronary artery bypass surgery. Am Heart J 123:866–872
19. Higgins TL, Estafanous FG, Loop FD, Beck GJ, Blum JM, Paranandi L (1992) Stratification of morbidity and mortality outcome by preoperative risk factors in coronary artery bypass patients: a clinical severity score. JAMA 267:2344–2348
20. Klein LW, Weintraub WS, Agarwal JB, Schneider RM, Seelaus PA, Katz RI, Helfant RH (1986) Prognostic significance of severe narrowing of the proximal portion of the left anterior descending coronary artery. Am J Cardiol 58:42–46
21. Lawrie GM, Morris GC Jr, Earle N (1991) Long-term results of coronary bypass surgery. Ann Surg 213:377–387
22. Loop FD, Lytle BW, Cosgrove DM, Stewart RW, Goormastic M, Williams GW, Golding LAR, Gill CC, Taylor PC, Sheldon WC, Proudfit WL (1986) Influence of the internal-mammary-artery graft on 10-year survival and other cardiac events. N Engl J Med 314:1–6
23. Loop FD, Lytle BW, Cosgrove DM, Mahfood S, McHenry MC, Goormastic M, Stewart RW, Golding LAR, Taylor PC (1990) Sternal wound complications after isolated coronary artery bypass grafting: early and late mortality, morbidity, and cost of care. J. Maxwell Chamberlain Memorial Paper. Ann Thorac Surg 49:179–187
24. Loop FD, Lytle BW, Cosgrove DM, Woods EL, Stewart RW, Golding LAR, Goormastic M, Taylor PC (1990) Reoperation for coronary atherosclerosis: changing practice in 2509 consecutive patients. Ann Surg 212:378–386
25. Loop FD, Higgins TL, Panda R, Pearce G, Estafanous FG (1992) Myocardial protection during cardiac operations: decreased morbidity and lower cost with blood cardioplegia and coronary sinus perfusion. J Thorac Cardiovasc Surg 104:608–618
26. Lorenz RL, Weber M, Kotzur J, Theisen K, Schacky CV, Meister W, Reichardt B, Weber PC (1984) Improved aortocoronary bypass patency by low-dose aspirin (100 mg daily). Lancet 1:1261–1264
27. Luscher TF, Diederich D, Siebenmann R, Lehmann K, Stulz P, von Segesser L, Yang Z, Turina M, Gradel E, Weber E, Buhler FR (1988) Difference between endothelium-dependent relaxation in arterial and in venous coronary bypass grafts. N Engl J Med 319:462–467
28. Lytle BW, Loop FD, Cosgrove DM, Ratliff NB, Easley K, Taylor PC (1985) Long-term (5 to 12 years) serial studies of internal mammary artery and saphenous vein coronary bypass grafts. J Thorac Cardiovasc Surg 89:248–248
29. Lytle BW, Loop FD, Taylor PC, Simpfendorfer C, Kramer JR, Ratliff NB, Goormastic M, Cosgrove DM (1992) Vein graft disease: the clinical impact of stenoses in saphenous vein bypass grafts to coronary arteries. J Thorac Cardiovasc Surg 103:831–840
30. Lytle BW, Loop FD, Taylor PC, Goormastic M, Stewart RW, Novoa R, McCarthy P, Cosgrove DM (1993) The effect of coronary reoperation on the survival of patients with

stenoses in saphenous vein bypass grafts to coronary arteries. J Thorac Cardiovasc Surg 105:605–612
31. Mills NL, Everson CT (1991) Atherosclerosis of the ascending aorta and coronary artery bypass: pathology, clinical correlates, and operative management. J Thorac Cardiovasc Surg 102:546–553
32. Morris JJ, Smith LR, Jones RH, Glower DD, Morris PB, Muhlbaier LH, Reves JG, Rankin JS (1991) Influence of diabetes and mammary artery grafting on survival after coronary bypass. Circulation 84 [Suppl III]:275–284
33. Quist WC, Haudenschild CC, LoGerfo FW (1992) Qualitative microscopy of implanted vein grafts. J Thorac Cardiovasc Surg 103:671–677
34. Rahimtoola SH, Fessler CL, Grunkemeier GL, Starr A (1993) Survival 15 to 20 years after coronary bypass surgery for angina. J Am Coll Cardiol 21:151–157
35. Ribakove GH, Katz ES, Galloway AC, Grossi EA, Esposito RA, Baumann FG, Kronzon I, Spencer FC (1992) Surgical implications of transesophageal echocardiography to grade the atheromatous aortic arch. Ann Thorac Surg 53:758–763
36. Sergeant P, Lesaffre E, Flameng W, Suy R, Blackstone E (1991) The return of clinically evident ischemia after coronary artery bypass grafting. Eur J Cardiothor Surg 5:447–457
37. Sisto T (1990) Atherosclerosis and the wall structure of the internal mammary artery. Acta Universitatis Tamperensis, series A, vol 286. University of Tampere, Tampere, Finland
38. Smith LR, Harrell FE Jr, Rankin JS, Califf RM, Pryor DB, Muhlbaier LH, Lee KL, Mark DB, Jones RH, Oldham HN, Glower DD, Reves JG, Sabiston DC Jr (1991) Determinants of early versus late cardiac death in patients undergoing coronary artery bypass graft surgery. Circulation 84 [Suppl III]:245–253
39. Solymoss BC, Madeau P, Millette D, Campeau L (1988) Late thrombosis of saphenous vein coronary bypass grafts related to risk factors. Circulation 78 [Suppl I]:140–143
40. Stewart WJ, Goormastic M, Healy BP, Lytle BW, Hoogwerf BJ, Cressman MD, Sheldon WC, Loop FD (1988) Clinical outcome 10 years after coronary bypass: effects of cholesterol and triglycerides in 4913 patients. J Am Coll Cardiol 11:7A
41. Veterans' Affairs Coronary Artery Bypass Surgery Cooperative Study Group (1992) Eighteen-year follow-up in the Veterans Affairs Cooperative Study of Coronary Artery Bypass Surgery for Stable Angina. Circulation 86:121–130
42. Wareing TH, Davila-Roman VG, Barzilai B, Murphy SF, Kouchoukos NT (1992) Management of the severely atherosclerotic ascending aorta during cardiac operations. J Thorac Cardiovasc Surg 103:453–462
43. Willard JE, Lange RA, Hillis LD (1992) The use of aspirin in ischemic heart disease. N Engl J Med 327:175–181

Newer Arterial Coronary Bypass Conduits: Right Gastroepiploic and Epigastric Artery

H. Suma

Following general recognition of the superiority of the internal thoracic artery graft on long-term patient outcome [1], an aggressive investigation was undertaken to find a new arterial conduit which is equally reliable to the internal thoracic artery. In the past 5 years the right gastroepiploic artery (GEA) and the inferior epigastric artery (IEA) have emerged as suitable arterial conduits for coronary artery bypass grafting (CABG), and their clinical application is expanding.

Right Gastroepiploic Artery

GEA was used for indirect myocardial revascularization (Vineberg's procedure) for posterior or inferior wall of the heart in the late 1960s by Bailey et al. [2] and Hirose et al. [3]; its angiographic patency was demonstrated in 1969. Vineberg [4] himself also attempted this procedure. With the development of CABG procedures, direct anastomosis of GEA to the right coronary artery was attempted by Sterling Edwards in early 1970s, as reported by Mills and Everson [5], but there was no exact documentation of the procedure. About 15 years later interest in GEA revived as a new arterial conduit as a result of reports from Pym et al. [6], Suma et al. [7], Carter [8], and Attum [9] in 1987. At the same time, Buffolo et al. [10] reported their use of the left GEA for CABG. Since then the frequency of GEA grafting has been increasing in several countries.

Anatomy and Histology

The right GEA is the largest terminal branch of the gastroduodenal artery, which originates from the common hepatic artery (Fig. 1). Occasionally, the GEA arises from the superior mesenteric artery. It runs along the greater curvature of the stomach from right to left and reaches beyond one-half of the greater curvature in a majority of cases. The GEA diameter is 3 mm or more at its origin and is 1.5–2 mm in the middle of the greater curvature [11].

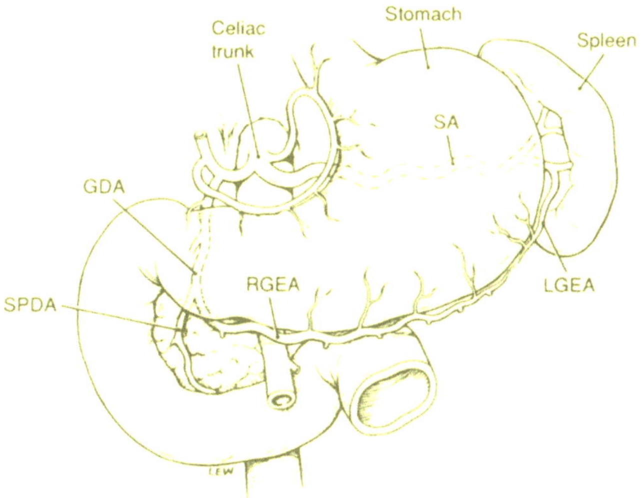

Fig. 1. Anatomy of the GEA. *GDA*, Gastroduodenal artery; *SA*, splenic artery; *RGEA*, right gastroepiploic artery; *LGEA*, left gastroepiploic artery; *SPDA*, superior pancreaticoduodenal artery

Histologically, the media of GEA contains many smooth muscle cells. Van Son et al. [12] have reported that the thickness of the wall of GEA (291 ± 109 μm) is similar to that of the internal thoracic artery (350 ± 92 μm) and the left anterior descending artery (320 ± 63 μm). There are some fenestrations in the internal elastic lamina of the GEA, but arteriosclerosis of GEA is observed less frequently. Larsen et al. [13] investigated the frequency of arteriosclerosis in elderly autopsied persons and have reported that 95 (93%) of 102 gastroduodenal arteries were normal or slightly arteriosclerotic while as few as 14 (14%) out of 103 left coronary arteries were normal and 56 (54%) severely arteriosclerotic.

From our study [14], the severity of arteriosclerosis of the GEA and the internal thoracic artery used for CABG, graded in three degrees, (normal to mild, moderate, and severe) was 92%, 6%, and 2% in the GEA and 99%, 1%, and 0% in the internal thoracic artery. Thus, GEA appears to be a little more susceptible to arteriosclerosis than the internal thoracic artery, but taking into account the finding that all patients studied had severe coronary artery diseases, GEA is not considered liable to develop arteriosclerosis.

Surgical Procedure

A midsternal incision is extended to the middle between the xyphoid process and the umbilicus. The GEA is detached as a pedicle along with the surrounding tissues from the greater curvature of the stomach. The length of the GEA pedicle required for the anastomosis varies according to the target coronary artery. Usually the GEA is taken down to one- to two-thirds of the greater curvature. Detachment of the GEA at the proximal site should be limited to the lower margin of the pylorus, and it is not necessary to extend it to the posterior region of the duodenum. Endoscopic Doppler flow study has shown no ischemia in the greater curvature after detachment of the GEA from the stomach [15]. Prior to the anastomosis 3–4 ml diluted papaverine hydrochloride (40 mg in 10 ml physiological saline) is injected into the GEA lumen from the distal cut end to relieve spasm. Because the GEA is a muscular artery, strong spasms frequently occur by manipulation for take-down. Intraluminal papaverine is an essential procedure to obtain good caliber and flow for successful anastomosis.

The GEA pedicle is then introduced into the pericardial space through the hole in the diaphragm made by electrocautery, passing the anterior surface of the stomach and the liver (anterior route) through the posterior surface of these organs (posterior route) or through the posterior surface of the stomach and the anterior surface of the liver (crossing route) [16]. I always use the anterior route (Fig. 2).

Anastomosis between the GEA and the coronary artery is made by 7-0 or 8-0 suture under a cardioplegic arrest similar to that of the internal

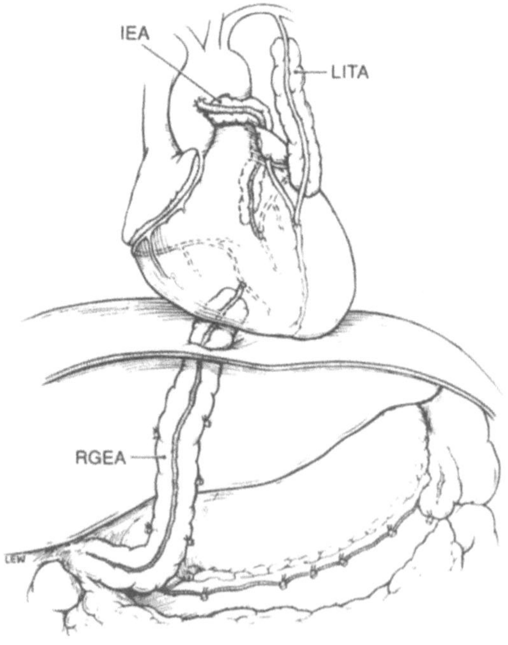

Fig. 2. Scheme of triple arterial grafts. *RGEA*, Right gastroepiploic artery; *IEA*, inferior epigastric artery; *LITA*, left internal thoracic artery

thoracic artery. The direction of the anastomosis depends on the site of the anastomosis. When the target is the posterior descending or low main right coronary artery, the GEA is anastomosed in antegrade fashion putting the heel to the proximal site of the anastomosis. On the other hand, the anastomosis is made in retrograde fashion by putting the heel to the distal site of the anastomosis when the target was the anterior descending or, rarely, the high main right coronary artery. For the circumflex artery, we prefer the antegrade anastomosis, but this should be decided by the relationship between the site of the anastomosis and the course of the graft to be natural and straight.

After the anastomosis is completed and no leakage is found by perfusing GEA flow, the pedicle is fixed to the epicardium appropriately without kinking or twisting. No drainage tube is necessary into the abdominal cavity.

The GEA is occasionally used as a free graft. The harvesting technique is the same as that of an in site GEA graft as described above. The technique for the anastomosis is basically the same as that of the IEA described below.

Indication

The indication for a GEA graft is not yet clearly established. Some are aggressive while others are conservative, as in many other procedures. At many institutes, GEA has initially been utilized for patients who had no suitable saphenous veins available, young patients who definitely need long term patency of the graft in addition to the internal thoracic artery, who had deseased ascending aorta which necessitates in situ arterial grafts for aortic no-touch technique [17, 18], or who had previous coronary artery surgery. However, it becomes utilized more freely at primary coronary artery bypass grafting since we found favourable early and mid-term results in GEA grafting [19].

In our GEA experience with 243 patients since 1986 to July 1992, GEA has been utilized not only in those patients mentioned above, but also in patients with impaired cardiac function, combined cardiac disease (valve or aneurysm), hemodialysis for chronic renal failure, previous abdominal surgery, or aneurysm or occlusive disease of the abdominal aorta, successfully. There are, however, unfavorable conditions for GEA grafts; such as obese or elderly patients, unstable hemodynamics at emergency situation, and/or proposed future abdominal surgery. While we must still await the global recognition of liberal use of the GEA graft until the long-term patency of the GEA and its clinical impact on patient outcome are clarified, it will be a great advantage to have a basic understanding and technical skill with the the GEA graft for treating complicated ischemic heart patients successfully.

Surgical Results

In 1987 Pym et al. [6] reported nine patients with GEA graft anastomosed to the circumflex or right coronary artery. All successfully opacified six GEAs were patent at early postoperative angiography. Suma and colleagues [7] used the GEA to bypass the left anterior descending artery at reoperation in two patients, and two GEAs were patent. Carter [8] performed GEA grafting in 30 patients, including five sequential grafts. Target arteries were all posterior descending or posterolateral arteries, and seven of nine GEAs were patent.

In 1989 extended experience was reported by Lytle et al. [20], Mills et al. [5], Suma et al. [21], and Verkkala et al. [22]. From the Cleveland Clinic, Lytle et al. [20] reported 36 patients with 17 in situ and 19 free GEA grafts. The majority of these were reoperation cases, and early angiography revealed that all nine restudied GEA grafts were patent. Mills and Everson [5] performed GEA grafting in 39 patients with 26 in situ and 15 free grafts. They found that all 29 GEA grafts were patent, and they pointed out that the free GEA graft is likely to have spasm more frequently than the in-situ graft. Suma et al. [21] reported 22 patients with combined use of the GEA and the internal thoracic artery with 14 of 15 GEA grafts patent, and Kusukawa et al. [23] showed the efficacy of the GEA graft by stress myocardial scintigraphy with their precise technique. Verkkala et al. [22] reported 11 patients with GEA grafts and 9 of 11 GEAs were patent.

In 1990 Beretta and associates [24] reported 20 patients with all free GEA grafts including seven sequential grafts. Because they were concerned about future abdominal surgery after in situ GEA grafting and thought a free graft to be more accessible to any coronary arteries than a in situ graft, they attempted to use a free GEA graft in all patients. Early angiography revealed that all 20 GEA grafts were patent. Pym et al. [25] reported their extended experience with the GEA graft in 57 patients at the annual meeting of the Society of Thoracic Surgeons in 1990. Imaging showed that 25 of 26 GEA grafts were patent. Two reports from Takeuchi et al. [26] and Isomura et al. [27] have shown successful use of the GEA graft in pediatric patients with Kawasaki's disease.

In 1991 Suma et al. [15] compared the surgical results between GEA and non-GEA CABG in 70 patients each and showed no increase in perioperative risk with use of the GEA graft. They also demonstrated that there is no gastric ischemia with devascularization of the greater curvature of the stomach using the endoscopic Doppler velocimetry. Suma et al. [14] also showed that the size, flow, and patency of GEA graft is comparable to those of the internal thoracic artery. The mean free flow after intraluminal papaverine was 91 ml/min in GEA and 81 ml/min in the internal thoracic artery, and their patency rate was 96% (n = 92) and 98% (n = 322), respectively.

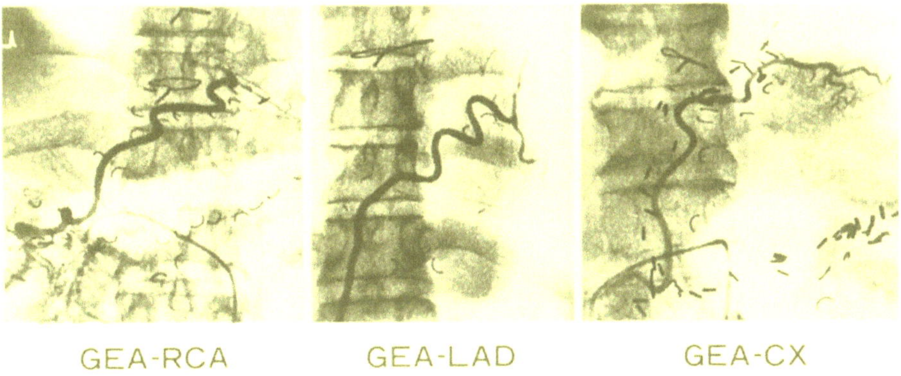

Fig. 3. Postoperative angiograms of in situ GEA grafts at 2 postoperative years

In 1992 Suma et al. [19] reported the midterm results of GEA grafting in 200 patients. Early mortality was 3%, and early patency rate was 96% in 140 in situ and 75% in 12 free GEA grafts (95% in overall). Among those who underwent early angiographic restudy, 40 patients underwent the second postoperative study; 38 of 40 in situ grafts (95%) were patent without any signs of focal stenosis at the mean of 2–5 years after surgery (Fig. 3). In stress myocardial scintigraphy performed sequentially before and after surgery in 11 patients, the washout ratio of the grafted area was significantly increased from 35% ± 10% preoperatively to 45% ± 15% immediately after surgery, and it was maintained satisfactorily at 43% ± 6% and 48% ± 9% at 1 year and 2 years after surgery.

In summary, the reported operative mortality ranges from 0% to 7.7%, and the early patency rate varies from 78% to 100% in the GEA graft. Although the procedure may be technically somewhat demanding, perioperative morbidity and duration of surgery do not increase with experience. The long-term patency and its clinical impact are still unclear, but the midterm results with the GEA graft are excellent.

Physiological and Biochemical Findings

As the GEA has been used increasingly for CABG, various studies have been carried out. For responses to various drugs, Koike et al. [28] have reported that the GEA shows contraction to ergonovine, serotonin, and phenylephrine similarly to the internal thoracic artery. Dignan et al. [29] stated that the GEA is more strongly contracted by potassium chloride, serotonin, and norepinephrine than the internal thoracic artery and suggested that it is important to prevent spasm of the GEA provoked by platelet aggregators, adrenergic stimulation, or depolarizing agents at clinical situation.

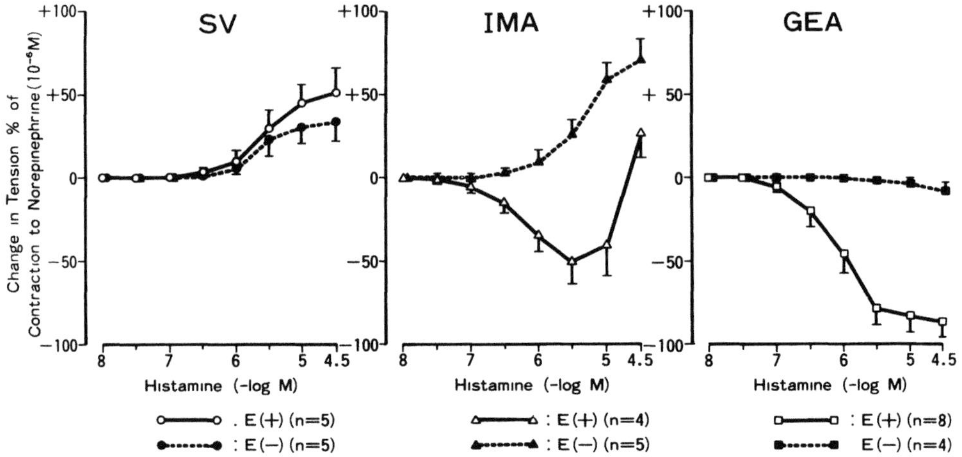

Fig. 4. Different responses to histamine in saphenous vein (*SV*), internal thoracic artery (*ITA*), and gastroepiploic artery (*GEA*) with and without endothelium. Note a dilatation of GEA with endothelium by histamine (*right*, *open square*) while SV and ITA showed constriction. (From [31])

O'Neil et al. [30] and Ochiai et al. [31] also compared responses of GEA and the internal thoracic artery and found a difference in response to histamine. This agent caused contraction of the internal thoracic artery and dilated the GEA (Fig. 4). Toda et al. [32] have reported that the GEA at the proximal site is contracted by dopamine in a dose-dependent manner, but at the distal site it is dilated at low concentrations and contracted at high concentrations. This finding indicates that GEA contains mainly α-adrenoreceptors at the proximal site and has both α-adrenoreceptors and α-dopaminergic receptors at the distal site.

Our recent clinical investigation using an implantable ultrasonic Doppler miniprobe demonstrated that GEA blood flow is increased after a meal [33]. This finding is in good agreement with the above-mentioned response to histamine, that is, there may be an organ-specific reaction in which the GEA is dilated by histamine released after a meal to increase blood supply to the digestive tract. This biological response is clearly observed in the GEA graft connected to the coronary artery early after operation.

With regard to biochemical products, the GEA shows greater prostacyclin production than the saphenous vein [34], and this finding is similar to that for the internal thoracic artery [35].

Inferior Epigastric Artery

With arterial grafts obtaining superior reliability for CABG, the IEA has become seen as a suitable conduit for myocardial revascularization. In 1990

Puig et al. [36] first reported use of the IEA for CABG, and its clinical trial is expanding (Fig. 2).

Anatomy and Histology

The IEA arises from the medial side of the external iliac artery and ascends between the transversalis fascia and peritoneum passing the ductus deferens (male) or the round ligament (female) medially. The IEA runs up toward the umbilicus and terminates with or without communications with the superior epigastric artery, which is the downstream of the internal thoracic artery by piercing the rectus muscle (Fig. 5).

Histologically, the IEA is a muscular artery, similarly to the GEA. In the study by Van Son et al. [12] the wall thickness of the IEA (249 ± 87 μm) was similar to that of the GEA, internal thoracic artery, and coronary artery. Puig et al. [36] reported that there is no interruption of the internal elastic lamina in the IEA, but Van Son et al. [12] showed some fenestration in it. Barner [37] noted that the continuity of the internal elastic lamina in

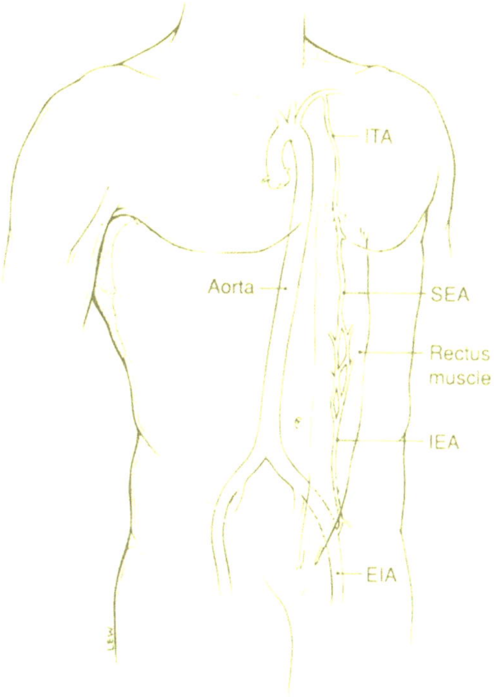

Fig. 5. Anatomy of the IEA. *ITA*, Internal thoracic artery; *SEA*, superior epigastric artery; *IEA*, inferior epigastric artery; *EIA*, external iliac artery

IEA is similar to that in the internal thoracic artery. Systematic study for incidence of arteriosclerosis of the IEA has not been made yet.

Surgical Procedure

From the description by Mills and Everson [38], harvest of the IEA is made through the paramedian incision angled as a "hockey sitck" toward the point at which the femoral artery arises from under the inguinal ligament. The lower end of the incision must be ended above 5 cm of the inguinal ligament. By incising the rectus sheath and retracting the rectus muscle laterally, the IEA is taken down along its course accompanying two inferior epigastric veins.

Vincent and colleagues [39] recommended excising the proximal IEA with the part of the external iliac artery as an oval cuff to facilitate its proximal anastomosis to the aorta. Mills and Everson [38], however, disagreed with this technique because of reluctancy of heparinization for this procedure at this point and possible atherosclerois in the iliac artery.

The obtained IEA length varied from 11 to 20 cm. Intraluminal papaverine may be helpful in relieving spasm and obtaining good caliber. The diameter of the IEA ranges from 2.5 to 3.5 mm at a proximal site and from 1.5 to 2.5 mm at a distal site and seems to be unrelated to the body surface area of the patients [38].

The distal anastomosis to the coronary artery is basically the same as that of the GEA or the internal thoracic artery. Precise anastomosis with 7-0 or 8-0 suture is necessary. The proximal anastomosis of the IEA graft is a matter of concern. Direct anastomosis to the thickened or diseased aortic wall is unfavorable for obtaining good patency. As shown in Fig. 6, there are several choices for the proximal anastomotic site of the free arterial graft. The correct choice gives a good result. Before closing the abdominal wall, drains are left in place behind the rectus muscle to avoid hematoma and infection.

There is no report of rectus muscle necrosis, but one case from Barner et al. (N.L. Mills 1991, on discussion in [40]) even if the internal thoracic artery and IEA were dissected at the same side.

Indication

As is mentioned in reference to the GEA, the indication for the IEA remains unclear. Because the history of using this conduit is shorter than that of the GEA, its midterm results are still unknown. As a rule, new conduits were used initially in limited situations such as patients whose saphenous veins or internal thoracic arteries were unavailable or insufficient to perform a complete revascularization. Although its indication is gradually

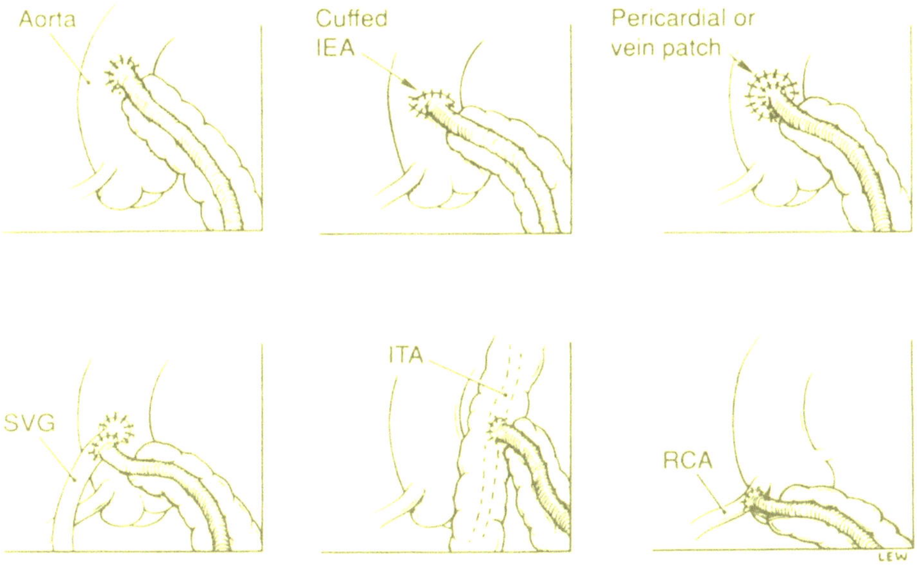

Fig. 6. Choice of proximal anastomotic site for IEA graft. *IEA*, Inferior epigastric artery; *SVG*, saphenous vein graft; *ITA*, internal thoracic artery; *RCA*, right coronary artery

expanding into an ordinary primary CABG, we must have further knowledge about the nature of the free arterial graft.

Surgical Results

In 1990 Puig and coworkers [36] reported IEA grafting in 22 patients, including two bilateral IEAs. The sites of the IEA anastomosis were 16 anterior descending, 5 diagonal, 2 obtuse marginal, and 1 right coronary artery. Early angiography revealed 15 of 17 IEAs were patent 8–10 days after surgery. All proximal anastomoses were made to the aorta, and they recommended vein or pericardial patch to the aorta for IEA anastomosis to improve the patency. Vincent and associates [39] reported two patients with IEA graft, anastomosed to the obtuse marginal artery in both cases. Postoperative angiography was not carried out, but these two patients are alive and well.

In 1991 Mills and Everson [38] reported 18 patients with IEA, including one natural Y graft. Sixteen IEA grafts were anastomosed to diagonal or circumflex artery, and the remaining three were used to bypass the right coronary artery. In three patients who had postoperative angiography within 10 days all IEAs were patent. However, they later noted two occlusions and two stringlike narrowings out of seven restudied IEAs (N.L. Mills 1991, on discussion in [40]) within 3 postoperative months. While they noted each one of abdominal wound hematoma and late wound infection, these wound complications were prevented by use of infrarectus muscle drains. Barner and coworkers [40] reported 47 patients with IEA, including ten bilateral and five natural Y grafts. More than one-third of the patients had previous coronary bypass procedures. Sites of IEA anastomosis were 19 anterior descending, 17 diagonal (including intermediate branch), 19 obtuse marginal, and 7 right coronary arteries. Excluding one operative death, all 46 patients were alive without ischemic events at follow-up within 10 months. No angiographic study was undertaken. They noted rectus muscle necrosis requiring surgical débridement in one patient of 16 having bilateral internal thoracic and inferior epigastric arteries harvesting.

In 1992 Milgalter et al. [41] from UCLA reported 38 patients with IEA, including four bilateral harvesting. Distal anastomoses were to 2 anterior descending, 27 diagonal, 9 marginal, and 4 right coronary arteries. Proximal anastomoses were to the aorta in 17, the vein graft hood in 20, and onto the internal thoracic artery graft in 5. All patients were alive without angina pectoris. No postoperative angiography was performed. They recommended preoperative Duplex scanning for IEA evaluation. Buche and colleagues [42] reported 73 patients with IEA graft, including three sequential and one natural Y grafts; 78 distal anastomoses with IEA were made to 35 main right coronary, 18 posterior descending or posterolateral, 22 obtuse marginal, 2 diagonal, and 1 anterior descending arteries. In 69 survivors 59 (97%) of 61 IEAs (63 of 65 distal anastomoses) were patent at early postoperative angiography at 10 days, and 17 (89%) of 19 IEAs, including one string sign, were patent 6 months after surgery. We have used the IEA graft in ten patients since March 1992. Sites of anastomosis were two anterior descending, two diagonal, three circumflex, and three right coronary arteries. Early postoperative angiography showed good patency in all six IEA grafts restudied (Fig. 7). But one of these anastomosed to the circumflex artery

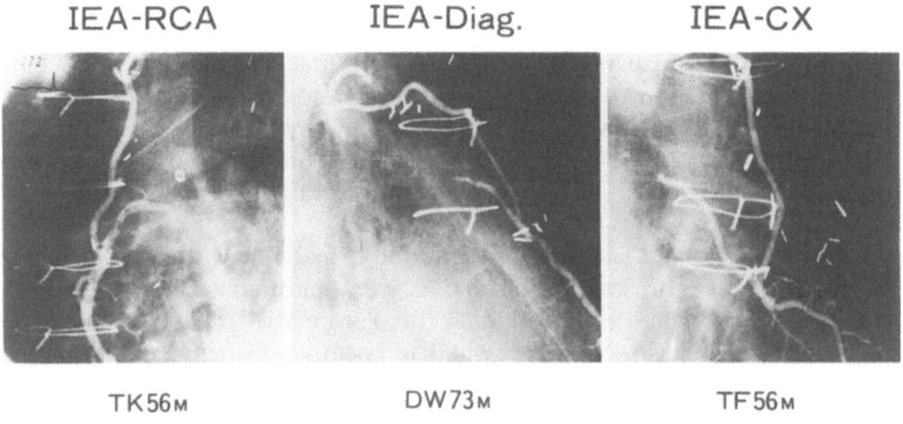

Fig. 7. Postoperative angiograms of IEA grafts at 2 postoperative weeks

turned out to be stringlike without any evidence of increased native flow or anastomotic stenosis 2 months later.

Summary

The GEA and IEA are new arterial conduits for CABG. While long-term data are yet not available to compare with the saphenous vein and the internal thoracic artery grafts, the midterm result of GEA graft is favorable. Whereas a liberal use of these new conduits at the primary myocardial revascularization is still contraversial, these two arteries are advantageous at coronary reoperation because they can be easily harvested before sternal reentry.

The in situ GEA graft is also convenient to perform as CABG with aortic no-touch technique for patients with diseased ascending aorta.

The understanding of basic knowledge and technical skill of these new conduits may be enormously advantageous for cardiac surgeons who manage complicated ischemic heart patients.

References

1. Loop FD, Lytle BW, Cosgrove DM, Stewart RW, Goormastic M, Williams GW, Golding LAR, Gill CC, Taylor PC, Sheldon WC, Proudfit WL (1986) Influence of the internal-mammary-artery graft on 10 year survival and other cardiac events. N Engl J Med 314:1–7
2. Bailey CP, Hirose T, Brancato R, Aventura A, Yamamoto N (1966) Revascularization of the posterior (diaphragmatic) portion of the heart. Ann Thorac Surg 2:791–805
3. Hirose T, Yaghmai M, Vera CA (1969) Cineangiographic visualization technique of the implanted right gastroepiploic artery of the posterior myocardium. Vasc Surg 3:61–67
4. Vineberg A, Afridi S, Sahi S (1975) Direct revascularization of acute myocardial infarction by implantation of left internal mammary artery into infarcted left ventricular myocardium. Surg Gynecol Obstet 140:44–52
5. Mills NL, Everson CT (1989) Right gastroepiploic artery: a third arterial conduit for coronary bypass. Ann Thorac Surg 47:706–711
6. Pym J, Brown PM, Charrette EJP, Parker JO, West RO (1987) Gastroepiploic-coronary anastomasis: a viable alternative bypass graft. J Thorac Cardiovasc Surg 94:256–259
7. Suma H, Fukumoto H, Takeuchi A (1987) Coronary artery bypass grafting by utilizing in situ right gastroepiploic artery: basic study and clinical application. Ann Thorac Surg 44:394–397
8. Carter MJ (1987) The use of the right gastroepiploic artery in coronary artery bypass grafting. Aust NZ J Surg 57:317–321
9. Attum AA (1987) The use of the gastroepiploic artery for coronary artery bypass grafts: another alternative. Tex Heart Inst J 14:289–292
10. Buffolo E, Maluf M, Barone B, Andrade JCS, Gallucci C (1987) Direct myocardial revascularization with the left gastroepiploic artery. A new alternative to aortocoronary bypass (a case report). Arq Bras Cardiol 48:167–171

11. Saito T, Suma H, Terada Y, Wanibuchi Y, Fukuda S, Furuta S (1992) Availability of the in situ right gastroepiploic artery for coronary artery bypass. Ann Thorac Surg 53:266–268
12. Van Son JAM, Smedts F, Vincent JG, van Lier HJ, Kubat K (1990) Comparative anatomic studies of various arterial conduits for myocardial revascularization. J Thorac Cardiovasc Surg 99:703–707
13. Larsen E, Johansen Aa, Andersen D (1969) Gastric arteriosclerosis in elderly people. Scand J Gastroenterol 4:387–389
14. Suma H, Wanibuchi Y, Furuta S, Isshiki T, Yamaguchi T, Takanashi R (1991) Comparative study between the gastroepiploic and the internal thoracic artery as a coronary bypass graft. Size, flow, patency, histology. Eur J Cardiothorac Surg 5:244–247
15. Suma H, Wanibuchi Y, Furuta S, Takeuchi A (1991) Does use of gastroepiploic artery graft increase surgical risk? J Thorac Cardiovasc Surg 101:121–125
16. Mills NL, Everson CT (1989) Technical considerations for use of the gastroepiploic artery for coronary artery surgery. J Cardiac Surg 4:1–9
17. Suma H (1989) Coronary artery bypass grafting in patients with calcified ascending aorta; aortic no touch technique. Ann Thorac Surg 48:728–730
18. Mills NL, Everson CT (1991) Atherosclerosis of the ascending aorta and coronary artery bypass, pathology, clinical correlates, and operative management. J Thorac Cardiovasc Surg 102:546–553
19. Suma H, Wanibuchi Y, Terada Y, Fukuda S, Takayama T, Furuta S (1993) The right gastroepiploic artery graft; clinical and angiographic mid-term results in 200 patients. J Thorac Cardiovasc Surg 105:615–623
20. Lytle BW, Cosgrove DM, Ratliff NB, Loop FD (1989) Coronary artery bypass grafting with the right gastroepiploic artery. J Thorac Cardiovasc Surg 97:826–831
21. Suma H, Takeuchi A, Hirota Y (1989) Myocardial revascularization with combined arterial grafts utilizing the internal mammary and the gastroepiploic arteries. Ann Thorac Surg 47:712–715
22. Verkkala K, Jarvinen A, Keto P, Virtanen K, Lehtala A, Pellinen T (1989) Right gastroepiploic artery as a coronary bypass graft. Ann Thorac Surg 47:716–719
23. Kusukawa J, Hirota Y, Kawamura K, Suma H, Takeuchi A, Adachi I, Akagi H (1989) An assessment of the efficacy of aorta-coronary bypass surgery using gastroepiploic artery with thallium 201 myocardial scintigraphy. Circulation 80 [Suppl I]:135–140
24. Beretta L, Lemma M, Vanelli P, Botta M, Antonacci C, Bevilacqua M, Monopoli A, Santoli C (1990) Gastroepiploic artery free graft for coronary bypass. Eur J Cardiothorac Surg 4:323–328.
25. Pym J, Parker JO, West RO (1990) The right gastroepiploic artery as a coronary artery bypass graft. Abstract from 27th annual meeting of the Society of Thoracic Surgeons, San Francisco, p 68
26. Takeuchi Y, Gomi A, Okamura Y, Mori H, Nagashima M (1990) Coronary revascularization in a child with Kawasaki disease; use for right gastroepiploic artery. Ann Thorac Surg 50:294–296
27. Isomura T, Hisatomi K, Asoh S, Ohyama K, Kosuga K, Ohishi K, Inoue O, Kato H (1990) Revascularization with the right gastroepiploic artery in Kawasaki's disease. J Thorac Cardiovasc Surg 100:796–798
28. Koike R, Suma H, Kondo K, Oku T, Satoh H, Fukuda S, Takeuchi A (1990) Pharmacological response of internal mammary artery and gastroepiploic artery. Ann Thorac Surg 50:384–386
29. Dignan RJ, Yeh T, Dyke CM, Lee KF, Lutz III HA, Ding M, Wechsler A (1992) Reactivity of gastroepiploic and internal mammary arteries; relevance to coronary artery bypass grafting. J Thorac Cardiovasc Surg 103:116–123
30. O'Neil GS, Chester AH, Schyns CI, Tadjkarimi S, Pepper JR, Yacoub MH (1991) Vascular reactivity of human internal mammary and gastroepiploic arteries. Ann Thorac Surg 52:1310–1314

31. Ochiai M, Ohno M, Taguchi J, Hara K, Suma H, Isshiki T, Yamaguchi T, Kurokawa K (1992) Responses of human gastroepiploic arteries to vasoactive substances – differences to internal mammary arteries and saphenous veins. J Thorac Cardiovasc Surg 104:453–458
32. Toda N, Okunishi H, Okamura T (1989) Responses to dopamine of isolated human gastroepiploic arteries. Arch Int Pharmacodyn Ther 297:86–97
33. Takayama T, Suma H, Wanibuchi Y (1992) Physiological and pharmacological response of the arterial graft flow after coronary artery bypass grafting. Circulation 86 [Suppl II]:217–223
34. Oku T, Yamane S, Suma H, Satoh H, Koike R, Sawada Y, Takeuchi A (1990) Comparison of prostacyclin production of human gastroepiploic artery and saphenous vein. Ann Thorac Surg 49:767–770
35. Chaikhouni A, Crawford FA, Kochel PJ, Olanoff LS, Halushka PV (1986) Human internal mammary artery produces more prostacyclin than saphenous vein. J Thorac Cardiovasc Surg 92:88–91
36. Puig LB, Ciongolli W, Cividanes GVL, Dontos A, Kopel L, Bittencourt D, Assis RVC, Jatene AD (1990) Inferior epigastric artery as a free graft for myocardial revascularization. J Thorac Cardiovasc Surg 99:251–255
37. Barner HB, Fischer VS (1992) Comparative study between the gastroepiploic and the internal thoracic artery as a coronary bypass. Eur J Cardiothorac Surg 6:224
38. Mills NL, Everson CT (1991) Technique for use of the inferior epigastric artery as a coronary bypass graft. Ann Thorac Surg 51:208–214
39. Vincent JG, Van Son AM, Skotnicki SH (1990) Inferior epigastric artery as a conduit in myocardial revascularization: the alternative free arterial graft. Ann Thorac Surg 49: 323–325
40. Barner HS, Naunheim KS, Fiore AC, Fisher VW, Harris HH (1991) Use of the inferior epigastric artery as a free graft for myocardial revascularization. Ann Thorac Surg 52: 429–437
41. Milgalter E, Pearl JM, Laks H, Elami A, Louie HW, Baker D, Buckburg GD (1992) The inferior epigastric arteries as coronary bypass conduits. Size preoperative duplex scan assessment of suitability, and early clinical experience. J Thorac Cardiovasc Surg 103: 463–465
42. Buche M, Schoevaerdts JC, Louagie Y, Schroeder E, Marchandise B, Chenn P, Dion R, Verhelst R, Deloos M, Gonzales E, Chalant CH (1992) Use of the inferior epigastric artery for coronary bypass. J Thorac Cardiovasc Surg 103:665–670

Diagnosis of Graft Failure

The Role of Radionuclide Imaging in the Diagnosis of Coronary Bypass Graft Failure

F.J.T. Wackers

Noninvasive diagnostic methods are particularly attractive to monitor success or failure of surgical revascularization. Using radionuclide imaging, three well-established approaches are considered here: (a) assessment of global or regional left ventricular function, (b) assessment of acute myocardial tissue damage, and (c) assessment of myocardial perfusion.

Assessment of Cardiac Function

Cardiac function can be assessed noninvasively either by first-pass radionuclide angiocardiography (FPRNA) or by equilibrium radionuclide angiocardiography (ERNA). FPRNA requires specialized gamma cameras with high-count sensitivity. The advantage of this technique is that is allows determination of left ventricular ejection fraction during the short time period, 15–30 s, when a rapidly injected radioactive bolus travels through the central circulation [1]. Although this method has been well validated, the required optimal equipment is not widely available. Therefore this specific method is not discussed further.

Widely available, is the regular gamma camera used to perform ERNA [2]. This technique is commonly also referred to as gated blood-pool imaging or radionuclide ventriculography. For this method the patient's own red blood cells are labeled with radioactive technetium-99m [3]. Because of the relatively stable binding of ^{99m}Tc within the red cells, radioactivity is contained within the vascular space. Externally measured changes in radioactivity are proportional to changes in blood volume. In order to determine cardiac function the gamma camera is positioned over the patient's chest, and data are acquired synchronized with the R wave of the QRS complex of the electrocardiogram [4]. ERNA data are recorded throughout the cardiac cycle (R-R interval) and stored separately in computer memory depending upon the relationship to each R wave. Imaging is continued for 5–8 min, accumulating data over several hundred cardiac cycles. Since radioactivity is in equilibrium within the blood pool, imaging can be performed over an extended period of time. For complete analysis of all cardiac chambers, images are acquired in multiple projections. Usually three views are obtained: the anterior, left anterior oblique, and left lateral views. For interpretation these images are displayed on computer screen as an endless loop movie. Each cardiac chamber can then be analyzed in terms of relative size and global and regional contraction pattern [5].

Left ventricular ejection fraction (LVEF) is calculated from the left anterior oblique view. In this projection radioactivity from the right ventricle is well separated from that of the left ventricle. By choosing a variable region of interest over the left ventricle, a time-activity curve corresponding to volume changes in the left ventricle can be generated [7]. LVEF is calculated from background-corrected enddiastolic (ED) and endsystolic (ES) counts as follows: (ED − ES)/ED. Most computers now have automated or semiautomated software to rapidly calculate LVEF, regional ejection fraction, and diastolic filling parameters. Right ventricular ejection fraction (RVEF) cannot be determined reliably from an ERNA study because of unavoidable overlap of radioactivity of the right atrium and left ventricles [6]. The technique of choice for the assessment of RVEF is ECG-gated list-mode FPRNA, which can be performed using regular gamma cameras. The lower limit of normal LVEF is 50%, whereas the lower limit of normal for RVEF is 40%.

A major advantage of radionuclide assessment of RVEF and LVEF is the relative ease of acquisition. These measurements can be obtained either in the outpatient laboratory or at the bedside of critically ill patients. Moreover, it is feasible to obtain diagnostic quality ERNA studies in virtually all patients. A most important aspect of ERNA is the excellent reproducibility of calculating ejection fraction [7]. In our laboratory calculation of LVEF is reproducible within 3% (ejection fraction units), whereas RVEF has slightly greater variability and is accurate within 6% (ejection fraction units).

ERNA allows detailed analysis of the chambers of the heart and adjacent structures. We usually report on the size of right and left atria, the size and contraction pattern of right and left ventricle, the presence of left ventricular hypertrophy, and the size and configuration of the pulmonary artery and ascending aorta [5].

Because of the excellent reproducibility of assessment of global and regional LVEF, ERNA is ideally suited for following patients after bypass surgery. In many patients improvement in regional and global left ventricular function is observed after successful revascularization. When perioperative infarction is suspected, deterioration of regional wall motion and a decrease in global LVEF is strong evidence of perioperative or postoperative graft failure and infarction (Fig. 1).

Although ERNA has been used extensively in the past in conjunction with supine bicycle exercise, at the present time this methodology is employed less often. It has become evident that an abnormal response of LVEF during exercise (failure to increase >5%) may be nonspecific and is not necessarily evidence of exercise-induced myocardial ischemia.

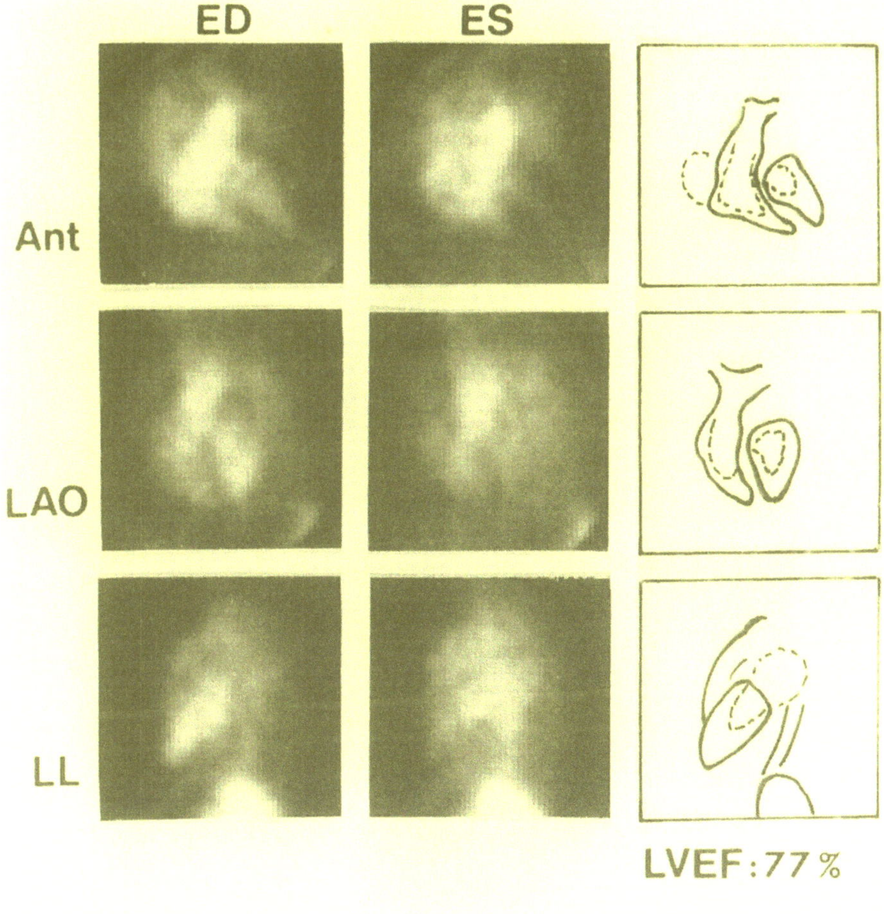

Fig. 1a,b. Equilibrium radionuclide angiocardiography (ERNA) in a patient before and after coronary bypass surgery. **a** The patient had closure of the graft to the LAD with perioperative infarction. Three ERNA views are shown: anterior (*Ant*), left anterior oblique (*LAO*), and left lateral (*LL*). The enddiastolic (*ED*) and end-systolic (*ES*) frames are shown. *Right*, a schematic drawing of right and left ventricle in ED (*continuous line*) and ES (*stippled line*). **a** Before coronary bypass surgery. Preoperatively the right and left ventricular functions were normal. LVEF was 77%. **b** (p. 90) After coronary bypass surgery the patient was in failure. Elevated enzymes and anterior electrocardiographic changes suggested perioperative infarction. The ERNA study shows a normal right ventricle. However, the left ventricle is enlarged and shows an extensive new regional wall motion abnormality in both the anterior, apical, and septal regions (*arrows*). Global left ventricular ejection fraction was severely depressed at 33%

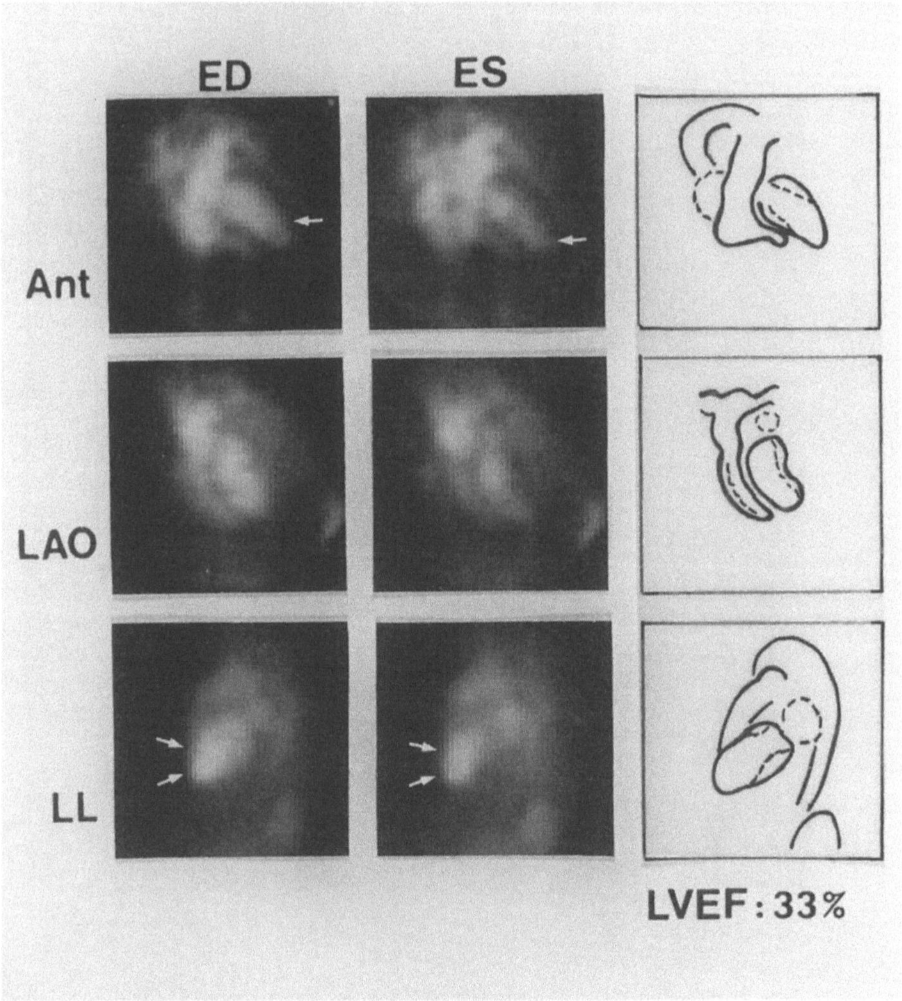

b

Fig. 1. *Continued*

Typical ERNA Images After CABG

After coronary bypass surgery typical changes can be observed on ERNA studies. In all patients without exception paradoxical motion of the septum is noted. This is a normal finding after surgical procedures involving opening of the pericardium. This does not indicate perioperative myocardial damage.

Shortly after CABG the quality of ERNA studies may be suboptimal, with relatively poor definition of cardiac blood pool and surrounding structures. This is probably due to accumulation of fluid and disturbance of normal anatomy. Over a period of several weeks the quality of images usually improves. Although these images are esthetically of lesser quality, LVEF can usually still be assessed reliably.

ERNA during the immediate postsurgery period can be helpful to detect slow leakage of blood. Since the blood is radioactive, leakage of blood can be recognized as slowly accumulating radioactivity adjacent to the heart.

Infarct Imaging

Noninvasive imaging of acute and recent myocardial necrosis with ^{99m}Tc-labeled Sn-pyrophosphate was one of the earliest practical applications of nuclear imaging in cardiac patients [8]. However, at the present time ^{99m}Tc-labeled Sn-pyrophosphate infarct imaging is performed only rarely in most laboratories. The sensitivity of ^{99m}Tc-labeled Sn-pyrophosphate imaging for non-Q-wave infarction is only moderate and is associated with relatively poor specificity. Moreover, significant skeletal uptake often rendered planar images difficult to interpret. Recently it has been suggested that tomographic imaging may improve the diagnostic quality of these images.

In recent years a monoclonal antibody (FAB fragment) against cardiac myosin, indium-111 antimyosin, has been developed [9]. Experimental studies have shown that irreversible myocyte membrane damage is required for antimyosin antibody binding with cardiac myosin. This imaging agent is highly sensitive and specific for the detection for myocardial necrosis. Antimyosin is particularly attractive because it has been shown to be useful for the detection of small myocardial infarcts (Fig. 2). At the present time indium-111 antimyosin is not widely available and has not yet been approved by the United States Food and Drug Administration. On the other hand, gamma camera imaging with indium-111 is not easy and requires special technical skills. Another inconvenience is the required delay of at least 24–36 h between the injection of the radiotracer and acquisition of images.

Recently, preliminary results have been reported on ^{99m}Tc-labeled antimyosin. The ^{99m}Tc label is considerably better suited for imaging with standard gamma cameras than indium-111. ^{99m}Tc-labeled antimyosin would be a significant advance and allow good quality images to be obtained within 4–6 h after injection. Still it remains to be seen whether positive infarct imaging will be clinically useful in the postsurgical patients [10].

Myocardial Perfusion Imaging

Myocardial perfusion imaging is probably the most useful imaging modality after coronary bypass surgery. Myocardial perfusion imaging is usually

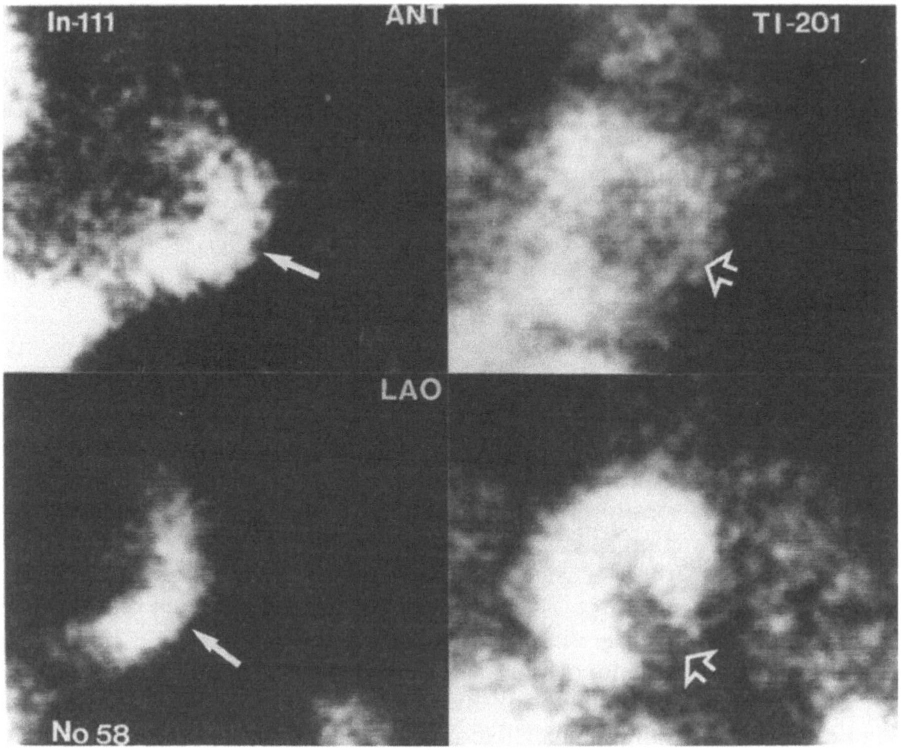

Fig. 2. Indium-111 antimyosin (*left*) and thallium-201 (*right*) imaging at rest in a patient with recent perioperative myocardial infarction. The thallium-201 images show an inferolateral (*LAO* view) and anterolateral (*Ant* view) perfusion defect (*open arrows*). The indium-111 antimyosin images show intense uptake (*arrows*) in the same anatomic area as the thallium-201 defect. Antimyosin uptake is consistent with recent acute infarction. Note that the area of antimyosin uptake is larger than that of the thallium-201 perfusion defect. The latter pattern is consistent with reperfusion of the infarct artery and suggests the presence of viable myocardium in the peripheral zone of infarction

performed in conjunction with either physical exercise or pharmacological stress. The basic principle of myocardial perfusion imaging is the visualization of heterogeneity of blood flow in patients with coronary artery disease [4]. At rest, coronary blood flow is generally not decreased until the coronary stenosis is greater than 90% of luminal diameter. However, coronary reserve, that is the ability to increase coronary blood flow in response to increased metabolic demand, is decreased when coronary stenosis exceeds 50%. Consequently, in most patients with coronary artery disease resting regional myocardial blood flow usually is homogeneous even in the presence of a significant coronary stenosis. However, the same narrowing results in decreased coronary reserve during exercise or pharmacological vasodilatation. This results in heterogeneity of regional myocardial perfusion during exercise or pharmacological stress. This heterogeneity of regional myocardial blood flow can be visualized with radiolabeled myocardial perfusion imaging agents that are distributed in proportion to myocardial blood flow. Presently, two myocardial perfusion imaging agents are widely used, ^{201}Tl- and ^{99m}Tc-labeled sestamibi. Both imaging agents accumulate in the myocardium proportional to the distribution of coronary blood flow. ^{201}Tl is unique in that it demonstrates redistribution over time. After initial myocardial accumulation (according to regional blood flow), ^{201}Tl washes out of the myocardial cells and ultimately distributes evenly throughout the myocardium according to the distribution of the intracellular potassium pool. On the other hand, sestamibi is relatively stably bound to intracellular mitochondria, and no significant washout or redistribution occurs. Both imaging agents require viable myocardial cells for accumulation. However, since sestamibi uptake is importantly determined by regional blood flow, and ^{201}Tl demonstrates in addition redistribution, ^{201}Tl conceivably is a more complete marker of myocardial viability than sestamibi.

Exercise myocardial perfusion imaging is performed as follows. The patient exercises on a treadmill or bicycle in stages of increasing workload. At peak exercise the radiotracer is injected, and the patient continues to exercise for another 1–2 min. Pharmacological stress can be performed with either dipyridamole [11], a potent coronary vasodilator which creates heterogeneity of myocardial blood flow by maximal recruitment of coronary reserve, or with dobutamine [12], which increases myocardial metabolic demand and secondarily may create heterogeneity of blood flow.

Once the radiotracer is injected, myocardial imaging is performed by either planar technique or single photon emission computed tomography (SPECT) [4]. Planar images show the projection of cardiac radioactivity on multiple views. Therefore various vascular territories are superimposed. For SPECT imaging the heart is reconstructed from multiple images acquired in a 180° arc around the patient. After computer reconstruction, the heart is displayed in multiple tomographic slices perpendicular to the anatomic axis of the heart. Usually short-axis, vertical and horizontal long axis slices are displayed. A major advantage of SPECT imaging over planar imaging is the ability to separate various coronary territories by careful analysis of tomographic slices [13]. The latter is particularly relevant in patients who had coronary bypass surgery, and in whom precise anatomic localization of a perfusion abnormality is of importance.

Images are analyzed for homogeneity of tracers accumulation. A normal image shows homogeneous uptake throughout the heart. A perfusion defect is an myocardial area with less localized uptake of radiotracer. Such defects may be fixed, that is, no change on rest imaging, or reversible, that is, on the rest or delayed images the defect is no longer present or has substantially improved. A fixed defect, in particular when present after resting injection of ^{201}Tl, indicates myocardial scar. A reversible defect indicates exercise-induced myocardial ischemia and significant coronary stenosis [4].

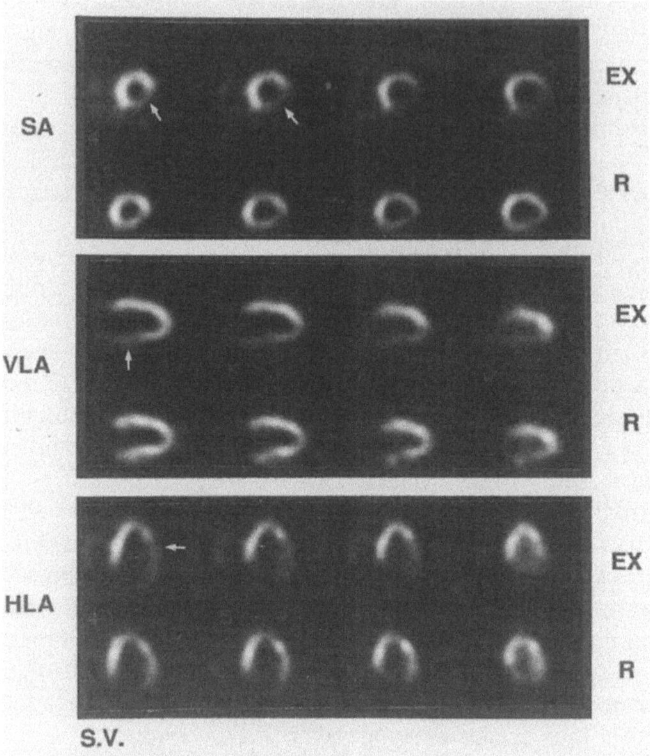
SA
EX
R
VLA
EX
R
HLA
EX
R
S.V.

a

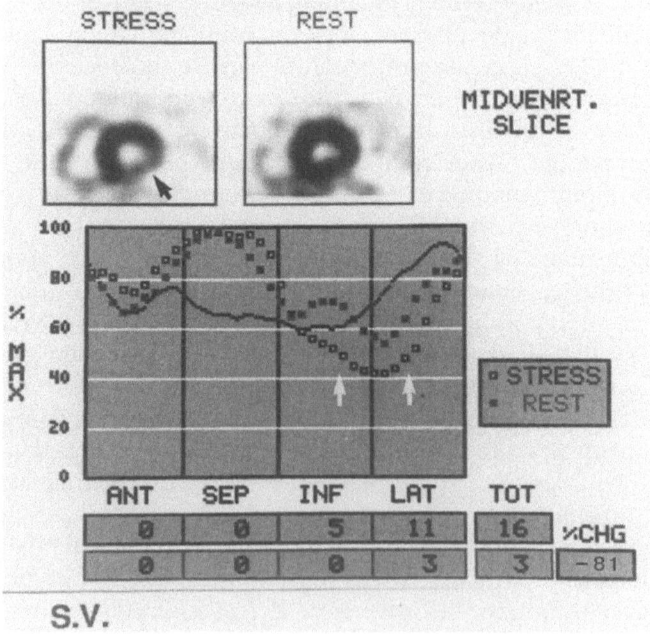
STRESS
REST
MIDVENRT.
SLICE
100
80
60
40
20
0
% MAX
STRESS
REST
ANT
SEP
INF
LAT
TOT
0
0
5
11
16
%CHG
0
0
0
3
3
-81
S.V.

b

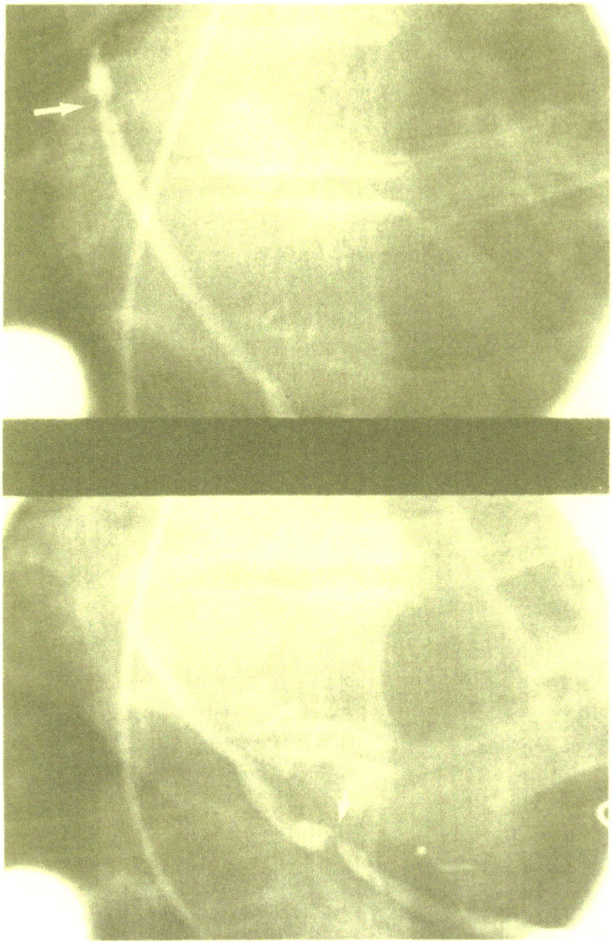

Fig. 3. a SPECT myocardial perfusion imaging at rest and exercise with ^{99m}Tc-labeled sestamibi, in a patient with recurrent chest pain after coronary bypass surgery. Tomographic images are shown in short-axis slices (*SA*), vertical long-axis slices (*VLA*), and horizontal long-axis slices (*HLA*). *Above*, exercise images; *below*, rest images. The exercise images show a large inferolateral myocardial perfusion defect (*arrows*). This perfusion defect is largely reversible on the rest images. This SPECT study suggests exercise-induced myocardial ischemia in the left circumflex territory. **b** Quantification of the image in **a**. *Above*, representative midventricular stress/rest short-axis slices with reversible inferolateral defect (*arrow*). *Middle*, circumferential count profiles. The patient's relative distribution of count activity in a midventricular slice is shown. The lower limit of normal sestamibi count distribution is shown as a continuous line. The stress profile is below the lower limit of normal in the inferolateral segment (*arrow*). The rest profile shows significant improvement. *Below*, quantification of defect reversibility. The stress defect is 5 in the inferior segment and 11 in the lateral segment. At rest the defects improve to 0 and 3, respectively. Total defect reversibility is −81%. **c** Coronary angiogram of the same patient. *Above*, a significant stenosis (*arrow*) developed in the venous graft to the left circumflex artery. *Below*, a second stenosis developed at the site of anastomosis (*arrow*) with the circumflex artery

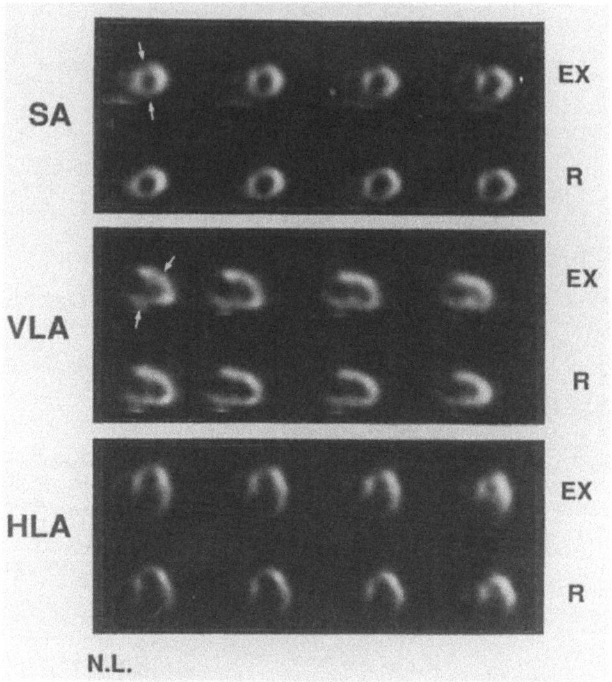
SA
VLA
HLA
EX
R
EX
R
EX
R
N.L.

a

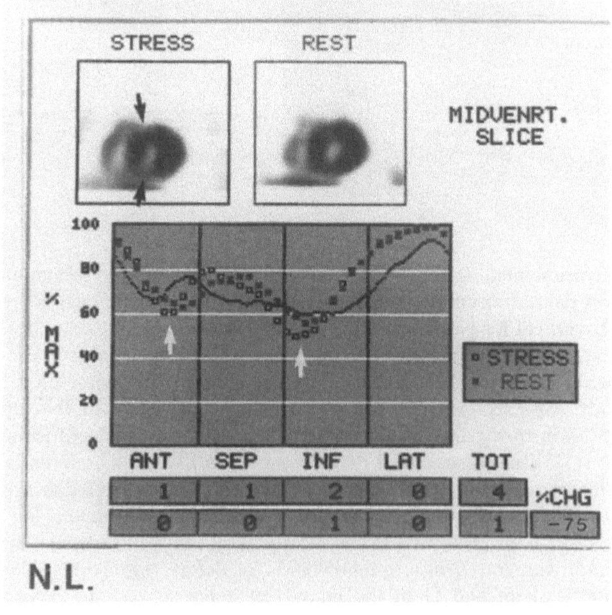
STRESS
REST
MIDVENRT.
SLICE
100
80
60
40
20
0
% MAX
STRESS
REST
ANT
SEP
INF
LAT
TOT
1
1
2
0
4
%CHG
0
0
1
0
1
-75
N.L.

b

The sensitivity of planar and tomographic imaging to detect coronary artery disease is similar, in the range of 80%–90%, with a specificity ranging from 80% to 95%. Several studies have specifically addressed the ability of ^{201}Tl myocardial perfusion imaging to demonstrate noninvasively improvement of myocardial perfusion after coronary bypass surgery. Consequently, myocardial perfusion imaging with either ^{201}Tl- or ^{99m}Tc-labeled sestamibi is the method of choice to localize and quantify recurrent myocardial ischemia after bypass surgery (Figs. 3, 4).

Conclusion

Radionuclide techniques are ideally suited to follow patients noninvasively after coronary bypass surgery. Graft closure and infarction can be detected on ERNA by either a new regional wall motion abnormality and/or a significant decrease in global LVEF. Graft stenosis or progression of disease in native coronary arteries is best evaluated by stress myocardial perfusion imaging using SPECT technique. This methodology can not only predict the anatomic location and coronary artery likely to be involved but also provides insight in the magnitude of recurrent myocardial ischemia.

References

1. Marshall RC, Berger HJ, Reduto L, Gottschalk A, Zaret BL (1978) Variability in sequential measures of left ventricular performance assessed with radionuclide angiocardiography. Am J Cardiol 41:531–536
2. Zaret BL, Strauss HW, Hurley PJ, Natarajan TK, Pitt B (1991) A noninvasive scintiphotographic method for detecting regional ventricular dysfunction in man. N Eng J Med 284:1165–1170
3. Rocco TP, Dilsizian V, Fischman AJ, Strauss HW I (1989) Evaluation of ventricular function in patients with coronary artery disease. J Nucl Med 30:1149–1165

Fig. 4. **a** SPECT myocardial perfusion imaging at rest and exercise with ^{99m}Tc-labeled sestamibi. The patient had recent coronary bypass surgery but had continued to have anginal symptoms. The format is the same as in Fig. 2. On the exercise images a small anteroapical myocardial perfusion defect (*arrow*) is present. In addition, there is a second small inferoseptal perfusion defect. Both defects are almost completely reversible on the rest images. **b** Circumferential count profile of a representative midventricular slice. The format is the same as in Fig. 2. Quantification confirms graphically the presence of a small anterior and a small inferior defect. Both defects improve quantitatively at rest. Defect reversibility is −75%. Coronary angiography in this patient showed four patent grafts. However, residual stenoses were present in the native anterior diagonal artery and in the right posterior descending artery. SPECT myocardial perfusion imaging indicates that the stenoses are functionally significant. After PTCA of both stenoses the patient was asymptomatic with normal exercise myocardial perfusion imaging

4. Zaret BL, Wackers FJT, Soufer R (1991) Nuclear cardiology. In: Braunwald E (ed) Heart disease, a textbook of cardiovascular medicine, vol 1, 4th edn. Saunders, Philadelphia, pp 276–311 (chap 10)
5. Wackers FJT, Jaffe CC, Lynch PJ (1992) Equilibrium and gated first pass radionuclide angiocardiography. Image PSL, St Paul, MN Image Disc Library
6. Wackers FJT, Mattera JA (1988) Evaluation of cardiac function by radionuclide angiocardiography: in particular of the right ventricle. Dynam Cardiovasc Nucl Imaging 1(4): 292–301
7. Wackers FJT, Berger HJ, Johnstone DE, Goldman L, Reduto LA, Langou RE, Gottschalk A, Zaret BL (1979) Multiple gated cardiac blood pool imaging for left ventricular ejection fraction: validation of the technique and assessment of variability. Am J Card 43:1159–1166
8. Sharpe DN, Botvinick EH, Shames DM, Norman A, Chatterjef K, Parmely WW (1978) The clinical estimation of acute myocardial infarct size with ^{99m}technetium pyrophosphate scintigraphy. Circulation 57:307–313
9. Takeda K, LaFrance ND, Weisman HF, Wagner HN, Becker LC (1991) Comparison of indium-111 antimyosin antibody and technetium-99m pyrophosphate localization in reperfused and nonreperfused myocardial infarction. J Am Coll Cardiol 17:519–526
10. Van Vlies B, van Royen EA, Visser CE, Meyne NG, van Buul MMG, Peters RJ, Dunning AJ (1990) Frequency of myocardial indium-111 antimyosin uptake after uncomplicated coronary artery bypass grafting. Am J Cardiol 66:1191–1195
11. Gould KL, Sorenson SG, Alboro P, Caldwell JH, Chaudhuri T, Hamilton GW (1986) Thallium-201 myocardial imaging during coronary vasodilation induced by oral dipyridamole. J Nucl Med 27:31–37
12. Pennel DJ, Underwood R, Swanton RH, Walker M, Ell FJ (1991) Dobutamine thallium myocardial perfusion tomography. J Am Coll Cardiol 18:1417–1479
13. Hecht HS, Shaw RE, Bruce TR, Ryan C, Stertzer SH, Myler RK (1990) Usefulness of tomographic thallium-201 imaging for detection of restenosis after percutaneous transluminal coronary angioplasty. Am J Cardiol 66:1314–1318

Coronary Artery Graft Disease: Diagnosis of Graft Failure by Magnetic Resonance Imaging

P.T. Buser and C.B. Higgins

Introduction

An increasing number of patients with previous coronary artery bypass graft (CABG) surgery suffer from chest pain due to ischemic or nonischemic causes. Ischemic pain may be caused by the occlusion or the stenotic narrowing of one or more bypass grafts or the progression of atherosclerotic disease of the native coronary arteries. The assessment of bypass graft patency in patients after CABG surgery with a noninvasive diagnostic modality is therefore of potential importance and may help to evaluate the need for repeat invasive coronary X-ray angiography. Since 1983, when successful imaging of a CABG by means of magnetic resonance imaging (MRI) was first reported, several studies on the diagnostic accuracy of CABG patency have been published. Nevertheless, today's commercially available MRI techniques for the evaluation of CABGs still suffer from several methodological shortcomings, but thc rapid improvement in hard- and software of MRI scanners, coils, and image processing makes MRI a very promising technique for the noninvasive assessment of CABG and even the native coronary vessels.

This chapter presents the present state of the art and provides some insight into the ongoing, very active research in the field of assessing CABG by MRI and magnetic resonance angiography (MRA).

Technical Aspects

MRI depends upon radiofrequency (RF) signals which result from the interaction of protons (hydrogen nuclei) with a strong magnetic field and intermittently applied RF pulses. The combined effect of the magnetic field and the RF pulses causes protons to resonate at a characteristic frequency. Spatial identification of the resonating protons is achieved by an intermittently applied weak magnetic gradient. This causes slight variations in resonant frequency, depending upon the site of the proton within the magnetic gradient, because of the proportionality between the resonant frequency and the local magnetic field strength.

Effect of Moving Blood

During an imaging sequence the motion of nuclei through the region that is being imaged greatly influences signal intensity. Although the influence of blood flow on MR images is complex, motion of the excited nuclei during the MR sequence generally causes a loss of signal intensity. Consequently, moving blood in the lumina of vessels appears dark (no signal), providing considerable inherent contrast for visualization of the internal surfaces of the blood vessels and the walls of the cardiac chambers. Since contrast media are not required to mark the blood pool, MRI is a totally noninvasive technique for cardiovascular diagnosis. Using standard spin-echo sequences, the time between the initiation of a pulse sequence and the sampling of the spin-echo signal – the so called echo delay time (TE) – is usually 15 ms for the first image. When blood velocity is such that protons move through the thickness of the tomogram (usually 5–10 mm) in this time, the signal is lost from the blood. On the other hand, with the fast imaging techniques recently introduced, TE may be reduced to 3 ms, and consequently signal is received from blood flowing at normal velocities in the cardiac chambers and all blood vessels. In this circumstance, blood appears substantially brighter than the myocardium. High velocity jets, however, produced by stenotic lesions or regurgitant valves can be recognized as a signal void within the signal-filled lumina of vessels and cardiac chambers.

Techniques for Magnetic Resonance Imaging of the Heart

Cardiac imaging requires some form of physiologic gating of the imaging sequence. Acquisition of MR signals of the thorax without gating results in poor cardiac image quality owing to loss of the signal from moving structures and to the variable position of the cardiac structure relative to imaging pixels when data are acquired indiscriminately throughout the cardiac cycle. Therefore, conventional cardiac imaging must be performed using some form of ECG gating. Current MRI exists in two basic forms: spin-echo imaging and gradient-echo imaging.

Spin-Echo Imaging

With a spin-echo imaging sequence images are produced after an initial 90° RF pulse followed by one or more 180° RF pulses. This sequence provides high-resolution images with clear definition of the intracardiac and intravascular structures in the presence of a low signal intensity of the blood pool. Up to 14 parallel two-dimensional tomographic slices of 5–10 mm thickness can be obtained at a time in any desired anatomical plane. The acquisition of such a slice set requires 4–6 min depending on the desired image quality (number of acquisitions) and the patient's heart rate. Spin-echo imaging is the technique of choice in assessing cardiac and vascular anatomy, myocardial mass, and the dimensions of cardiac chambers and myocardial walls.

Gradient-Echo Imaging

Gradient-echo imaging employs 16 or more images of the cardiac cycle which can be played in a cine loop to show cardiac function, the so-called cine MRI. With gradient-echo imaging the normal blood pool shows high signal intensity throughout the cardiac cycle within the heart and the vessels. Intravascular signal loss does occur in those circumstances where there is turbulence or high velocity flow such as in stenotic lesions or regurgitant valvular disease. This phenomenon has been used to assess the severity of valvular regurgitation.

Echo-Planar Imaging

The echo-planar sequence allows very rapid imaging with acquisition of a complete image in tens of milliseconds. Because of this speed, cardiac images can be obtained without ECG gating. Because of the very rapidly switched gradients this technique is very demanding on imaging hardware and can be applied only in newer generation MRI scanners.

Safety Considerations

Regarding imaging of patients with coronary artery disease a major concern regarding safety considerations has been the production of severe ventricular arrhythmias through induction of a current into the patient by rapidly changing magnetic fields. However, in canine studies the threshold rate of change of the magnetic field to produce ventricular fibrillation was found to be approximately 500 T/s [18], and the currently used clinical magnets do not exceed a maximum rate of field change of about 3 T/s, thus indicating an enormous safety margin for the investigation of patients.

Contraindications for MRI include patients with metallic implants in the CNS and patients with cardiac pacemaker systems. A small number of 2%–5% can not be investigated in a superconducting electromagnet because of claustrophobia.

Magnetic Resonance Imaging of Venous Coronary Artery Bypass Grafts

The coronary arteries are small, tortuous, and rapidly moving structures. These are properties which make successful imaging with tomographic techniques rather difficult [1, 17]. CABGs are depicted more easily mainly because they are less mobile on their proximal segments than coronary arteries. The vessel diameter of the saphenous vein grafts is larger, at least as long as the graft is not arterialized.

Bypass grafts are generally recognized by their anatomic location in relation to the ascending aorta, common pulmonary artery, cardiac chambers, and native coronary arteries. It is therefore important to be familiar with the positioning of the grafts used by the surgeon because this may be very variable. The appearance of CABG in MRI was first described in 1983 [9]. Using ECG-gated spin-echo sequence in an axial tomographic view, bypass grafts were depicted as signal intense circular structures with low intraluminal signal intensity (black). With the spin-echo multislice technique CABG can be identified by their anatomic location and course. The origin of the right coronary artery (RCA) graft is placed most inferiorly on the ascending aorta by most cardiovascular surgeons. This sometimes complicates its differentiation from the native RCA at the level of the myocardium which takes its further course in the right atrioventricular grove. In contrast, in more caudal images at the ventricular level RCA grafts are usually seen lateral to the native RCA, depending on the site of their distal anastomosis.

Left anterior descending (LAD) grafts originate anterior from the ascending aorta at the level of the common pulmonary artery. Their course can be followed around the common pulmonary artery down to the interventricular grove where they usually insert to the native LAD or to diagonal branches (Fig. 1).

The left circumflex artery (LCX) grafts usually originate most cephalic on the ascending aorta, pass over the common pulmonary artery, and descend along the left pulmonary artery into the region of the left atrioventricular grove.

A successful approach involves imaging of an entire volume of the thorax, encompassing most of the length of the grafts, from near its aortic insertion to the epicardial surface of the heart near the receiving vessel. It is suitable to start imaging in the axial plane placing the most cranial slice high on the ascending aorta and the most caudal below the midventricular level. A slice thickness of 5–7 mm would be ideal, although at lower field strengths thicker slices may be required in which case it is useful to interleave two acquisitions to acquire 10-mm slices with a gap of 5 mm. Additional images in the sagittal plane or in an obligue coronal plane parallel to the left ventricular long axis often allow the identification of LAD grafts arising anteriorly from the ascending aorta passing around the pulmonary artery

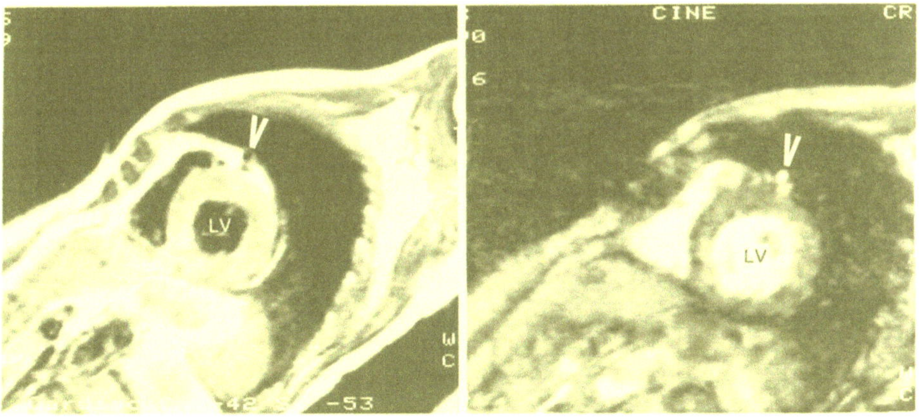

Fig. 1a,b. MRI of the left ventricle (*LV*) in a short-axis view perpendicular to the left ventricular long axis. **a** Using the spin-echo technique, the venous coronary bypass graft to the LAD (*arrow*) is depicted as a circular structure with no signal in its lumen. **b** Using the gradient-echo technique, the lumen of the graft appears with a bright signal (*arrow*), thus indicating a patent graft

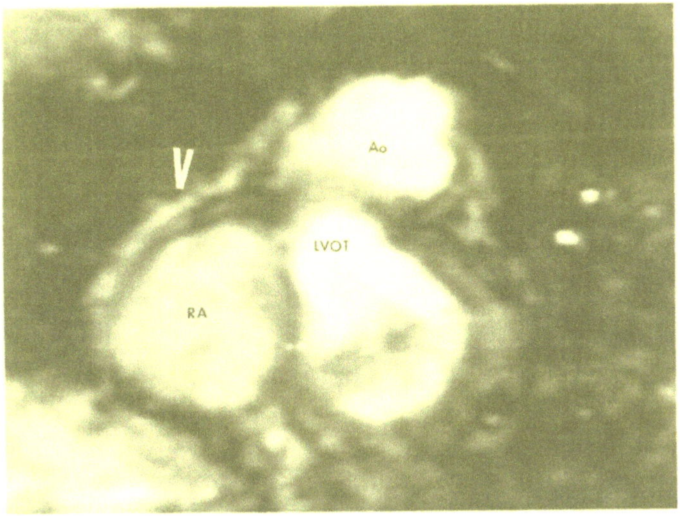

Fig. 2. Gradient-echo MRI of a saphenous venous bypass graft to the RCA in a short-axis view. The graft (*arrow*) originates at the ascending aorta (*Ao*), and its course is shown along the right atrioventricular groove. Because of the bright signal within its lumen, the graft is considered patent. *RA*, Right atrium; *LVOT*, left ventricular outflow tract

down to their epicardial insertion. The course of RCA and LCX grafts may be depicted in a short axis plane dissecting the region of the right or left atrioventricular grove (Fig. 2). Depending on the patients heart rate and the number of acquisitions the assessment of bypass grafts with spin-echo technique in one imaging plane can be completed within 4–6 min. Thus, the maximal imaging time for three different imaging planes would require 18 min with the patients remaining in the MRI scanner for approximately 30 min. Such a dwell time within the magnet is usually well tolerated.

The appearance of intraluminal signal void contrasting with the high signal of surrounding fat or other soft tissue implies that the graft contains blood which is moving at normal flow rates and is therefore patent. If a graft cannot be identified, or if its origin is seen but cannot be followed distally, this graft may be considered occluded or at least significantly obstructed. The criteria for the designation of the patency state of CABG has been described by White et al. [25]. They proposed that a CABG is judged to be patent if the normal signal void of flowing blood in the expected region of the CABG was seen at two or more anatomic levels. If it is seen only at one level, the patency state is judged indeterminate. If there is no evidence of signal void at any level, the graft is judged occluded.

One of the earlier studies [7] was addressed to the detection of CABG using spin-echo technique with a slice thickness of 9–12 mm in axial, coronal, and oblique coronal planes. A total of 64 grafts including 53 saphenous vein grafts and 11 internal mammary artery (IMA) grafts were investigated, however, patency of the graft was not addressed. When the investigators looked for CABG without knowledge of the number and site of operated grafts 54/64 grafts were detected and 3 "new grafts" were described erroneously. When reviewing the MR images individually with correlation of the angiographic and operative reports two more grafts were detected. However, only 5/11 IMA grafts were detected correctly, although the native internal mammary arteries are readily seen with appropriate imaging.

Seven studies have addressed the diagnostic accuracy of spin-echo techniques performed with whole-body coils using a slice thickness of 8–11 mm. The most frequently used imaging plane was axial, and in some of the studies additional coronal, oblique coronal, or sagittal planes were performed. In all of these studies the findings of MRI readings were compared to angiographic assessment of CABG patency state. Sensitivity defined as patent CABG correctly diagnosed by MRI relative to angiographically patent CABG and specificity defined as occluded CABG correctly diagnosed by MRI relative to angiographically occluded CABG varied in a total of 329 CABG between 73%–90% and 56–74%, respectively (Table 1). The positive predictive value for patent CABG was 83%–91% and for occluded CABG 42%–81%. Thus, when bypass grafts can be depicted at least on two levels at their usual location as a circular or tubular structure with a very low signal intensity of its lumen, there is a high confidence that this bypass graft is patent. However, when the site of CABG insertion is considered, the accuracy for the determination of CABG status varies according to the site. Three studies have demonstrated that the overall accuracy for the correctly classified status is 79%–88% for RCA grafts, 71–90% for LAD grafts, and 68%–85% for LCX grafts. In all studies the assessment of patent grafts

Table 1. Sensitivity and specificity of MRI for the definition of CABG patency as compared to conventional X-ray angiographic findings

	MRI sequence	CABG (*n*)	Sensitivity (%)	Specificity (%)
Rubinstein [19]	SE	42	90	72
White [25]	SE	78	86	59
Jenkins [12]	SE	60	89	73
Theissen [20]	SE	92	83	56
Wicke [27]	SE	52	73	74
White [26]	Cine MRI	28	93	86
Aurigemma [2]	Cine MRI	45	88	100

Table 2. Sensitivity and specificity of MRI for the definition of CABG patency as compared to conventional X-ray angiographic findings (discrimination according to the site of the CABG)

	Site	CABG (*n*)	Sensitivity (%)	Specificity (%)
Rubinstein [19]	LAD	20	92	86
	LCX	13	88	80
	RCA	14	88	67
White [25]	LAD	31	88	50
	LCX	25	73	88
	RCA	16	100	68
Theissen [20]	LAD	49	85	20
	LCX	28	67	69
	RCA	15	100	75

was more confident with a high sensitivity of 88%–100% for RCA grafts, 85%–92% for LAD grafts, and 67%–88% for LCX grafts (Table 2). The reliable detection of occluded grafts, however, was less confident, with an overall specificity ranging from 56% to 78%.

With the use of spin-echo techniques, the accuracy of MRI for the assessment of CABG patency versus occlusion appears to be sufficiently high that it can serve as a valuable adjunct in the management of CABG patients. However, it must be noted that MRI with today's routinely available techniques does not provide adequate information on hemodynamically relevant stenoses of CABG. Although a spine surface coil, a slice thickness of 5 mm, and a multi-echo spin-echo sequence was used, the sensitivity to identify a patent but stenotic CABG was only 25% [19].

It has been emphasized that the use of gradient-refocused sequences with the image display in a cinematic format – the so-called cine MRI – would have major theoretical advantages for the evaluation of bypass graft patency: (a) blood flow is imaged as a positive bright signal; (b) blood flow signal is qualitatively present over the entire range of flow velocities arising in patent grafts; and (c) images are obtained throughout the cardiac cycle and can be viewed in a cine loop format to display pulsatile flow. Two studies applying cine MRI for the evaluation of CABG patency found a sensitivity of 88% and 93% and a specificity of 86% and 100% [2, 26]. Therefore, the assessment of patent grafts seems to be comparable using spin-echo sequences and cine MRI. On the other hand, occluded grafts can be identified with a high accuracy using cine MRI. In addition, blood flow within side arms of jump grafts could be depicted allowing definition of the patency of such complex grafts. However, the differentiation of normal, patent grafts, and stenotic grafts was not possible.

Factors Causing Inaccuracies

Several potential problems and sources of error must be recognized when CABG status is assessed using cine MRI and spin-echo sequences. Metal hemostatic clips produce signal void which makes them resemble flowing blood in a vascular structure [20]. Their diameter appears usually in the range of 10–20 mm. Such metal clips therefore present a major cause for misinterpretation of the CABG status using MRI. In fact, 50% of false-positive diagnosis could be attributed to metal articfacts. These artifacts are seen only exceptionally on more than one anatomic level, and the depiction of an open CABG at the typical location on several anatomic levels may reduce the misinterpretation due to metal artifacts. Other sources of error include bands of mediastinal fibrosis, thickened pericardium, small pericardial collections of air or fluid, especially early after surgery, and confusing CABG with native coronary arteries or veins. CABG can be differentiated from native coronary vessels by their site of origination at the ascending aorta and following their course level by level down to their site of insertion at the native vessel. CABGs are often complex ("jump grafts") with side arms to multiple branches. The diagnostic accuracy for the patency state of such side arms with spin-echo sequences is uncertain. This specific problem has been addressed in only one study. Because of interactions with metal clips and sutures at the site of insertion and motion artifacts patency of complex CABG was evaluated only between the aortic anastomosis and the first insertion at the native coronary artery.

Magnetic Resonance Imaging of Arterial Coronary Bypass Grafts

Six of the above studies included analysis of IMA grafts [2, 6, 16, 20, 25, 26]. Generally it seems much more difficult to determine the graft status because the pedicule of this arterial graft is usually surrounded with metal clips used for the occlusion of side branches and graft localization. Therefore, the predictive accuracy varies considerably among the studies (45%–88%). In one study using spin-echo sequences the evaluation of the patency of all IMA grafts remained undetermined. On the other hand, neither study in which cine MRI was applied reported specific problems with respect to IMA graft patency. In a recent report the assessment of the patency state in 14 patients who had received a CABG using the right gastroepiploic artery (RGEA) with combined spin-echo and cine MRI techniques was described [16]. In all patients the RGEA graft was seen as a tubular structure with luminal signal void with spin-echo sequences. In all patients in whom cine MRI was performed (13/14) the graft was visualized with high intraluminal signal intensity, thus suggesting a functionally normal patent graft.

Measurement of Blood Flow in Coronary Artery Bypass Grafts

Blood flow velocity and volume flow can be measured using MR techniques [14]. Two techniques have been applied most frequently; time-of-flight and phase-shift techniques. The time-of-flight, or bolus-tracking technique, monitors the displacement of a slab of tagged spins (saturation of signal) during blood flow in a vessel of interest [5]. The motion of the tagged slab is imaged at multiple times using sequential gradient-echo images, so that the distance traversed by the tagged spins between the acquisition of sequential images can be measured. The slab of tagged spins appears as a signal void in the vessel of interest. The velocity is measured as the distance traversed between acquisitions divided by the time between acquisitions. Alternately, the velocity can be calculated on a single acquisition by dividing the displacement distance of the bolus by the time between tagging and readout of the signal. The initial position of the saturation band used for tagging a slab of tissue is recorded on the stationary tissue so that displacement can be measured as the distance between the slab in the vessel and the stationary tissue.

The phase-shift technique depends upon the principle that spins in stationary tissue experience no phase shift when a bipolar magnetic gradient is applied, whereas spins flowing in a gradient accumulate a net phase shift [15]. The phase shift is proportional to flow velocity according to the equation: phase shift = G V T Ag, a gyromagnetic ratio which is a constant, where V is the velocity, T is the time between the centers of the two gradient lobes, and Ag is the area of one lobe of the bipolar gradient pulse. Because T and Ag are known and G is a constant, phase shift can be directly related to velocity.

Use of the phase-shift technique with the cine GRE technique is termed velocity encoded cine GRE (VEC). For each acquisition at each time in the cardiac cycle, the VEC technique provides magnitude (anatomical image) and phase (velocity or flow image) images. With the VEC technique, usually

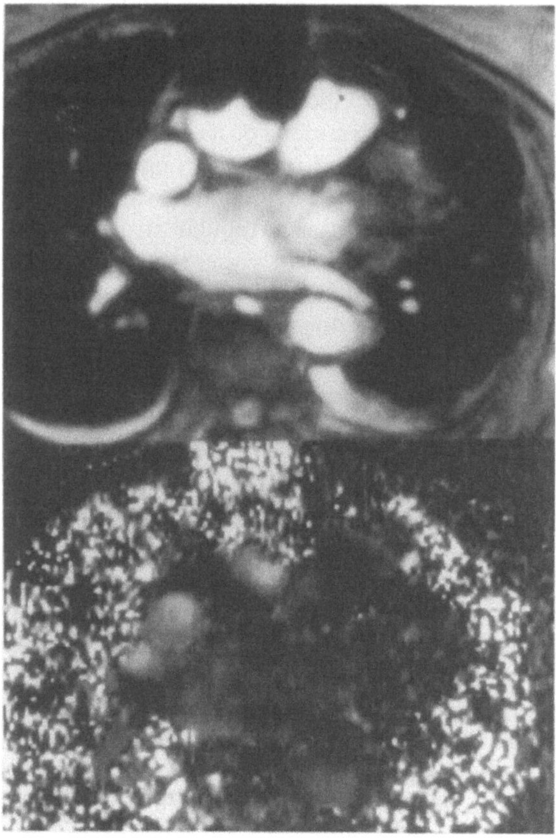

Fig. 3. Magnitude and phase images of the chest in a patient after aortocoronary arterial bypass graft. The graft is indicated (*arrow*) on the magnitude and phase images, which are used to measure instantaneous blood flow

16 images are acquired, corresponding to evenly spaced intervals during an average cardiac cycle. From the phase-shift GRE data, velocity can be measured for each pixel or the average velocity within a region of interest encircling the entire vessel. Instantaneous flow is calculated as the product of the cross-sectional area of the vessel (measured on the magnitude image) and the average velocity in the vessel. Integration of the flow measurement for all images during the cardiac cycle provides a measurement of net blood flow per cardiac cycle. In vitro and in vivo validation studies have documented the accuracy of phase shift measurements of blood flow up to velocities of 600 cm/s [13, 21].

The phase-shift technique has been used to measure flow velocities in aortocoronary bypass grafts and in the internal mammary artery [11]. Figure 3 demonstrates magnitude and phase images, showing an aortocoronary bypass graft. Figure 4 demonstrates the velocity-time curve for vessels in the

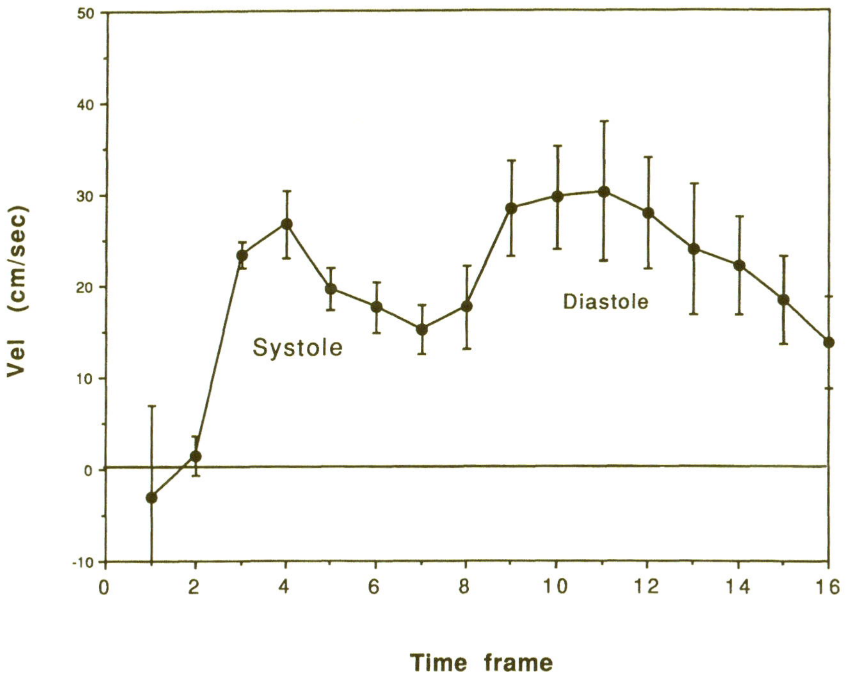

Fig. 4. Velocity versus time curve for a CABG. Note that peak velocity of the bypass graft occurs in diastole while the peak flow velocity occurs in early systole in noncoronary arteries. Reproduced from Duerinckx et al. [4]

mediastinum, including this aortocoronary bypass graft. Flow velocity in noncoronary arteries is during early systole, while peak velocity in the bypass graft is recorded in diastole. Surface coils can be employed in order to improve the resolution of small arteries such as the internal mammary artery (Fig. 5).

Summary

Current MRI implementations are inadequate for morphologic evaluation of the native coronary circulation, although approaches to evaluation of coronary flow have been described [23]. Several major advances in cardiac-gated gradient-echo methodology are required to permit noninvasive coronary artery imaging with the use of this approach. Even at present, however, spin-echo and cine MRI are methods for a noninvasive imaging of CABG. High flow rate in the graft produces a signal void in the lumen of the graft using spin-echo MRI and thus indicates patency of the graft. With cine MRI

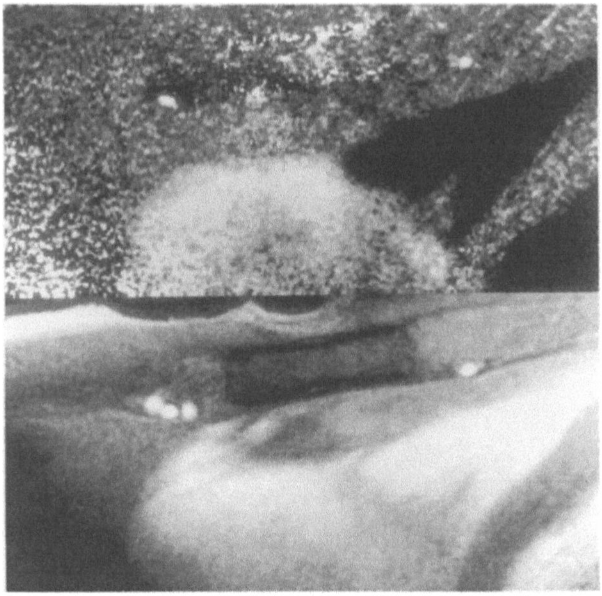

Fig. 5. Phase (velocity; *top*) and magnitude (*bottom*) images of the internal mammary artery. High-resolution image was acquired using a surface coil

flowing blood causes bright signal intensity; therefore, bright signal rather than flow void indicates graft patency with this technique. Using these techniques, graft patency can be defined with an accuracy of 80%–90%. In addition, using cine MRI with slices encompassing the heart, especially in a short-axis view, global and regional contractile performance of the ventricles, left ventricular enddiastolic, endsystolic volumes, stroke volume, and ejection fraction can be assessed with high accuracy [3].

Morphologic and functional consequences of ischemic heart disease such as previous or acute myocardial infarctions, thrombus within a cardiac chamber, and left ventricular aneurysm formation can be depicted [10]. Thus, MRI provides the means for a comprehensive evaluation of patients with ischemic heart disease after CABG surgery.

In clinical cardiology it is not usually sufficient simply to know whether a graft is patent or occluded. Stenotic grafts and hemodynamic relevant stenosis of the native vessel distal of the anastomosis may limit myocardial perfusion. This answer cannot be given with today's routinely available MRI techniques. MR velocity mapping is a possible technique for the measurement of blood flow within the graft. Velocity measurements have been achieved in vein grafts. Peak flow velocities lower than 0.1 m/s are indicative of poor graft function [23]. Velocity measurements can be obtained in approximately 50% of grafts, and the factors which prevent a more complete assessment are the artifacts originating from metal clips, sternal sutures, and the long-imaging times. It is possible that echo-planar velocity mapping may overcome some of the problems of imaging rapidly moving structures. Given the remarkable advances in MRI hardware and software over the past few years, high-quality imaging of CABG and flow quantitation within grafts may be achieved, thus making MRI an excellent, noninvasive modality for the assessment of the morphology and function of CABG.

References

1. Alfidi RJ, Masaryk TJ, Haacke EM, Lenz GW, Ross JS, Modic MT, Nelson AD, LiPuma JP, Cohen AM (1987) MR angiography of peripheral, carotid, and coronary arteries. AJR 149:1097–1109
2. Aurigemma GP, Reichek N, Axel L, Schiebler M, Harris C, Kressel HY (1989) Noninvasive determination of coronary artery bypass graft patency by cine magnetic resonance imaging. Circulation 80:1595–1602
3. Buser PT, Auffermann W, Holt WW, Wagner S, Kircher B, Wolfe C, Higgins CB (1989) Noninvasive evaluation of the global left ventricular function with use of cine nuclear magnetic resonance. J Am Coll Cardiol 13:1294–1300
4. Duerinckx AJ, Higgins CB, Pettigrew G (1993) The cardiovascular MRI reading file. Raven, New York
5. Edelman RR, Matte HP, Kleefield J, Silver MS (1989) Quantitation of blood flow with dynamic MR and presaturation bolus tracking. Radiology 171:551–556
6. Frija G, Schouman-Claeys E, Lacombe P, Bismuth V, Ollivier JP (1989) A study of coronary artery bypass graft patency using MR imaging. J Comput Assist Tomogr 13: 226–232
7. Gomes AS, Lois JF, Drinkwater DC, Corday SR (1987) Coronary artery bypass grafts: visualization with MR imaging. Radiology 162:175–179
8. Grossmann W (1986) Cardiac catheterization and angiography, 3rd edn. Lea and Febiger, Philadelphia, p 31
9. Herfkens RJ, Higgins CB, Hricak M, Lipton MJ, Crooks LE, Lanzer P, Brundage B, Shelton PE, Kaufman L (1983) Nuclear magnetic resonance imaging of the cardiovascular system: normal and pathologic findings. Radiology 147:749–759
10. Higgins CB (1988) MR of the heart: anatomy, physiology and metabolism. AJR 151: 239–248
11. Higgins CB, Caputo GR (1993) Role of MR imaging in acquired and congenital heart disease. AJR 161:13–22
12. Jenkins JPR, Love HG, Foster GJ, Isherwood I, Rowlands DJ (1988) Detection of coronary artery bypass graft patency as assessed by magnetic resonance imaging. Br J Radiology 61:2–4
13. Kondo C, Caputo GR, Semelka R, Shimakawa A, Higgins CB (1991) Right and left ventricular stroke volume measurements with velocity encoded cine NMR imaging: in vitro and in vivo evaluation. AJR 157:9–16
14. Mostbeck GW, Caputo GR, Higgins CB (1992) MR measurement of blood flow in the cardiovascular system. AJR 159:453–461
15. Nayler GL, Fermin DN, Longmore DB (1986) Blood flow imaging by cine magnetic resonance. J Comput Assist Tomogr 10:715–722
16. Nishimura F, Yoshino Y, Ichikawa S, Hayama Y, Toyama M (1992) MRI of the gastro-epiploic artery used as a bypass graft. J Comput Assist Tomogr 16:549–552
17. Pascal CB, Haacke EM, Adler LP, Finelli DA (1992) Magnetic resonance coronary artery imaging. Cardiovasc Intervent Radiol 15:23–31

18. Roy OZ (1980) Technical note: summary of cardiac fibrillation thresholds for 60 Hz currents and voltages applied directly to the heart. Med Biol Eng Comput 18:657–662
19. Rubinstein RI, Askenase AD, Thickman D, Feldman MS, Agarwal JB, Helfant RH (1987) Magnetic resonance imaging to evaluate patency of aortocoronary bypass grafts. Circulation 76:786–791
20. Theissen P, Sechtem U, Langkamp S, Jungehülsing M, Hilger HH, Schicha H (1989) Nichtinvasive Beurteilung aortokoronarer Venenbrücken mit Kernspintomographie. Nucl Med 28:234–242
21. Underwood SR, Firmin DN, Klipstein RH, Rees RSD, Longmore DB (1986) The assessment of CABGs using oblique magnetic resonance imaging and flow mapping (abstract). Medicine 47–48 (Society of Magnetic Resonance Imaging, Book of abstracts)
22. Underwood SP, Firmin DN, Klipstein RH et al. (1987) Magnetic resonance velocity mapping. Clinical application of a new technique. Br Heart J 57:5
23. Underwood SP, Firmin DN, Klipstein RH, Rees RSO, Longmore DD (1987) The assessment of coronary artery bypass grafts using magnetic resonance imaging with velocity mapping. Br Heart J 57–93 (abstract)
24. Wagner S, Auffermann W, Buser PT, Lim TW, Kircher B, Pflugfelder P, Higgins CB (1989) Diagnostic accuracy and estimation of the severity of valvular regurgitation from the signal void on Cine MR. Am Heart J 118:760
25. White RD, Caputo GR, Mark AS, Modin GW, Higgins CB (1987) Coronary artery bypass graft patency: noninvasive evaluation with MR imaging. Radiology 164:681–686
26. White RD, Pflugfelder PW, Lipton MJ, Higgins CB (1988) Coronary artery bypass grafts: evaluation of patency with cine MR imaging. AJR 150:1271–1274
27. Wicke K, Mühlberger V, Judmaier W, Moes N, zur Nedden D (1991) Die Wertigkeit von CT und MRT bei der Erfassung von aortokoronaren Venenbrücken im Vergleich zur Koronarangiographie. Fortschr Rontgenstr 154:306–309

Positron Emission Tomography: Evaluation of Myocardial Blood Flow and Viability Before and Following Coronary Revascularization

S.G. Sawada and M. Schwaiger

Introduction

Various noninvasive cardiac imaging modalities have been employed in patients who present with myocardial ischemia following coronary artery bypass grafting (CABG). The high frequency of multivessel disease makes accurate identification of graft or native vessel obstruction particularly challenging. The presence of graft or native vessel stenosis can be determined by coronary angiography, but noninvasive imaging techniques combined with stress testing are required to determine the functional significance of anatomic disease. Analysis of left ventricular wall motion during exercise or pharmacologic stress and assessment of perfusion by single photon emission computerized tomography (SPECT) are routinely employed for this purpose. SPECT has a high sensitivity for detection of coronary artery disease. However, it provides primarily qualitative information and has limited specificity because of imaging artifacts which may not be readily distinguished from true abnormalities of perfusion.

The high frequency of regional asynergy in previously revascularized patients complicates the interpretation of exercise wall motion studies. In addition, a significant proportion of asynergic regions contain viable but functionally depressed myocardium that will regain function after restoration of blood flow. Detection of viable myocardium is of utmost importance in patients with prior revascularization and reduced left ventricular function because of the increased morbidity and mortality associated with repeat surgical revascularization.

Positron emission tomography (PET) is an imaging modality that overcomes many of the limitations of other noninvasive techniques. PET has demonstrated both a high sensitivity and a high specificity for the detection of coronary artery disease. Myocardial perfusion can be accurately measured using positron-emitting tracers of blood flow. Finally, the ability of PET to image tracers of myocardial metabolism permits the unique assessment of myocardial viability at the cellular level. This chapter discusses the clinical role of PET imaging after surgical revascularization for (a) the detection of graft and coronary artery disease, (b) quantitation of myocardial perfusion, and (c) determination of myocardial viability.

General Principles of Positron Emission Tomography

PET imaging employs radionuclides that decay by emission of a positron, a positively charged particle with a mass equivalent to an electron. An emitted positron travels a few millimeters in tissue before combining with an electron. The total mass of the two particles is converted to energy in the form of two 511 KeV photons that leave the site of "annihilation" in directions 180° opposite from each other. An annihilation event is recorded when the two photons simultaneously strike a pair of detectors positioned 180° apart. Scanners composed of circular arrays of scintillation detectors connected by coincidence circuitry enable detection of multiple annihilation events. Cross-sectional transverse images of the heart are produced following application of the reconstruction algorithm. The transverse images can be reoriented with respect to the major and minor axes of the heart for display of horizontal and vertical long-axis and short-axis views. The images represent the distribution and concentration of the positron emitter in cardiac tissue. Quantitation of myocardial tracer concentrations is made possible by correction of the emission images for photon attenuation, which represents an important advantage over single photon emission computed tomography (SPECT).

The spatial resolution of PET is uniform with depth and is primarily determined by the resolution of the system and the positron range of the isotope employed. The in-plane resolution of current systems is less than 10 mm [58]. This resolution is superior to that of most SPECT systems. However, it is less than optimal for absolute quantitation of tissue tracer concentrations. Limited spatial resolution imposes two sources of error in the quantitation of tracer activity in the myocardium. The "partial volume effect" results in underestimation of myocardial tissue activity because the thickness of the myocardium (8–11 mm) is less than twice the spatial resolution (6–10 mm). "Spillover" or assignment of some activity in the blood pool to the myocardium occurs early after tracer injection. Various methods have been developed for correction of these resolution distortions [29].

Qualitative Evaluation of Myocardial Perfusion for Detection of Coronary Artery and Bypass Graft Disease

Table 1 summarizes the physical characteristics of positron-emitting tracers used for assessment of blood flow. These radioisotopes are either generator or cyclotron produced. The employment of generator-produced tracers eliminates the need for an on-site cyclotron, but this advantage may be offset by the periodic need for generator replacement. An ideal blood flow tracer should have a stable and high extraction by myocardial tissue over a

Table 1. Extraction fraction, biological and physical half-life, and emitted positron energy of PET tracers used for assessment of myocardial blood flow

	Extraction fraction (%)	Biological half-life	Physical half-life	Emitted positron energy
Generator-produced				
Rubidium-82	65	Long (hours)	76 s	3.3
Copper-62 PTSM	65	Long (hours)	9.8 min	2.9
Cyclotron-produced				
[^{13}N]Ammonia	>90	Long (hours)	10 min	1.2
[^{15}O]Water	100	Short (seconds)	2 min	1.72

wide range of blood flows, be avidly retained in myocardial tissue, and have a short enough physical half-life so that serial studies can be performed within a reasonable time span. Rubidium-82 and nitrogen-13 ammonia fulfill most of these requirements and are the most commonly used tracers for qualitative assessment of myocardial blood flow. Rubidium-82 has the advantage of a brief half-life (76 s) which permits completion of a rest and stress study within 60 min. This tracer has the disadvantages of a reduced extraction fraction with elevated blood flows and production of higher energy positrons that potentially reduce image resolution. [^{13}N]Ammonia has a uniformly high extraction over a wide range of flows and slow tissue clearance as a result of myocardial conversion of the tracer to [^{13}N]glutamine, yielding excellent image quality.

The results of studies investigating the sensitivity and specificity of rubidium-82 and [^{13}N]ammonia PET for detection of coronary artery disease are shown in Table 2. Perfusion imaging is most often used in combination with pharmacologic stress rather than exercise stress for two reasons. The degree of coronary vasodilation achieved by infusion of dipyridamole or adenosine is greater than that achieved during vigorous exercise. Additionally, patient motion within the scanner is minimized with pharmacologic stress. Static images of the heart are obtained at rest and during stress following separate tracer injections at rest and during peak stress. The PET studies summarized in Table 2 all employed static imaging which limited analysis to the comparison of relative distributions of tracer activity such as that performed with SPECT.

All of the studies report a uniformly high sensitivity for PET perfusion imaging. When patients with prior myocardial infarction are excluded, the sensitivity declines to values reported for SPECT imaging [59]. An example of a rest and stress rubidium-82 study in a patient without a previous infarction is shown in Fig. 1. The sensitivity of PET flow imaging in surgically revascularized patients has not been investigated.

In studies comparing PET and SPECT in the same patients with and without infarction (Table 2), PET demonstrated greater specificity for the

Table 2. Detection of coronary artery disease using PET and SPECT

Reference	PET						SPECT			
	n	Tracer	Stress	Sens	Spec	Acc	n	Sens	Spec	Acc
Schelbert [50]	32	$[^{13}N]NH_3$	Dip	97	100	98				
Tamaki [60]	51	$[^{13}N]NH_3$	Bike ex	98	100	98	48	96		
Demer [17]	193	$[^{13}N]NH_3$ ^{82}Rb	Dip	94	95	94				
Go [23]	132	^{82}Rb	Dip	82	82	92	135	76	76	78
Stewart [59]	81	^{82}Rb	Dip	84	88	85	81	84	53	79

Acc, Accuracy; Bike ex, bicycle exercise; Dip, dipyridamole; *n*, number of patients; Sens, sensitivity; Spec, specificity.

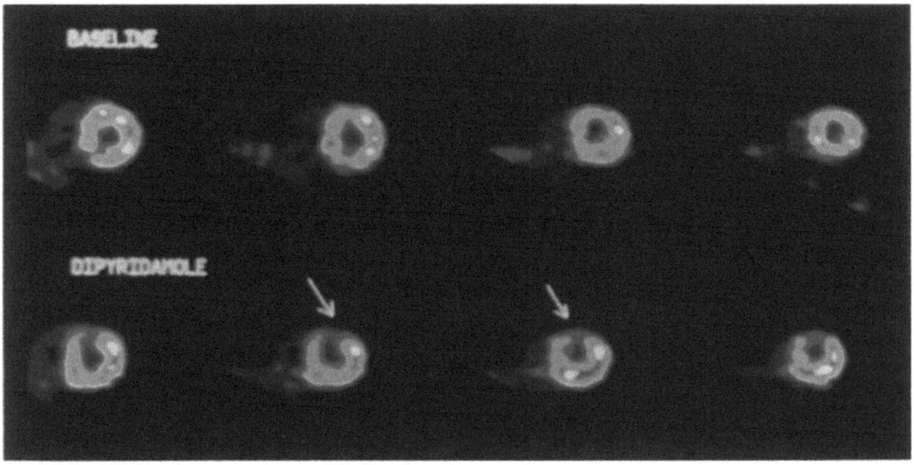

Fig. 1. Oblique (short-axis) tomograms of the left ventricle at baseline (*top*) and during dipyridamole stress (*bottom*) in a patient with significant stenosis of the left anterior descending artery. The baseline study demonstrates homogeneous uptake of rubidium-82. An anterior perfusion defect (*arrow*) is induced by the vasodilator

detection of coronary disease. This improved specificity of PET is most likely a result of attenuation correction which eliminates the artifacts caused by tissue interposed between the heart and the detector system.

Perfusion imaging is routinely employed for determining the location of significantly diseased vessels in patients with previous CABG. The high prevalence of multivessel disease in patients presenting more than 5 years after CABG makes accurate localization of obstructed vessels difficult when qualitative analysis of myocardial tracer activity is employed [43]. In some studies PET has demonstrated better accuracy than conventional perfusion imaging for localization of disease to regional vascular beds [50]. The

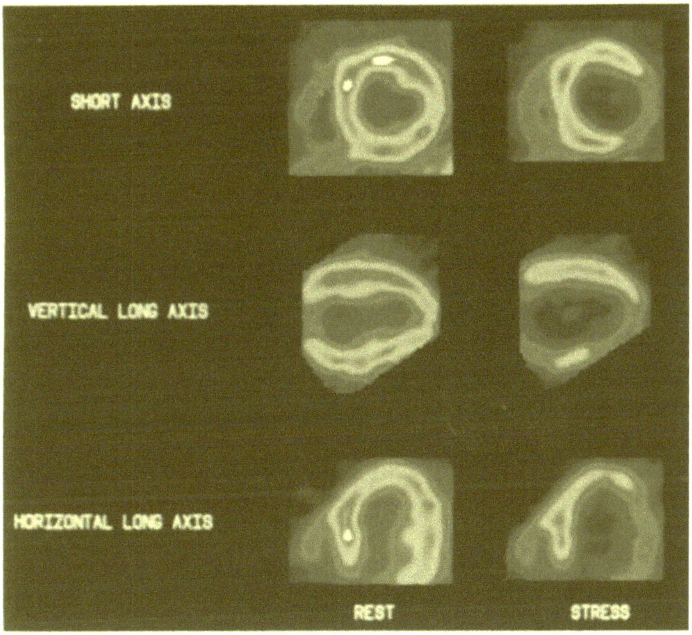

Fig. 2. Rest and pharmacologic stress study demonstrating an extensive dipyridamole-induced posterior and lateral perfusion defect in a patient with obstruction of the left circumflex artery

enhanced accuracy of PET is in detection of disease involving the posterior circulation (right coronary and left circumflex ateries). Correction of diaphragm attenuation improves the specificity of PET for disease detection in the posterior circulation. PET has also been shown to have greater sensitivity compared to SPECT for detection of disease in this region. Go et al. [23] correctly identified disease of the right coronary or left circumflex arteries in 21 cases incorrectly diagnosed as negative by SPECT. In post-CABG patients the accuracy of thallium scintigraphy for localization of disease to the posterior circulation has been reported to be as low as 50% [47]. Figure 2 depicts a rest and stress PET perfusion study in a patient with obstruction of the left circumflex artery.

Further studies are required to determine the accuracy of PET perfusion studies for detection and localization of disease in patients with prior revascularization. In cases where the results of SPECT or other noninvasive tests are equivocal, PET perfusion imaging can provide additional diagnostic information. A cost-effective strategy for the routine use of PET perfusion imaging may be achieved with rubidium-82. In busy stress laboratories, the use of this short-lived tracer permits acquisition of high-quality rest and stress images within 1 h. A high patient throughput may offset the higher cost of PET instrumentation.

Quantitative Evaluation of Myocardial Perfusion

Estimates of stenosis severity, derived by visual analysis of coronary angiograms, do not accurately predict the effects of atherosclerosis on coronary flow [63]. The physiologic significance of coronary artery disease is more precisely described by measurement of coronary flow reserve, which is the ratio between flow at maximal coronary vasodilation and at rest.

The noninvasive measurement of myocardial blood flow is particularly valuable in patients with prior CABG because of the additional shortcomings of coronary angiography in this population. Flow to regions of the myocardium supplied by more than one conduit may not be predicted by observation of the coronary anatomy. Flow through a patent graft may actually increase after occlusion of the artery proximal to the graft insertion. A reduction in coronary flow reserve may be observed in patients who have no angiographic evidence of bypass graft disease [2]. This reduction in vasodilatory capacity may be due to diffuse atherosclerotic disease involving bypass grafts and native vessels [68]. In the absence of discrete stenoses this condition may not be detected by angiography. Finally, the adequacy of the collateral circulation can only be determined by measurement of blood flow.

Quantitative evaluation of myocardial perfusion using PET is a subject of intensive experimental and clinical investigation. Assessment of regional myocardial blood flow was made possible by the development of tomographs with improved spatial resolution and multislice imaging capacity. Using suitable blood flow tracers (Table 1), dynamic image acqusition provides data which permit generation of blood and tissue time-activity curves. A mathematical model describing the known kinetic behavior of the tracer is applied to the data and solved for variables that include absolute blood flow expressed in milliliters per minute per 100 g of tissue.

The two most widely investigated tracers for quantitation of myocardial blood flow are [^{15}O]water and [^{13}N]ammonia [53]. Diagrams of the kinetic models for these two tracers are shown in Fig. 3. [^{15}O]Water is a freely diffusable tracer that has almost 100% extraction over a wide range of flows. Its brief physical half-life facilitates serial determinations of blood flow (Table 1). The tissue kinetics of [^{15}O]water, with rapid myocardial uptake and washout, resemble blood kinetics, and this results in low contrast images. Identification of myocardial tissue requires blood pool subtraction using [^{15}O]carbon monoxide [65].

[^{13}N]Ammonia has a higher than 90% extraction even at high blood flows (Table 1). However, retention of the tracer is not linearly related to flow and decreases with hyperemic flows. A three-compartment model is used to describe the kinetics of [^{13}N]ammonia [28] (Fig. 3). The initial extraction of the tracer into the extravascular space (K1) provides an accurate estimate of blood flow. The [^{15}O]water and [^{13}N]ammonia methods have been validated as accurate techniques for the measurement of myocardial blood flow in the animal laboratory [5, 45]. Kinetic models have recently

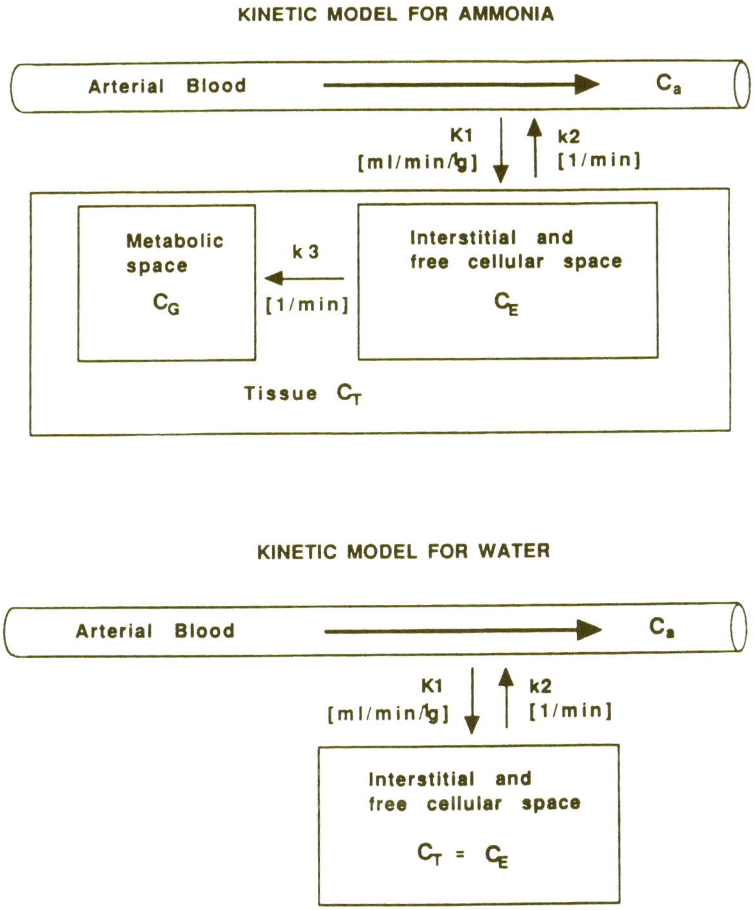

Fig. 3. Kinetic models of [^{13}N]ammonia and [^{15}O]water used for determination of myocardial blood flow. C_a, C_T, C_E, C_G, tracer concentration in blood, tissue, interstitial and free cellular space, and metabolically trapped compartments, respectively; *K1*, *k2*, *k3*, rate constants for the tracer's initial extraction, back diffusion, and retention, respectively. A three-compartment model is used for ammonia. K1 provides an accurate estimate of myocardial blood flow. The model for water consists of two compartments, and blood flow is computed from the washout rate constant k2

been developed for rubidium-82 and copper-62 PTSM. Preliminary evidence suggests that these generator-produced tracers may also be used for quantitation of flow [3, 27].

The water and ammonia methods have been applied to the measurement of coronary flow reserve in humans without coronary artery disease (Table 3). Administration of the potent coronary vasodilator dipyridamole produces a four- to fivefold increase in baseline flow in these subjects. Similar values for coronary flow reserve in normals have been reported using other

Table 3. Measurement of myocardial blood flow in normal subjects

Reference	Tracer	Stress method	Rest flow (ml min^{-1} 100 g^{-1})	Stress flow (ml min^{-10} 100 g^{-1})	Perfusion reserve
Bergmann [6]	$[^{15}O]H_2O$	Dipyridamole	90 ± 22	355 ± 112	4.10
Krivokapich [34]	$[^{13}N]NH_3$	Bicycle exercise	70 ± 17	132 ± 22	1.97
Hutchins [28]	$[^{13}N]NH_3$	Dipyridamole	88 ± 17	417 ± 112	4.80
Araujo [1]	$[^{15}O]H_2O$	Dipyridamole	84 ± 9	352 ± 112	4.19

methodologies [67]. Krivokapich et al. [34] obtained lower values for perfusion reserve when supine bicycle exercise was used as the stimulus for coronary vasodilation (Table 3).

PET quantitation of myocardial blood flow has not been evaluated in patients who have undergone surgical revascularization. However, recent studies have investigated the utility of PET for detecting regional changes in coronary flow. Araujo et al. [1] employed a modified $[^{15}O]$water method to measure regional flow in normals and in patients with coronary artery disease. The flow during dipyridamole infusion in regions supplied by vessels with greater than 75% diameter stenosis was significantly lower at 1.32 ml min^{-1} g^{-1} compared to the flow (3.52 ml^{-1} min^{-1} g^{-1}) in normal volunteers. Beanlands et al. [4] demonstrated that $[^{13}N]$ammonia imaging can be used to assess the severity of coronary disease. Mean values of regional flow reserve declined from 2.2 to 1.4 with increasing severity of coronary obstruction as measured by quantitative coronary angiography. These data indicate that PET determinations of coronary flow reserve can be used to assess the physiologic significance of coronary disease.

In patients who have undergone CABG, alterations in the coronary circulation create further difficulty in the evaluation of regional perfusion. Bypass grafting may change the size and location of the myocardial region perfused by the native vessel necessitating evaluation of flow throughout the left ventricle [32, 42]. Use of an appropriate tracer and multislice imaging capacity of currently available tomographs allows construction of flow maps encompassing the entire heart (Fig. 4).

As discussed above, coronary angiography may underestimate the extent and severity of disease in post-CABG patients who have diffuse atherosclerosis. In patients with coronary disease, both Araujo et al. [1] and Beanlands et al. [4] have reported a modest reduction in flow reserve in regions supplied by arteries without angiographic evidence of obstruction. This reduction in flow reserve is less severe (flow reserve of 2.9 versus 1.4) than that observed in regions suppled by arteries with discrete stenoses. This implies that PET measurements of flow may possess adequate sensitivity to detect small changes in vascular resistance caused by diffuse disease.

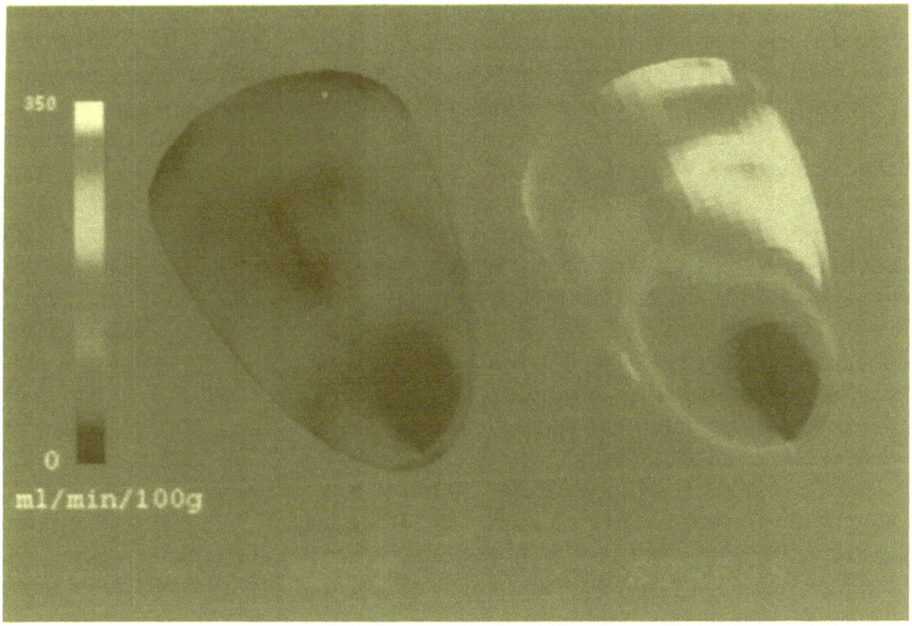

Fig. 4. Simulated three-dimensional flow map of the left ventricle at baseline (*left*) and during pharmacologic stress (*right*). At baseline the ventricle has homogeneous perfusion. A two- to threefold increase (*green*, *yellow*) in myocardial flow is observed in the proximal two-thirds of the ventricle during stress. No increase in flow is seen at the apex (*blue*) due to significant stenosis of the midportion of the left anterior descending artery

Microvascular disease may also complicate evaluation of perfusion in post-CABG patients. Prolonged hypertension with left ventricular hypertrophy, diabetes mellitus, and recent cardiopulmonary bypass may diminish flow reserve in the absence of coronary obstruction [68]. Quantitative PET flow studies have detected significant impairments in flow reserve in patients with suspected microvascular disease [14, 22].

The results cited thus far are sufficiently promising to encourage further development of PET as a tool for quantitation of blood flow. Additional clinical studies are needed to establish the accuracy of this method of noninvasive measurement of blood flow. Development of user-friendly, automated analysis techniques will be necessary before PET flow measurements can be widely applied.

Evaluation of Myocardial Function and Metabolism

The presence and severity of resting left ventricular dysfunction are both important predictors of survival in patients with coronary artery disease [8,

12]. It is now well recognized that global or regional left ventricular dysfunction may improve following revascularization. This improvement is attributed to restoration of blood flow to functionally depressed but viable myocardium. Depression of left ventricular contractility in the absence of tissue necrosis occurs in three situations. Acute ischemia produces transient wall motion abnormalities in regions deprived of blood flow. Prolonged or repeated episodes of ischemia may produce wall motion abnormalities that persist for hours to days after the acute insult before eventual recovery. This phenomenon has been termed "myocardial stunning," which is to be distinguished from chronic depression of myocardial contractility or "hibernating myocardium" [9, 10, 49]. Hibernating myocardium describes the phenomenon of reversible left ventricular dysfunction in the setting of persistent, severe reductions in blood flow. Coronary perfusion is sufficient to preserve tissue viability but not contractility. Contractility improves following restoration of blood flow.

Determination of myocardial viability is a problem of considerable magnitude in post-CABG patients. The frequency of regional wall motion abnormalities approaches 67% in patients presenting for repeat CABG [38]. Patients who have already had one operative procedure are also those most likely to have globally depressed ventricular function. In one-third of patients, ventricular function declines between the first and second surgeries [35].

The importance of detection of viable myocardium extends beyond the prediction of reversible dysfunction. The identification of viable myocardium provides valuable prognostic information in patients who present with infarction after their first CABG. Those patients who have viable myocardium remaining in the vascular bed at risk may be more likely to have reinfarction compared to those without residual viability [66].

Selection of therapy for patients with bypass graft disease is influenced by the presence, extent, and location of viable myocardium. The perioperative mortality of a second CABG ranges from 3.0% to 5.3%, representing a two- to fivefold increase over the mortality of the primary procedure [19, 36, 37]. Most of the increased mortality is related to an increase in perioperative myocardial infarction, ranging from 4% to 18% [15, 38]. Patients with reduced left ventricular function and substantial myocardium in jeopardy are those at increased risk for perioperative infarction. In some cases this risk may be reduced by changes in the operative procedure. Embolization of atherosclerotic debris through patent but diseased grafts is a major cause of infarction during reoperation [24]. In patients with significant myocardium at risk, ligation of vein grafts with administration of retrograde cardioplegia may reduce the risk of perioperative infarction.

Identification of viable tissue may serve as a guide for coronary angioplasty or repeat surgical revascularization. The goal of reoperation is complete revascularization. However, selection of sites to revascularize may be necessary if there is a limited number of available bypass conduits, or if

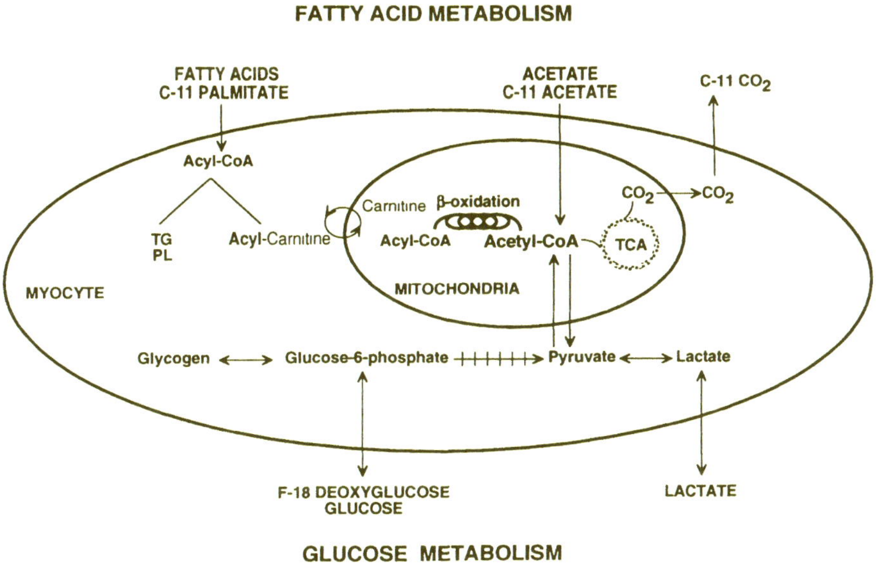

Fig. 5. Diagram of the metabolic pathways of myocardial substrate metabolism. The sites of entry are shown for fatty acid tracers of oxidative metabolism ([^{11}C]palmitate and [^{11}C]acetate) and for the glucose analogue F-18 deoxyglucose

excessively prolonged cardiopulmonary bypass is needed for complete revascularization.

The electrocardiogram and wall motion studies assessing the severity of regional dysfunction cannot be used to accurately distinguish viable from infarcted tissue. The unique ability of PET to provide information on myocardial metabolism has led to the rapid acceptance of this technique as the reference standard for detection of myocardial viability.

A diagram of cardiac metabolism and the tracers that serve as substrates are shown in Fig. 5. Fluorine-18 deoxyglucose (FDG) is the tracer most commonly employed for viability studies. FDG is a glucose analogue that undergoes cellular uptake and phosphorylation to FDG-6-phosphate. FDG-6-phosphate undergoes no additional metabolism, and is essentially trapped in the myocardium because of slow dephosphorylation [21]. Myocardial uptake of FDG reflects both glycolysis and glycogen synthesis. Under steady-state conditions equilibrium exists between glycogen formation and breakdown so that the myocardial accumulation of FDG reflects the extraction and phosphorylation rate of exogenous glucose [26, 33].

In ischemically injured tissue, myocardial uptake of glucose is enhanced, and oxidation of free fatty acids is impaired relative to normal tissue [54]. Elevation of glucose uptake occurs in acute ischemia and in stunned and hibernating myocardium [13, 40, 51]. The increase in glucose utilization may persist for hours to weeks after restoration of blood flow to ischemic tissue

[46, 54]. Fatty acid oxidation may also remain impaired for a substantial period of time after reperfusion.

Myocardial viability is assessed in regions of the left ventricle by evaluation of regional myocardial perfusion and FDG uptake. Analysis can be performed in a qualitative fashion by visual comparison of regional tracer distributions. Alternatively, the regional activity of a blood flow tracer and FDG can be quantified and compared to values generated from a normal population.

The perfusion and FDG images can be classified into three general categories. Normal blood flow and FDG uptake is observed in normally perfused myocardium without necrosis. Myocardial infarction without viable tissue demonstrates a second pattern of a concordant reduction in perfusion and FDG uptake. The third pattern of enhanced FDG uptake with a relative reduction in blood flow, designated as flow-metabolism mismatch, is indicative of viable but compromised myocardium. Enhanced FDG uptake may be present even with reductions in flow up to 70% of normal resting flow [30, 57]. Viable and necrotic tissue may coexist in a zone of ischemically injured myocardium that has maintained glucose metabolism [57]. Two patterns of mismatch have been described by Fudo et al. [20]. Diffuse mismatch, the most commonly observed pattern, occurs throughout the ischemically injured zone. Less commonly, border zones between normal and infarcted myocardium may exhibit a peripheral-type of mismatch pattern. Examples of a matched reduction in flow and FDG uptake and flow-metabolism mismatch are shown in Fig. 6.

In clinical studies the correlation of diffuse mismatch with myocardial viability was first established in patients evaluated after acute myocardial infarction [11, 51]. Flow-metabolism mismatch correlated with the presence of postinfarction angina, the site of ischemic electrocardiographic changes, and the presence of residual blood flow in severely diseased arteries [11, 39, 52]. With the passage of time improvement in wall motion was observed in some segments that exhibited mismatch but not in those with matched reductions in perfusion and FDG metabolism [55]. Subsequently, perfusion and FDG studies have been performed in patients undergoing CABG to determine the value of PET for predicting reversibility of regional wall motion abnormalities.

Table 4 summarizes the results of studies investigating the sensitivity, specificity, and predictive value of flow and FDG imaging for the detection of segments with reversible dysfunction. Differences in the methods em-

Fig. 6. Myocardial viability studies (*left*, perfusion; *right*, FDG images) demonstrating flow and metabolism mismatch (**A**), and a matched reduction in flow and metabolism (**B**). **A** A marked reduction in flow but preserved FDG uptake in the anterior wall consistent with viable, but compromised myocardium. **B** A severe reduction in both flow and FDG uptake in the posterolateral wall consistent with myocardial necrosis

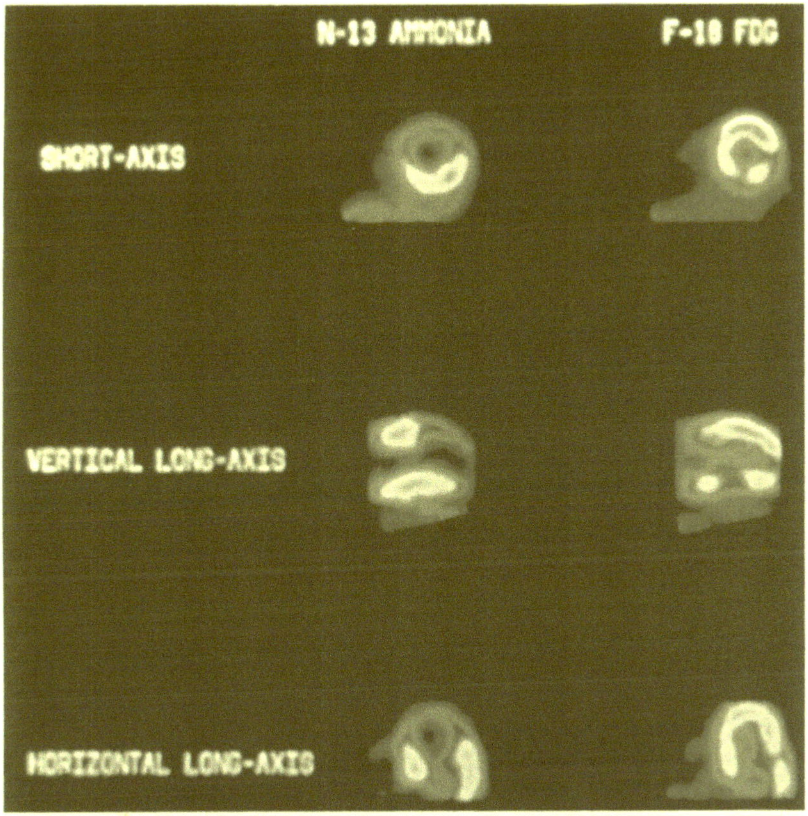
N-13 AMMONIA
F-18 FDG
SHORT-AXIS
VERTICAL LONG-AXIS
HORIZONTAL LONG-AXIS

A

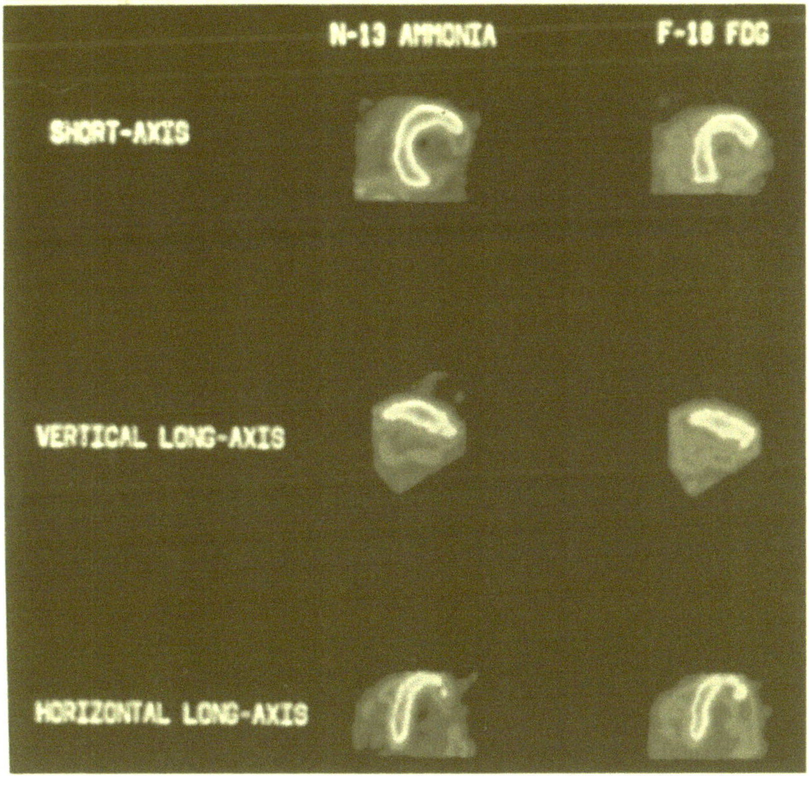
N-13 AMMONIA
F-18 FDG
SHORT-AXIS
VERTICAL LONG-AXIS
HORIZONTAL LONG-AXIS

B

Table 4. Prediction of improvement in regional wall motion by preoperative perfusion and FDG imaging

Study	*n*	FDG protocol	Criteria for predicting improved wall motion	Sensitivity		Specificity		Positive predictive value		Negative predictive value	
				(%)	*n*	(%)	*n*	(%)	*n*	(%)	*n*
Tillisch [62]	17	Glucose Load	N1 flow, N1 FDG Mismatch	94	35/37	80	24/30	85	35/41	92	24/26
Tamaki [60]	22	Fasted	Normal flow, FDG Mismatch	78	18/23	78	18/23	78	18/23	78	18/23
Marwick[a] [40]	23	Fasted	Mismatch	61	19/31	83	35/42	73	19/26	74	35/47
vom Dahl [64]	40	Glucose Load	N1 flow, N1 FDG	75	15/20	66	27/41	52	15/29	84	27/32
			Reduced flow, mildly reduced FDG								
			Mismatch	94[b]	15/16	53[b]	10/19	62[b]	15/24	91[b]	10/11

N1, Normal.
[a] 12 patients had coronary angioplasty.
[b] Results in segments with severe preoperative wall motion abnormal malities.

ployed in each study may account for the variability of the results. FDG imaging may be performed following glucose loading or in the fasting state. Glucose loading augments FDG uptake in normal myocardium, potentially reducing the sensitivity of the technique for ischemic myocardium by decreasing the difference in FDG activity between normal and ischemic tissue. In contrast, fasting diminishes FDG uptake in normally perfused myocardium, accentuating the difference in FDG activity between normal and ischemic tissue. In practice, glucose loading has not reduced the sensitivity of FDG imaging for detection of ischemic myocardium that demonstrates recovery of function. At the present time, glucose loading should be considered as the standard protocol for assessment of tissue viability before revascularization. The specific identification of ischemic myocardium may be less important than identification of all myocardial regions that are viable (normally perfused and ischemic tissue) because the perioperative outcome of the patient with advanced coronary disease is largely dependent on the quantity of residual viable myocardium.

In spite of the methodologic diversity, investigators have shown that flow and metabolic imaging with FDG predict reversible dysfunction with reasonable accuracy. Tillisch [62] demonstrated that the uptake of FDG is highly predictive of regional recovery of function when a segment is adequately revascularized. This finding was confirmed by Tamaki et al. [60], who demonstrated that the postoperative decline of FDG uptake to normal levels is always correlated with improvement in wall motion. However, FDG uptake was observed in a substantial number of segments that did not have functional recovery in a recent study by vom Dahl [64]. Revascularization may not restore function in segments with necrosis of a critical amount of the subendocardium in spite of improvement in blood supply to viable outer layers that demonstrate FDG uptake preoperatively. Even in the absence of improvement in function, revascularization of segments with epicardial viability may still be important for relief of ischemia and preservation of left ventricular geometry. Segments with partial necrosis can have mild reductions in FDG activity and may or may not exhibit improvement in function with revascularization. When FDG uptake is severely reduced or absent, revascularization rarely results in significant improvement in regional function. Small nonviable regions may appear to improve in wall motion because of tethering to adjacent viable segments.

Metabolic studies with FDG are now providing important prognostic information and shedding light on the mechanisms behind the long-term benefit of CABG in patients with reduced left ventricular function. Eitzman and colleagues [18] recently demonstrated the importance of detection of viable myocardium at risk. In this study a mismatch pattern in medically treated patients with a mean ejection fraction of 36% was associated with a 1-year cardiac event rate of 50%. The event rate was significantly lower (12.5%) in patients with mismatch and a similar degree of dysfunction who were treated surgically.

PET viability studies also show that the amount of myocardium demonstrating mismatch has direct effects on ejection fraction and exercise capacity, two of the most important prognostic indicators in patients with coronary artery disease. Tillisch et al. [62] found that significant improvement in ejection fraction occurs after CABG in patients who have preoperative evidence of viability in three or more dysfunctional segments. Marwick et al. [41] reported that patients with at least two mismatched regions exhibit improved exercise capacity after CABG, even in the absence of improvement in resting ejection fraction. Thus, the above studies provide a plausible explanation for the improved survival of revascularized patients with multivessel disease and ventricular dysfunction.

There are some disadvantages to the use of FDG in viability studies. Image quality is diminished in patients with diabetes mellitus. A reduction in myocardial uptake of FDG coupled with slower clearance of the isotope from blood both contribute to the reduced image quality [53]. However, images adequate for diagnosis can be obtained in most patients with administration of insulin prior to the FDG study.

The metabolic tracers [^{11}C]palmitate and [^{11}C]acetate are potential alternatives to the use of FDG for assessment of tissue viability [16, 31]. Improvement of [^{11}C]palmitate uptake immediately after revascularization is indicative of successful restoration of flow and predictive of eventual recovery of myocardial oxidative metabolism. Unlike [^{11}C]palmitate, the metabolism of [^{11}C]acetate is substrate independent and its clearance rate closely correlates with myocardial oxygen consumption. Preservation of oxidative metabolism in segments with reduced blood flow may identify viable segments that demonstrate recovery of wall motion after revascularization [25].

Recognition of the clinical importance of stunned and hibernating myocardium and the high cost and limited availability of PET have encouraged the development of alternative methods for detection of viable myocardium. Thallium-201 scintigraphy and assessment of the response of regional wall motion to pharmacologic stimulation are more widely available modalities and less costly compared to PET. Thallium-201 serves as an indicator of viability because its uptake requires active transport across cell membranes. A significant proportion of irreversible perfusion defects (40%–50%) on images acquired 3–4 h after stress demonstrate viability by uptake of thallium with more delayed imaging (8–24 h) [53]. The inconvenience of obtaining images 8–24 h after stress led to investigation of protocols that employ imaging after a second injection of thallium given immediately after completion of the 3-h delayed images. In correlative studies with PET the thallium reinjection technique detects the majority of segments (75%–89%) that demonstrate FDG uptake [7, 61]. Further comparative studies are needed to determine the clinical significance of this modest difference in sensitivity between the two methods.

In experimental studies, the improvement of regional wall motion during administration of inotropic drugs has been shown to be a marker of viablity.

Two-dimensional echocardiography and nuclear angiography combined with catecholamine infusion have been used for the preoperative detection of segments that demonstrate improved wall motion with revascularization [44, 48, 56]. These methods have the dual advantages of widespread availability and relatively low cost. However, use of these techniques restricts the determination of viability to those segments that have contractile reserve. The extent of myocardium at risk may be underestimated if metabolically active segments without contractile reserve are not detected.

At the present time there is insufficient evidence to draw conclusions about the relative value of PET, reinjection thallium, and wall motion techniques for detection of viable myocardium. Utilization of a specific technique is in part determined by the expertise of the laboratory or institution evaluating patients for revascularization. Until additional comparative studies are performed, PET will remain the gold standard for detection of viable myocardium.

Acknowledgements. This work was performed during the tenure of an established investigatorship of Dr. Schwaiger from the American Heart Association and was supported in part by the National Institute of Health, Bethesda, MD (R01 HL41047) and the Department of Energy (DE-FG02-9ER61091).

References

1. Araujo L, Lammertsma A, Rhodes C et al. (1991) Noninvasive quantification of regional myocardial blood flow in coronary artery disease with oxygen-15-labeled carbon dioxide inhalation and positron emission tomography. Circulation 83:875–885
2. Bates E, Aueron F, Legrand V et al. (1985) Comparative long-term effects of coronary artery bypass graft surgery and percutaneous transluminal coronary angioplasty on regional coronary flow reserve. Circulation 72:833–839
3. Beanlands R, Muzik O, Mintun M et al. (1992a) The kinetics of copper-62-PTSM in the normal human heart. J Nucl Med 33:684–690
4. Beanlands R, Muzik O, Sutor R et al. (1992b) Noninvasive determination of regional perfusion reserve in coronary artery disease using N-13 ammonia PET. J Nucl Med 33:826
5. Bergmann S, Fox K, Rand A et al. (1984) Quantification of regional myocardial blood flow in vivo with O-15 water. Circulation 70:724–733
6. Bergmann S, Herrero P, Markham J, Winheimer C, Walsh M (1989) Noninvasive quantification of myocardial blood flow in human subjects with oxygen-15-labeled water and positron emission tomography. J Am Coll Cardiol 14:639–652
7. Bonow R, Dilsizian V, Cuocolo A, Bacharach S (1991) Identification of viable myocardium in patients with chronic coronary artery disease and left ventricular dysfunction. Circulation 83:26–37
8. Bourassa M (1991) Left ventricular function after coronary bypass surgery. In: Waters D, Bourassa M (eds) Care of the patient with previous coronary bypass surgery. Davis, Philadelphia, pp 227–237 (Cardiovascular clinics, vol 21)
9. Braunwald E, Kloner R (1982) The stunned myocardium: prolonged, postischemic ventricular dysfunction. Circulation 66:1146–1149

10. Braunwald E, Rutherford J (1986) Reversible ischemic left ventricular dysfunction: evidence for the "hibernating myocardium." J Am Coll Cardiol 8:1467–1470
11. Brunken R, Tillisch J, Schwaiger M et al. (1986) Regional perfusion, glucose metabolism, and wall motion in patients with chronic electrocardiographic Q Wave infarctions: evidence for persistence of viable tissue in some infarct regions by positron emission tomography. Circulation 73:951–963
12. Bruschke A, Proudfit W, Sones F (1973) Progress study of 590 consecutive nonsurgical cases of coronary disease followed 5–9 years. II. Ventriculographic and other considerations. Circulation 47:1154–1163
13. Camici P, Araujo L, Spinks T et al. (1986) Increased uptake of F-18-deoxyglucose in postischemic myocardium of patients with exercise-induced angina. Circulation 74:81–88
14. Camici P, Chiriatti G, Lorenzoni R et al. (1991) Coronary vasodilation is impaired in both hypertrophied and non-hypertrophied myocardium of patients with hypertrophic cardiomyopathy: a study with nitrogen-13 ammonia and positron emission tomography. J Am Coll Cardiol 17:879–886
15. Carrier M, Perreault L, Pelletier L (1991) Reoperation for coronary bypass grafting. In: Waters D, Bourassa M (eds) Care of the patients with previous coronary bypass surgery. Davis, Philadelphia, pp 257–263 (Cardiovascular clinics, vol 21)
16. Czernin J, Porenta G, Brunken R et al. (1990) Oxidative and glycolytic metabolic tissue characterization in patients with acute infarction using dynamic PET. J Nucl Med 31:774
17. Demer L, Gould L, Goldstein R et al. (1989) Assessment of coronary artery disease severity by positron emission tomography. Comparison with quantitative arteriography in 193 patients. Circulation 79:825–835
18. Eitzman D, Al-Aouar Z, Kanter H et al. (1992) Clinical outcome of patients with advanced coronary artery disease following positron emission tomography viablity studies. J Am Coll Cardiol (in press)
19. Foster E, Fisher L, Kaiser G (1984) Comparison of operative mortality and morbidity for initial and repeat coronary artery bypass grafting: the Coronary Artery Surgery Study (CASS) Registry experience. Ann Thorac Cardiovasc Surg 38:563–569
20. Fudo T, Kambara H, Hashimoto T et al. (1988) F-18 deoxyglucose and stress N-13 ammonia positron emission tomography in anterior wall healed myocardial infarction. Am J Cardiol 61:1191–1197
21. Gallagher B, Fowler J, Gutterson N, Macgregor R, Wan C, Wolf A (1978) Metabolic trapping as a principle of radiopharmaceutical design: some factors responsible for the biodistribution of F-18-2-deoxy-2-fluoro-D-glucose. J Nucl Med 19:1154–1161
22. Geltman E, Henes C, Senneff M, Sobel B, Bergmann S (1990) Increased myocardial perfusion at rest and diminished perfusion reserve in patients with angina and angiographically normal coronary arteries. J Am Coll Cardiol 16:586–595
23. Go R, Marwick T, MacIntyre W et al. (1990) A prospective comparison of rubidium-82 PET and thallium-201 SPECT myocardial perfusion imaging utilizing a single dipyridamole stress in the diagnosis of coronary artery disease. J Nucl Med 31:1899–1905
24. Grondin C, Pomar J, Hebert Y et al. (1984) Reoperation in patients with patent atherosclerotic coronary vein grafts. A different approach to a different disease. J Thorac Cardiovasc Surg 87:379–385
25. Gropler R, Geltman E, Sampathkumaran J et al. (1992) The superiority of cardiac PET with C-11 acetate for prediction of functional recovery after revascularization. J Nucl Med 5:855
26. Halama J, Gatley J, DeGrado T, Bernstein D, Ng C, Holden J (1984) Validation of 3-deoxy-3-fluoro-D-glucose as a glucose transport analog in rat heart. Am J Physiol 246: H754–H759
27. Herrero P, Markham J, Shelton M, Weinheimer C, Bergmann S (1990) Noninvasive quantification of regional myocardial perfusion with rubidium-82 and positron emission tomography. Circulation 82:1377–1386

28. Hutchins G, Schwaiger M, Rosenspire KJ, Krivokapich J, Schelbert H, Kuhl D (1990) Noninvasive quantification of regional blood flow in the human heart using N-13 ammonia and dynamic positron emission tomographic imaging. J Am Coll Cardiol 15:1032–1042
29. Hutchins G, Schwaiger M, Wolfe E (1992) Quantitative evaluation of myocardial perfusion using positron emission tomography. Am J Cardiac Imaging (in press)
30. Kalff V, Schwaiger M, Nguyen N, McClanahan T, Gallagher K (1992) The relationship between myocardial blood flow and glucose uptake in ischemic canine myocardium determined with F-18 glucose. J Nucl Med (in press)
31. Knabb R, Bergmann S, Fox K, Sobel B (1987) The temporal pattern of recovery of myocardial perfusion and metabolism delineated by positron emission tomography after coronary thrombolysis. J Nucl Med 28:1563–1570
32. Kolibash A, Lewis R, Goodenow J (1980) Extensive myocardial blood flow distribution through individual coronary artery bypass grafts. Chest 77:17–23
33. Krivokapich J, Huang S, Selin C, Phelps M (1987) Fluorodeoxyglucose rate constants, lumped constant, and glucose metabolic rate in rabbit heart. Am J Physiol 252:H777–H787
34. Krivokapich J, Smith G, Huang S et al. (1989) N-13 ammonia myocardial imaging at rest and with exercise in normal volunteers. Quantification of absolute myocardial perfusion with dynamic positron emission tomography. Circulation 80:1328–1337
35. Loop F, Lytle B, Gill C et al. (1983) Trends in selection and results of coronary reoperations. Ann Thorac Surg 36:380–388
36. Lytle B, Loop F, Cosgrove D et al. (1987) Fifteen hundred coronary reoperations: results and determinants of early and later survival. J Thorac Cardiovasc Surg 93:847–859
37. Lytle B, Cosgrove D, Taylor P et al. (1989) Multiple coronary reoperations: early and late results. Circulation 89 [Suppl II]:II–626
38. Lytle B, Cosgrove D, Loop F (1991) Future implications of current trends in bypass surgery. In: Waters D, Bourassa M (eds) Care of the patient with previous coronary bypass surgery. Davis, Philadelphia, pp 265–278 (Cardiovascular clinics, vol 21)
39. Marshall R, Tillisch J, Phelps M (1983) Identification and differentiation of resting myocardial ischemia in man with positron computed tomography. F-18 labeled fluorodeoxyglucose and N-13 ammonia. Circulation 67:766–778
40. Marwick T, MacIntyre W, Lafont A, Nemec J, Salcedo E (1992) Metabolic responses of hibernating and infarcted myocardium to revascularization. A follow-up study of regional perfusion, function and metabolism. Circulation 85:1347–1353
41. Marwick T, Nemec J, Lafont A, Salcedo E, MacIntyre W (1992) Prediction by postexercise fluoro-18 deoxyglucose positron emission tomography of improvement in exercise capacity after revascularization. Am J Cardiol 69:854–859
42. McNamara J, Bjerke H, Chung G (1979) Blood flow in sequential vein grafts. Circulation 60 [Suppl I]:33
43. Miller D (1991) Evaluation of the patient with stable angina following coronary artery bypass surgery. In: Waters D, Bourassa M (eds) Care of the patient with previous coronary bypass surgery. Davis, Philadelphia, pp 137–167
44. Movahed A, Reeves W, Rose G et al. (1990) Dobutamine and improvement of regional and global left ventricular function in coronary artery disease. Am J Cardiol 66:375–377
45. Muzik O, Beanlands R, Hutchins G et al. (1991) Experimental validation of a tracer kinetic model for N-13 ammonia in comparison to O-15 water for quantification of myocardial blood flow. J Nucl Med 32:926
46. Nienaber C, Brunken R, Sherman C et al. (1991) Metabolic and functional recovery of ischemic human myocardium after coronary angioplasty. J Am Coll Cardiol 18:966–978
47. Pfisterer M, Emmenegger H, Schmitt E et al. (1982) Accuracy of serial myocardial perfusion scintigraphy with thallium-201 for prediction of graft patency early and late after coronary artery bypass surgery. Circulation 66:1017–1024
48. Pierard L, DeLandsheere C, Berthe C et al. (1990) Identification of viable myocardium by echocardiography during dobutamine infusion in patients with myocardial infarction after

thrombolytic therapy: comparison with positron emission tomography. J Am Coll Cardiol 15:1021–1031
49. Rahimtoola S (1985) A perspective on the three large multicenter randomized clinical trials of coronary bypass surgery for chronic stable angina. Circulation 8:V-123–V-135
50. Schelbert H, Wisenberg G, Phelps M et al. (1982) Noninvasive assessment of coronary stenosis by myocardial imaging during pharmacologic coronary vasodilation. VI. Detection of coronary artery disease in human beings with intravenous N-13 ammonia and positron computed tomography. Am J Cardiol 49:1197–1207
51. Schwaiger M (1986) Metabolism and blood flow as new markers of myocardial viability in the evolution of myocardial infarction. Eur J Nucl Med 12:S62–65
52. Schwaiger M (1987) Beneficial effect of residual anterograde flow on tissue viability as assessed by positron emission tomography in patients with myocardial infarction. Eur Heart J 8:981–988
53. Schwaiger M, Hicks R (1991) The clinical role of metabolic imaging of the heart by positron emission tomography. J Nucl Med 32:565–578
54. Schwaiger M, Schelbert H, Ellison D et al. (1985) Sustained regional abnormalities in cardiac metabolism after transient ischemia in the chronic dog model. J Am Coll Cardiol 6:336–347
55. Schwaiger M, Brunken R, Grover-McKay M et al. (1986) Regional myocardial metabolism in patients with acute myocardial infarction assessed by positron emission tomography. J Am Coll Cardiol 8:800–808
56. Smart S, Sawada S, Ryan T et al. (1990) Dobutamine echocardiography predicts recovery after thrombolysis in myocardial infarction. Circulation 82 [Suppl III]:75
57. Sochor H, Schwaiger M, Schelbert H et al. (1987) Relationship between Tl-201, Tc-99m (Sn) pyrophosphate and F-18 2-deoxyglucose uptake in ischemically injured dog myocardium. Am Heart J 114:1066–1077
58. Sorenson J, Phelps M (1987) Physics in nuclear medicine. Saunders, Philadelphia, pp 435–436
59. Stewart R, Schwaiger M, Molina E et al. (1991) Comparison of rubidium-82 PET and thallium-201 SPECT imaging for the detection of coronary artery disease. Am J Cardiol 67:1303–1310
60. Tamaki N, Yonekura Y, Yamashita K et al. (1989) Positron emission tomography using fluorine-18 deoxyglucose in evaluation of coronary artery bypass grafting. Am J Cardiol 64:860–865
61. Tamaki N, Ohtani H, Yamashita K et al. (1991) Metabolic activity in the areas of new fill-in after thallium-201 reinjection: comparison with positron emission tomography using fluorine-18-deoxyglucose. J Nucl Med 32:673–678
62. Tillisch J, Brunken R, Marshall R et al. (1986) Reversibility of cardiac wall-motion abnormalities predicted by positron tomography. N Engl J Med 314:884–888
63. Vogel R, Bates E, O'Neill W et al. (1984) Coronary flow reserve measured during cardiac catheterization. Arch Intern Med 144:1773–1777
64. vom Dahl J, Eitzman D, Al-Aouar Z et al. (1992) Relationship of regional function, perfusion and metabolism in patients with advanced coronary artery disease. Circulation (in review)
65. Walsh M, Bergmann S, Steele R et al. (1988) Delineation of impaired regional myocardial perfusion by positron emission tomography with O-15 water. Circulation 78:612–620
66. Waters D (1991) Myocardial infarction in patients with previous bypass surgery. In: Waters D, Bourassa M (eds) Care of the patient with previous coronary bypass surgery. Davis, Philadelphia, pp 193–209 (Cardiovascular clinics, vol 21)
67. White C, Wilson R, Marcus M (1988) Methods of measuring myocardial blood flow in humans. Prog Cardiovasc Dis 31:79–84
68. Wilson R, Marcus M, White C (1988) Effects of coronary bypass surgery and angioplasty on coronary blood flow and flow reserve. Prog Cardiovasc Dis 31:95–114

Transcutaneous Assessment of Blood Flow in Internal Thoracic Artery to Coronary Artery Grafts

D.P. de Bono

Introduction

The internal thoracic (internal mammary) artery is now the preferred conduit for aortocoronary bypass grafts to the left anterior descending coronary artery, and in many cases also to the right and left circumflex coronary arteries [1, 2]. The use of transcutaneous duplex ultrasound to study blood flow in internal thoracic to coronary artery grafts was pioneered by Fusejima and colleagues [3] and Kyo and colleagues [4]. It has also been studied by Sons and colleagues in Dusseldorf [5] and by our own group in Leicester [6]. Canver and colleagues [7] have used duplex ultrasound to assess internal thoracic artery patency before grafting. This chapter reviews the anatomical and technical aspects of ultrasound flow measurement in internal thoracic artery grafts, discusses the interpretation of the waveform patterns seen, and considers the possible uses of ultrasound flow measurement in studying the physiology and pathophysiology of the coronary circulation.

Anatomical and Technical Aspects of Internal Thoracic Artery Imaging

The internal thoracic artery originates from the first part of the subclavian artery just before the latter passes over the superior surface of the first rib. It then runs parallel to the sternal edge, posterior to the costal cartilages and just lateral to the costosternal joints. In performing an internal thoracic artery to coronary artery graft, the surgeon dissects the distal part of the artery away from the chest wall until a sufficient free length is created to allow anastomosis with the coronary artery (Fig. 1). The extent of the dissection depends on the shape of the thorax, the point at which the anastomosis is to be made, and the personal technique of the individual surgeon. It has a critical effect on the ease with which the grafted vessel can be imaged using transcutaneous ultrasound.

The two available ultrasound "windows" for imaging the internal thoracic artery are the supraclavicular and parasternal views (Fig. 2). The supraclavicu-

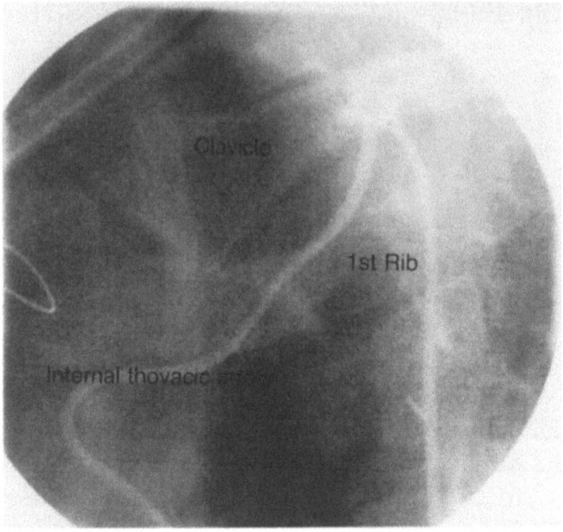

Fig. 1. Angiogram showing relationship of proximal part of a (grafted) left internal thoracic artery to the first rib, clavicle and chest wall

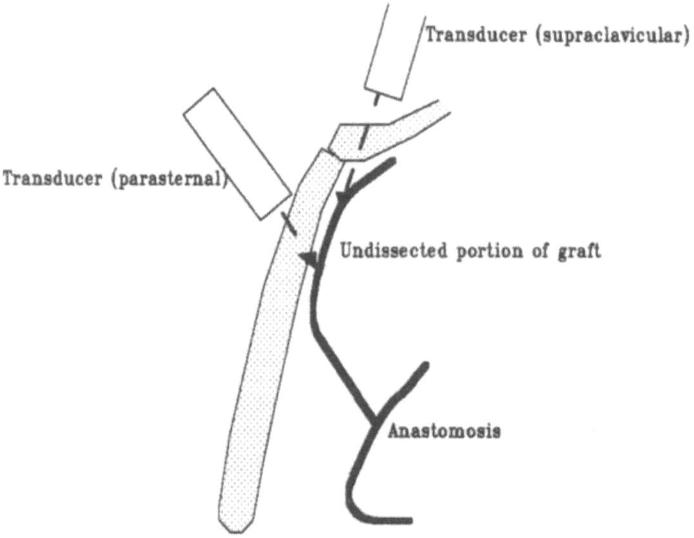

Fig. 2. Diagram showing the two possible routes, supraclavicular and parasternal, for examination of the internal thoracic artery by ultrasound

Fig. 3. Two-dimensional image (parasternal view; **a**) and Doppler sonogram (**b**) of an ungrafted right internal thoracic artery

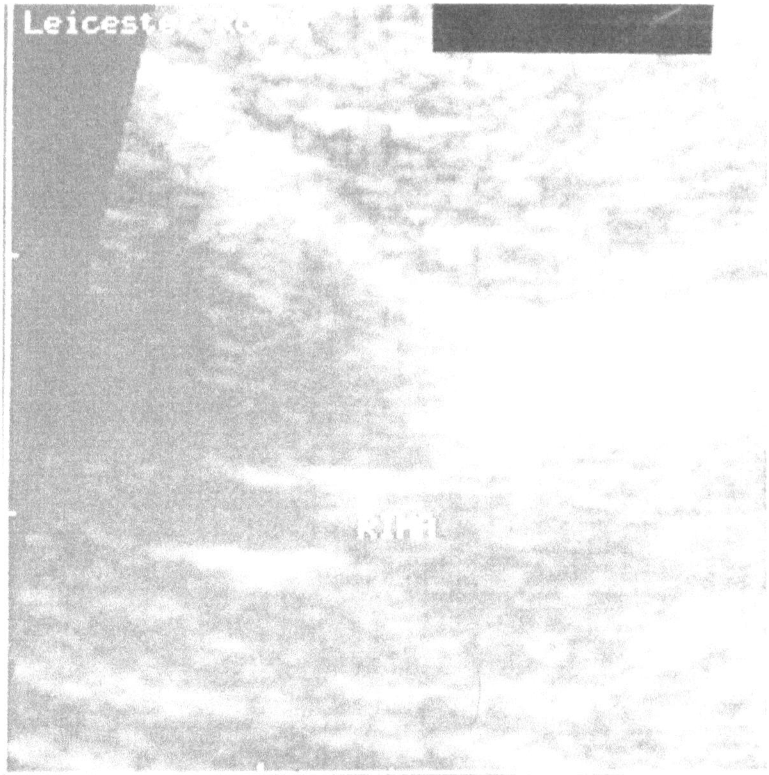
RIMA

a

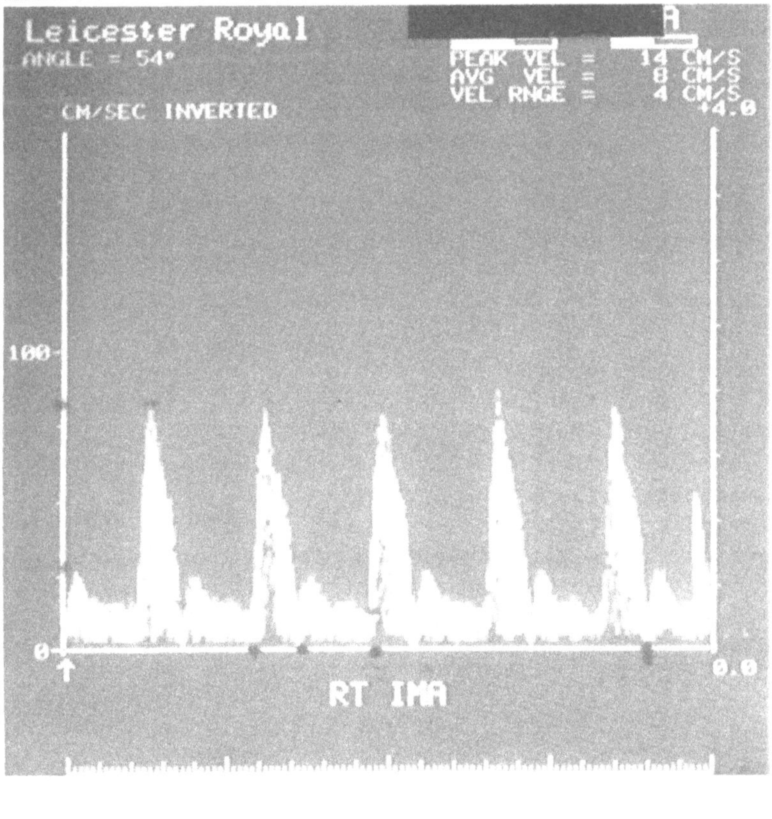
Leicester Royal
ANGLE = 54°
PEAK VEL = 14 CM/S
AVG VEL = 8 CM/S
VEL RNGE = 4 CM/S
+4.0
CM/SEC INVERTED
100
0
0.0
RT IMA

b

lar approach images the artery as it originates from the subclavian vessel. It is influenced less by surgical technique, but access can be difficult, especially in patients with short, thick necks. A small, angled transducer can be very useful, and colour Doppler imaging helps to locate the correct vessel. Since the ultrasound beam is roughly parallel to the direction of blood flow, velocity measurements are likely to be accurate, but, conversely, the accuracy with which vessel diameter can be measured is limited.

The parasternal approach has little difficulty in identifying the *ungrafted* internal thoracic artery (Fig. 3), and we have been able to image this in virtually 100% of cases, but high dissection of the artery by the surgeon may make this view impracticable. When the vessel can be imaged, its diameter can be measured with some accuracy, but velocity measurements must be corrected for the angle which the axis of the transducer makes with the axis of the vessel: ideally this should be less than 60°. In some patients the grafted vessel can be imaged from both supraclavicular and parasternal approaches; in others only one view is practicable. Serial measurements should as far as possible be made using a standardised transducer type and position. Ultrasound frequencies from 3.5 to 7.5 MHz have been used satisfactorily; higher frequencies provide more accurate measurement but less tissue penetration. Probes designed for peripheral vascular imaging are more satisfactory than cardiac probes.

Qualitative Analysis of the Internal Thoracic Artery Sonogram

The sonogram obtained from an ungrafted internal thoracic artery is similar to that obtained from other medium-sized peripheral arteries such as the external carotid (Fig. 3). It shows predominant flow in systole, with a peak systolic to peak diastolic velocity ratio of greater than 2.5:1. The sonogram from a grafted internal thoracic artery is different, usually with distinct systolic and diastolic peaks (Fig. 4). Peak systolic to peak diastolic velocity ratios are close to 1:1 (Table 1). In contrast, sonograms from native coronary coronary arteries and from coronary bypass grafts (Fig. 5) show flow almost entirely confined to diastole.

The simplest model to explain the biphasic flow pattern at the proximal end of the graft is to regard it as a compliant tube closed at the distal end during systole and open during diastole. During systole blood flows into the graft at a rate determined by its hydrodynamic resistance and the difference between aortic pressure and the pressure generated by radial and longitudinal stretch of the graft walls. During diastole, myocardial vessel conductance becomes large, the graft shortens and becomes smaller in diameter, and then becomes a passive conduit for blood flow between aorta and the myocardium. More rigorous treatment of this model to allow for wave propagation and for phase differences between aortic pressure and myocardial

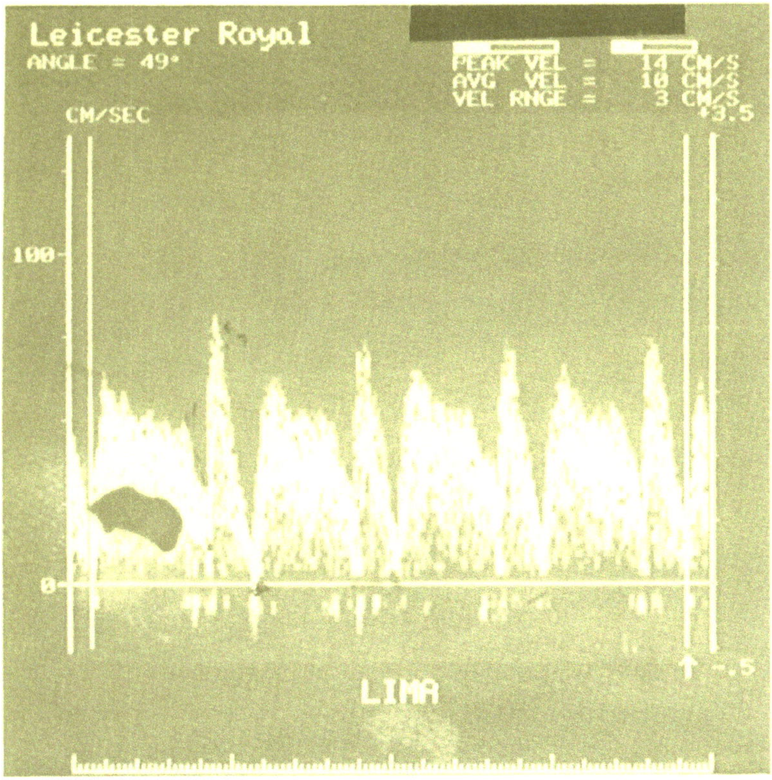

Fig. 4. Doppler sonogram of a left internal thoracic artery grafted to the left anterior descending and first diagonal coronary arteries. Resting graft flow was estimated at 79 ml/min

Table 1. Duplex ultrasound measurements on ungrafted and grafted internal thoracic arteries

	Ungrafted (n = 19)		Grafted (n = 16)	
	Mean	Range	Mean	Range
Diameter (mm)	2.2	1.6–2.5	2.3	1.6–2.9
Peak systolic velocity (cm/s)	94.1	68–197	56.7	25–90
Peak diastolic velocity (cm/s)	24.7	13–38	45.7	25–66
Peak S/peak D ratio	3.99	2.64–5.84	1.38	0.68–2.25
TAV systole (cm/s)	50.3	15–118	20.3	13–25
TAV diastole (cm/s)	11	3–18	20.7	16–30
TAV S/D ratio	3.9	2.1–7.7	1.07	0.67–1.6
Flow systole (ml/min)	23.7	15.0–33.8	15.2	8.6–23.7
Flow diastole (ml/min)	10.2	3.7–15.4	26.9	11.6–55.3
Total flow	33.7	22.0–53.0	42.1	17.0–79.0

Patients were examined a mean of 10 weeks after surgery.
TAV, Time-averaged velocity.

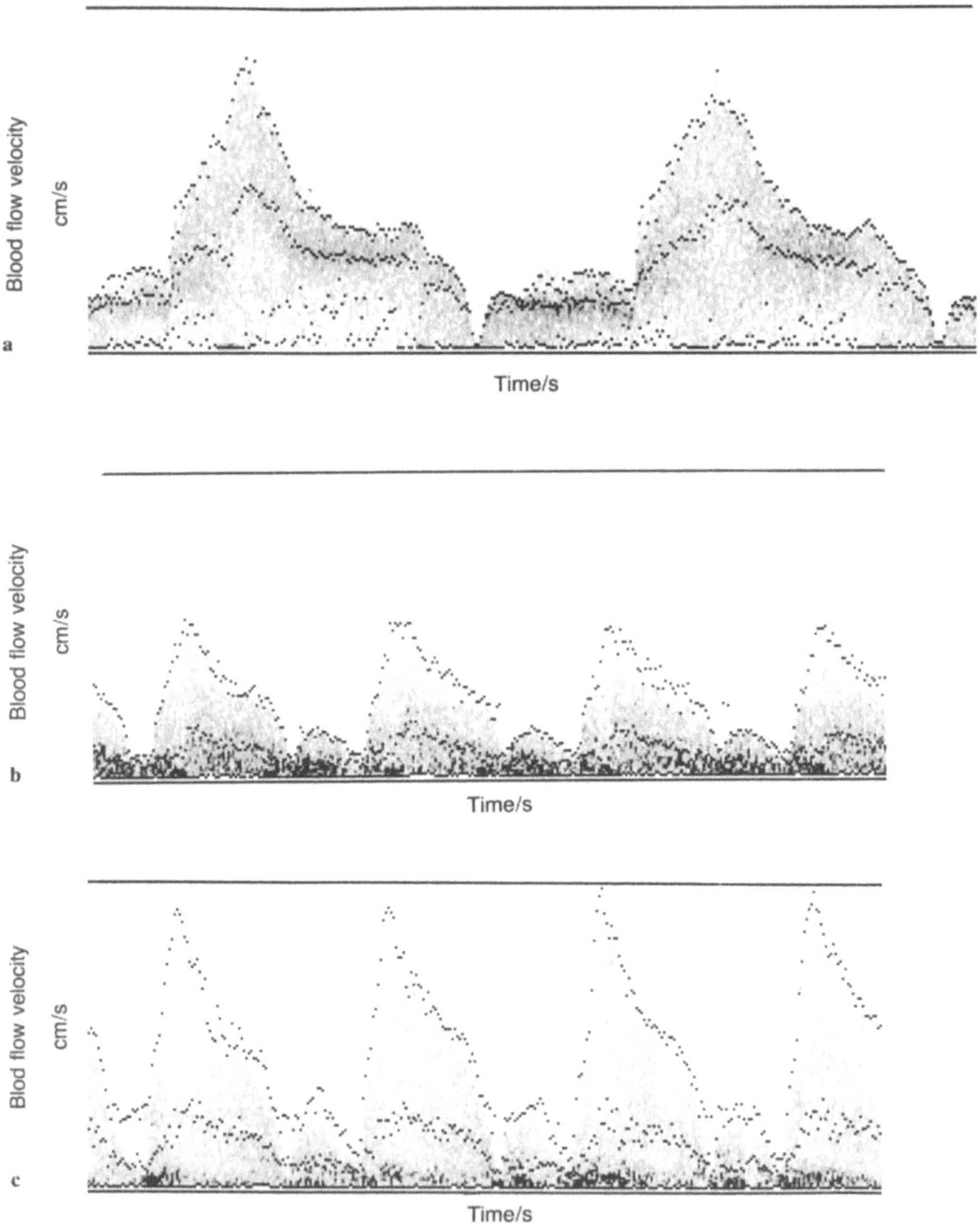

Fig. 5a–c. Doppler sonograms of native coronary artery (**a**), proximal (**b**) and distal (**c**) saphenous vein bypass graft to left anterior descending artery. Intravascular 20 MHz Doppler catheter (Schneider). Note predominant diastolic flow in all tracings

compliance becomes very complicated [8], but the simple model allows some important deductions to be made: (a) Myocardial runoff is the integral of systolic and diastolic flow observed in the proximal part of the graft (reversed flow for part of the cycle is theoretically possible, but we have never observed it). (b) Systolic flow is a function of graft compliance. This compliance is a major difference between internal thoracic grafts and saphenous vein grafts, which have little compliance and little systolic flow (Fig. 5). It also depends on the point at which flow is measured; as one moves distally the volume of the graft between the point of measurement and the (temporarily) closed end becomes smaller and its capacitance less. Flow measurements at the ostium of a large and healthy (i.e., compliant) right coronary artery may show a substantial systolic flow component, but this diminishes distally.

The possible relationship between flow patterns and graft malfunction are described below.

Quantitative Flow Measurements

When the intensity-weighted mean velocity of flow is multiplied by the cross-sectional area of the vessel, the result is volume flow per unit time. The use of transcutaneous ultrasound for measuring absolute graft flow is subject to a number of important limitations. True velocity is related to apparent velocity by the cosine of the angle of insonation: if this is known, a correction can be applied, but it is often difficult to measure accurately, especially from the parasternal approach. Accurate measurement of the diameter of a 1.5–2.5 mm vessel is close to the resolving ability of these ultrasound frequencies, and since area is related to the square of the radius any inaccuracy is much amplified. It is probably better therefore to regard flow measurements as approximations and to pay more attention to changes in flow than to absolute flow values.

Systolic and diastolic velocity values, estimated vessel diameters and approximate flow values for a series of patients studied within 12 weeks of grafting are listed in Table 1. Although systolic/diastolic velocity and flow ratios are clearly different in grafted and non-grafted vessels, there is no discernable relation between systolic/diastolic ratios and absolute flow measurements.

Myocardial flow in the territory supplied by the graft is actually given by total graft flow *minus* flow to non-myocardial branches *plus* flow from the native coronary vessel. Most internal thoracic artery grafts are made to vessels which are stenosed but not occluded, and at least at rest a substantial proportion of coronary flow may still be provided through the native vessel. In patients studied shortly after grafting, we were able to show a positive correlation between absolute graft flow and a "runoff score" calculated from

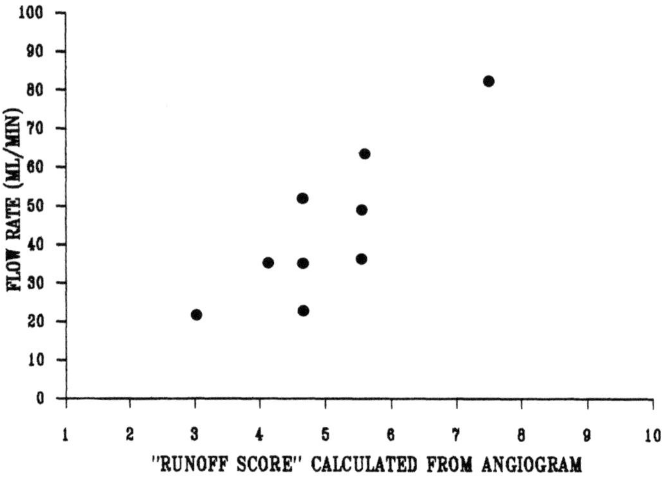

Fig. 6. Plot of total graft flow against "runoff score" calculated from the preoperative angiogram in nine patients with recent left internal thoracic artery grafts to the left anterior descending coronary artery

the distribution of the grafted vessels, with allowance made for the severity of any proximal stenosis (Fig. 6).

Effects of Physical and Pharmacological Intervention on Graft Flow

Mental arithmetic and physical exertion cause an increase in graft flow (Fig. 7). It is interesting that the systolic/diastolic velocity ratio does not change significantly, but in fact in the patients studied a change in heart rate accounted for a substantial part of the change in flow.

We studied the effects of glyceryl trinitrate (sublingual, 1 mg) on grafted internal thoracic artery flow in seven patients. All patients were at rest and angina free. In all patients nitrates produced a fall in systolic pressure and an increase in heart rate, which was mild in six but marked in one patient. Diastolic blood pressure fell in all except one patient. The rate pressure product remained constant in five patients and rose slightly in two. In all patients peak systolic velocity and time averaged systolic velocity diminished; in four patients there was an increase in both peak and time averaged

Fig. 7a,b. Effect of exercise (leg raising) on grafted left internal thoracic artery flow before (**a**) and after (**b**) exercise

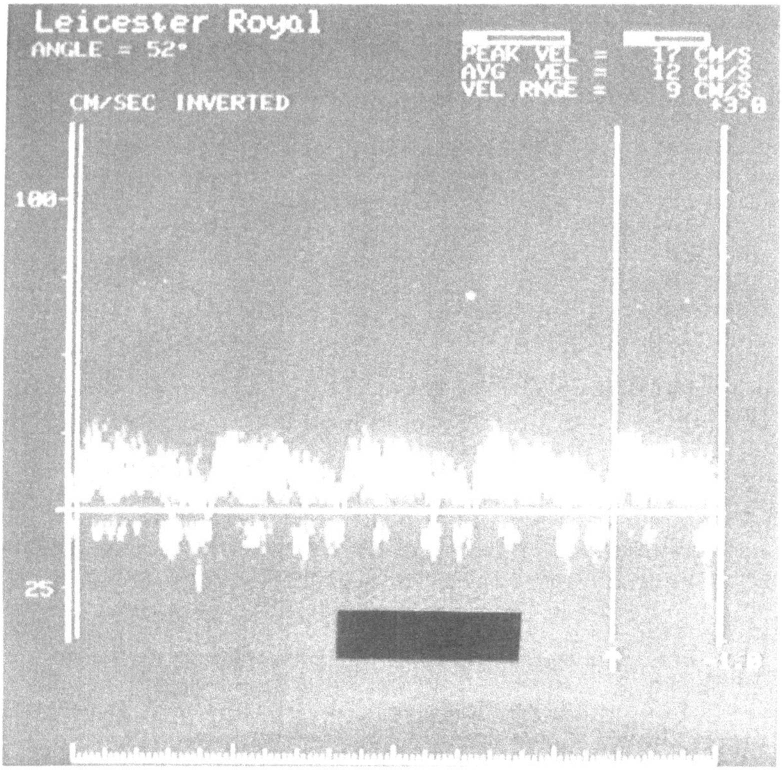
Leicester Royal
ANGLE = 52°
PEAK VEL = 17 CM/S
AVG VEL = 12 CM/S
VEL RNGE = 9 CM/S
CM/SEC INVERTED
+3.0
100
25
[redacted]
-1.0

a

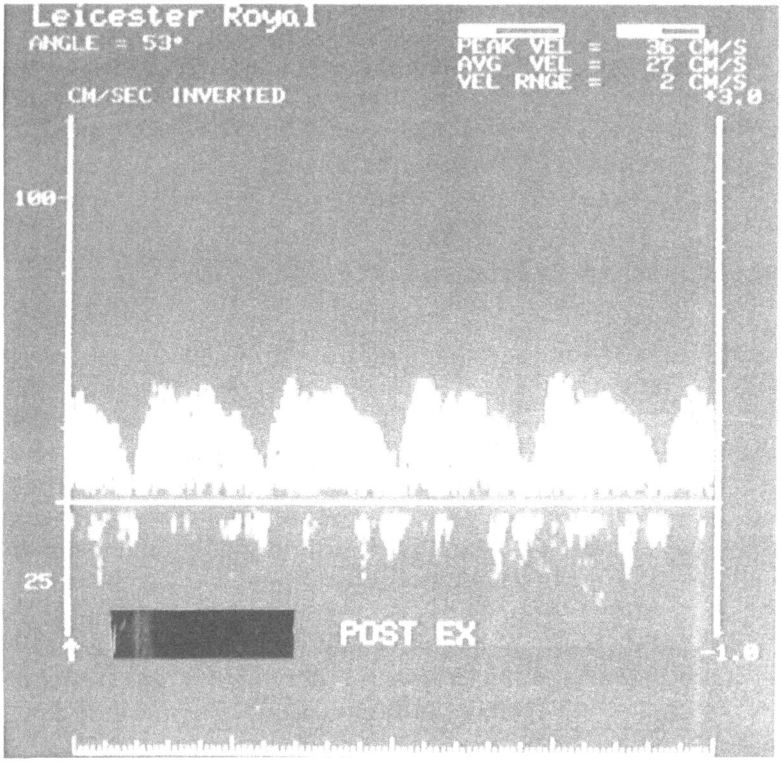
Leicester Royal
ANGLE = 53°
PEAK VEL = 36 CM/S
AVG VEL = 27 CM/S
VEL RNGE = 2 CM/S
CM/SEC INVERTED
+3.0
100
25
[redacted]
POST EX
-1.0

b

Table 2. Haemodynamic effects on ultrasound measurements of the grafted internal thoracic artery

	Average systolic velocity	Average diastolic velocity	Graft diameter	Systolic Flow	Diastolic Flow
Increase systolic BP	+	(+)	+	+	(+)
Decrease systolic BP	−	(−)	−	−	(−)
Increase diastolic BP		+	(+)		+
Decrease diastolic BP		−	(−)		−
Dilate graft	−	−	++	+	+
Reduce intramyocardial resistance		++			++
Increase heart rate	(−)	(−)	(−)	+	−

velocity in diastole, in one case reaching 150% of the resting value. In the other three patients diastolic peak and average velocity decreased slightly.

In attempting to interpret these results it is helpful to use a qualitative matrix relating changes in individual haemodynamic parameters to expected changes in ultrasound measurements (Table 2). It can be seen that the only likely causes for an increased flow velocity during diastole are increased diastolic pressure, a fall in heart rate, or a diminished graft/coronary/myocardial resistance. Since the first two were not observed, it seems that diminished resistance is the most likely cause. In the other three patients there was a slight fall in average diastolic velocity, but this does not necessarily indicated reduced flow, since it could be compensated by a small increase in graft diameter beyond the resolution of our measurements. The grafted internal thoracic artery is a potentially useful model for studying coronary pharmacology and physiology in a human model.

Ultrasound Measurement for Detecting Graft Problems

If a graft is successfully imaged, and displays both systolic and diastolic flow, it is likely to be patent. The converse is not necessarily true; we have sometimes failed to detect a graft using ultrasound but have subsequently demonstrated excellent graft function angiographically. Disappearance of a graft which had previously been demonstrable with ultrasound is more likely to be due to graft failure, but even this may sometimes result from minor alterations in the course of a graft as it matures. Within these limitations, duplex ultrasound is a helpful additional tool for studying graft function.

Graft obstruction proximally would be expected to lead to total loss of the Doppler signal. Distal graft obstruction would not affect systolic flow, but diastolic flow would be much reduced. This pattern was demonstrated by Krijne and colleagues in one of their patients [5]. Chronic graft atheroma would be expected to influence graft compliance and might affect systolic to diastolic flow ratios; this would be easier to detect in serial studies.

Acknowledgements. The collaboration of Dr. N.J. Samani, Prof. D.H. Evans, Dr. A. Thrush, Mr. T. Hartshorne, Mr. T.J. Spyt and Mrs. B. Lawrie is gratefully acknowledged. This work was supported by the British Heart Foundation.

References

1. Loop FD, Lytle BW, Cosgrove DM et al. (1986) Influence of the internal mammary artery graft on 10 year survival and other cardiac events. N Engl J Med 314:1–6
2. Barner HB, Swartz MT, Mudd JG, Tyras DH (1982) Late patency of the internal mammary artery as a coronary bypass conduit. Ann Thorac Surg 34:408–412
3. Fusejima K, Takahara Y, Sudo Y, Murayama H, Masuda Y, Inagaki Y (1990) Comparison of coronary haemodynamics in patients with internal mammary artery and saphenous vein coronary artery bypass grafts: a noninvasive approach using combined two dimensional and Doppler echocardiography. J Am Coll Cardiol 15:131–139
4. Kyo S, Matsumura M, Yokote Y, Takaomoto S, Omoto R (1990) Evaluation of patency of internal maamary artery grafts: a comparison of two dimensional Doppler echocardiography with coronary angiography. J Cardiol 20:607–616
5. Krijne R, Lyttwin RM, Holtgren R, Heinrich KW, Marx R, Sons H (1992) Combined two dimensional and doppler sonographic examination of internal mammary grafts from the supraclavicular fossa. Int J Cardiol 37:61–64
6. De Bono DP, Samani NJ, Spyt TJ, Hartshorne T, Thrush AJ, Evans DH (1992) Transcutaneous ultrasound measurement of blood flow in internal mammary artery to coronary artery grafts. Lancet 339:379–381
7. Canver CC, Ricotta JJ, Bhayana JN, Fiedler RC, Mentzer RM (1991) Use of duplex imaging to assess suitability of the internal mammary artery for coronary artery surgery. J Vasc Surg 13:294–301
8. Nichols WW, O'Rourke MF (1990) McDonald's blood flow in arteries, 3rd edn. Arnold, London, pp 270–282

Coronary Angiography in the Diagnosis of Graft Failure

P.R. Lichtlen and H. Hausmann

Despite its known limitations [1–3] coronary angiography has remained the standard technique to demonstrate alterations of coronary artery bypass grafts, especially so-called graft disease. This concerns above all those graft changes which lead to ischemic events such as stable and unstable angina pectoris or acute myocardial infarction. These alterations consist predominantly in localized, high-grade luminal narrowings (diameter stenoses ≥70%) of the graft body or the proximal or distal anastomoses or in occlusions of grafts due mainly to progressing atherosclerotic plaque formation with or without thrombotic occlusion. Graft angiograms are therefore always indicated when typical ischemic symptoms arise, or prophylactically when grafts approach the age at which the risk of vein graft disease increases significantly (5 and more years). This applies especially to patients with combined risk factors [4] and increased progression of graft atherosclerosis and plaque formation, as it is established that plaque rupture followed by thrombotic occlusion and myocardial infarction involves not only high-grade, symptomatic but also low-grade (<50%), clinically asymptomatic plaques not detectable by non-invasive means [2, 5, 6].

Limitations of Graft Angiography

Initially the atherosclerotic process is confined to the intima of the vessel wall [7–9]; it can therefore not be visualized by angiography, a technique demonstrating the silhouette of the vessel lumen, i.e., the inner contours of the vessel wall. Hence not only the development of the earliest lesions, the so-called fatty streaks [2, 10], but also of those atherosclerotic plaques initially "growing" towards the adventitia and not towards the vessel lumen [3, 11] is missed by angiography, both in native coronary arteries and in vein grafts. It is expected that intravascular ultrasound will be able to close this gap by demonstrating intramural changes with sufficient accuracy [12–14]. In addition, even when atherosclerotic lesions start to impinge on the vessel lumen and minimal localized narrowings become visible (diameter stenosis of approximately 10%–20%) [2], angiography has difficulties to distinguish between platelet thrombi adhering to the vessel wall and initial plaque "growing" or localized spasm, i.e., short segments with increased vasomotor tone [2]. Furthermore, in spite of improved sensitivity of angiograms [15, 16] in recent years (AD conversion, digital image acquisition), the lowest cutpoint for individual stenoses [2] to distinguish with high probability biologically "true" plaques from variability changes is at a diameter stenosis of approximately 10%–15%.

Finally, graft atherosclerosis must be distinguished from the "natural thickening" of grafts taking place in the first weeks and months after implantation, at a time before atherosclerotic changes start developing [17–19].

Limitations of Recognition of Graft Failures Due to Insufficient Technical Approach

There are several reasons for failures to recognize graft alterations. (a) The principal reason is an inadequate visualization technique. This concerns especially stenoses at the site of the proximal (Fig. 1) or peripheral graft

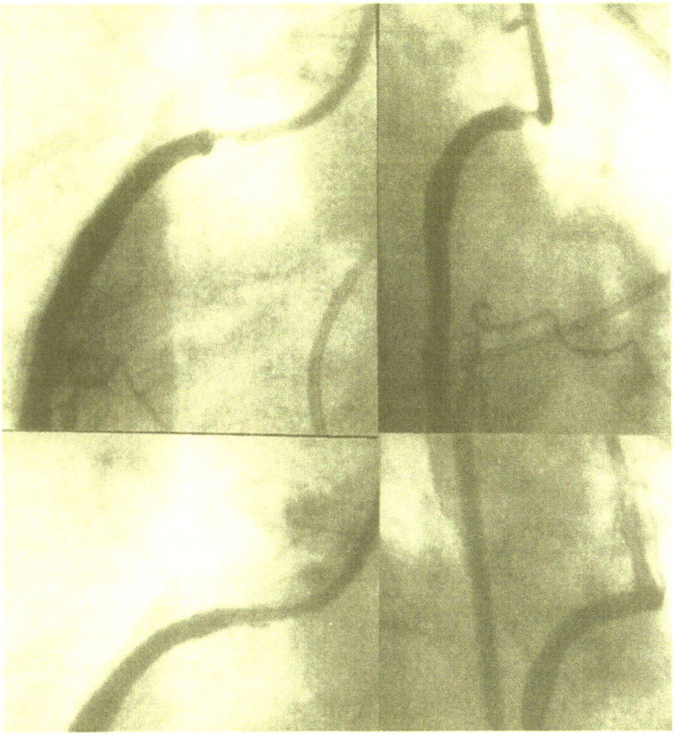

Fig. 1. High-grade stenosis at the proximal anastomosis of an RCA graft. *Above*, two RAO projections, approximately 30° and 10°, demonstrating the short, proximal stenosis. *Below*, two LAO projections where the stenosis – due to foreshortening – cannot be seen

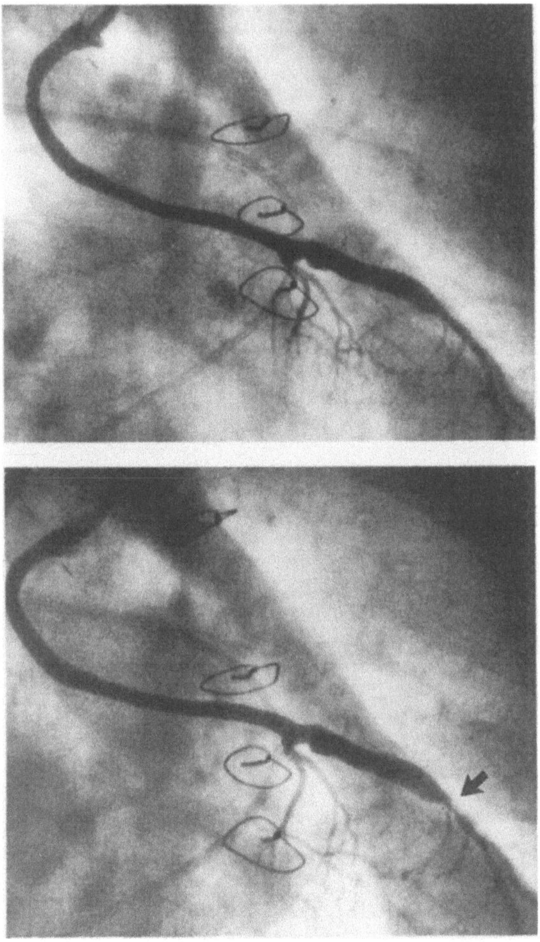

Fig. 2. High-grade stenosis at the distal anastomosis of a vein graft to the left anterior descending branch. Only one of the two RAO projections with slightly different angulations demonstrates the stenosis. The stenosis extends from the vein to the distal, poststenotic portion of the LAD

anastomoses (Fig. 2); here, special projections (half axial, oblique projections) must often be obtained within differences of a few degrees in angulation for optimal visualization of such stenoses. However, this is frequently also necessary for stenoses within the graft body, where due to inadequate projections the size of a stenosis is often underestimated. As graft visualization often needs an increased number of injections and larger amounts of contrast media, biplane cineangiograms with appropriate projections are advantageous. (b) Inadequate visualization of graft stenoses is frequently caused by insufficient amounts of contrast media, especially in situations of difficult intubations where nonselective injections are applied;

this often leads to an only partial visualization of grafts, especially when coronary blood flow is high (hypertension, administrations of drugs such as calcium entry blockers increasing flow) [20]. (c) An important problem is insufficient film quality due to less than optimal film development or under- or overexposure [1]. As graft angiography often has far reaching consequences (reoperation, PTCA), optimal image acquisition is mandatory.

Angiographic Approach to Vein Grafts

Projections for optimal visualization of grafts differ slightly from those for native coronary arteries. The angle of the course of the graft body to the image plane varies from the angle of the by-passed artery. Therefore, as mentioned above, graft stenoses, especially on anastomotic sites, are often observed only in special angles (Figs. 1, 2). In general, *RCA grafts* are best visualized in planar LAO and RAO projections (Figs. 3, 4), sometimes also in PA projection, rarely in RAO 20–60° caudocranial and cranio-caudal oblique projections of approximately 10°. The anastomotic site often needs additional projections. *LAD grafts* are best visualized in planar RAO and LAO projections and craniocaudal oblique RAO, as well as in straight left lateral projections (Figs. 5, 6). *LCX grafts* are best seen in planar RAO projections of 30°, RAO caudo-cranial oblique projections or planar LAO projections of 30° (Fig. 7). However, as mentioned above, due to the large variability in the course of grafts, depending on the implantation site on the aortic root as well as in the coronary artery and on the bypass technique (single or jump graft), optimal projections differ widely among patients.

Topology of Vein Grafts

The majority of vein grafts are implanted as single grafts, taking their origin from the anterior portion of the aortic root, usually a few centimeters above the origin of the coronary arteries; the site of the distal anastomosis depends on the location of the high-grade stenosis or occlusion to be by-passed. For *RCA grafts*, due to the long body of the RCA without important major side branches above the crux cordis (only right ventricular, rarely marginal branches), the distal graft anastomosis is often located in the periphery, beyond the crux cordis, on one of the major side branches; the location of the anastomosis depends on the site of the stenosis on the posterior and/or right posterolateral branch or the crux cordis itself (Figs. 3, 4). Hence, the distal anastomosis is often placed directly at the crux cordis (Fig. 4), i.e., at the bifurcation of the two major side branches, rarely above the crux cordis. In contrast, *LAD grafts* most often have their peripheral anastomosis in the

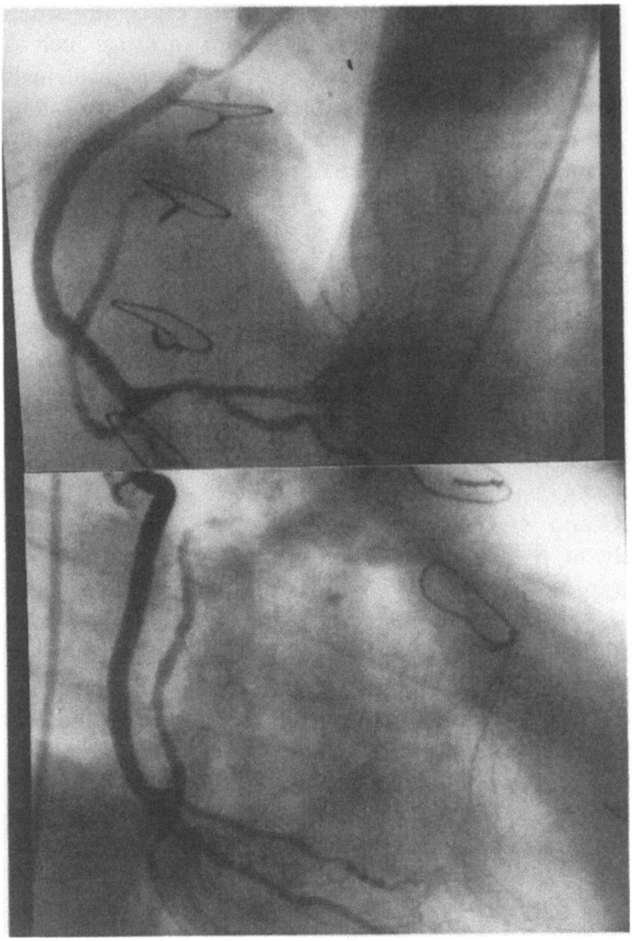

Fig. 3. Vein graft to the right coronary artery; the distal anastomosis is slightly above the crux cordis; there is retrograde filling of the distal right coronary artery showing diffuse disease and antegrade filling of the two major distal RCA branches, the right posterolateral, and the right posterior descending branch; in addition, there is faint retrograde filling of septal branches via the posterior descending branch (*below*). *Above*, RAO projection of approx. 10°; *below*, RAO projection of approx. 30°

middle third of the artery, below the first diagonal and first large septal branch (Fig. 5); again, this depends on the exact location of the stenosis, which, however, is preferentially located in the upper third of the vessel, above or below the take-off of the first diagonal branch, often in the area of the origin of the first large septal branch (Figs. 5, 6). *LCX grafts* are usually anastomosed on the first or second posterolateral branch, depending on the site of stenosis. The AV branch of the left circumflex system rarely serves for an anastomosis, due to its close proximity to the coronary sinus (Fig. 7).

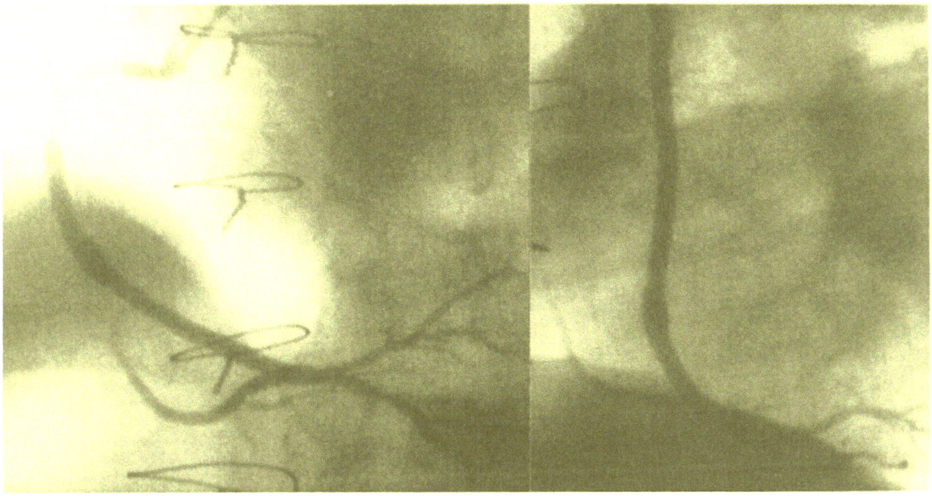

Fig. 4. Vein bypass graft to the distal RCA; the distal anastomosis is directly at the crux cordis, at the site of the bifurcation into the 2 major branches. *Left*, LAO projection of 10°; *right*, RAO projection of approx. 30°

To accelerate and simplify the procedure, so-called *jump* or *sequential* grafts were introduced [21], having only one aortic and two or more peripheral anastomoses; they often connect the proximal LAD and the diagonal branch (Fig. 5), the two posterolateral LCX branches or the two inferior RCA branches (posterior descending and right posterolateral branch). A special sequential graft approach is the so-called *snake graft*, where only one vein is implanted and provides all major arteries; the first anastomosis is usually at the distal RCA; from there the graft reaches one or two posterolateral branches, then a diagonal branch and finally joins the left anterior descending branch (Fig. 8). This type of graft is rarely performed today due to the increased risk of graft closure associated with steal phenomena; often only detached bridges, for example, between the second and first posterolateral branch being left.

Sequential and snake grafts, as ideal as they seem to be (fewer anastomoses, less time of extracorporeal circulation), are fraught with various problems. (a) They might lead to a "steal phenomenon", depending on different flow rates of the connected arteries; an anastomosis with a high flow providing a large myocardial area, might drain blood away from an anastomosis with a low flow, connected to a small vessel, providing only a small area which is then threatened by ischemia, especially during exercise, i.e., in situations of high flow demand. (b) Occlusions of various anastomoses, for example, of grafts segments between a distal RCA branch and a posterolateral branch of the left circumflex artery lead to ischemia of all subsequent myocardial areas; some vein bridges are then often perfused via

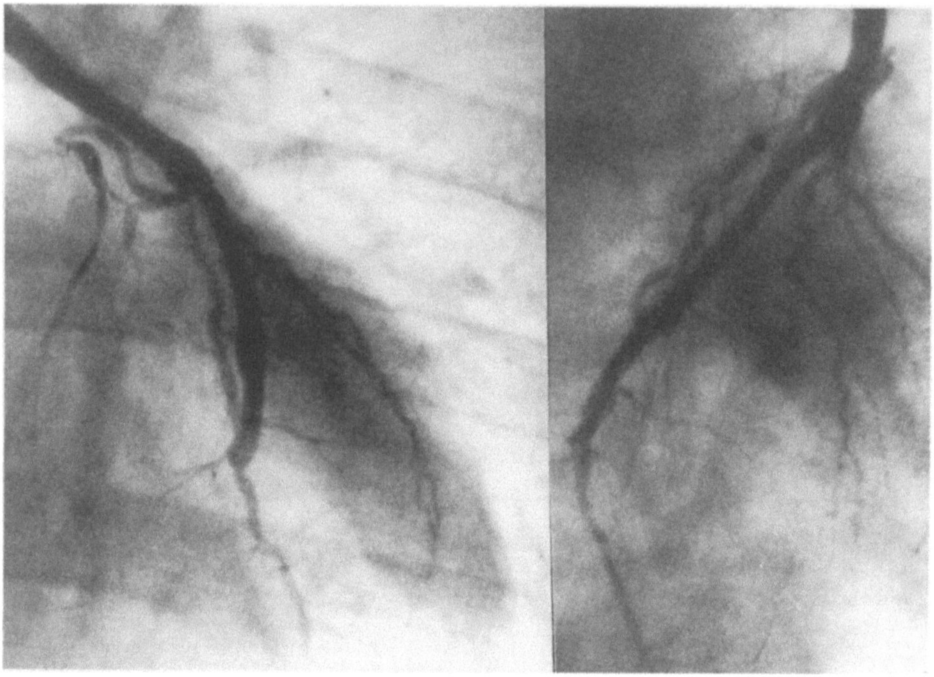

Fig. 5. Sequential vein graft first to the diagonal branch (side to side) and from there to the middle portion of the LAD branch (end to side). *Left*, in RAO projection of approx. 20°; *right*, in LAO projection of approx. 20°. There is retrograde filling of the proximal LAD, and of high septal branches, and antegrade filling of the distal LAD branch. The LAD and its side branches are diffusely diseased, shown as numerous irregularities of the contours. Note the smooth anastomotic sites

a native, previously by-passed coronary artery, however, in an insufficient way (Fig. 9).

Internal Mammary Artery Grafts

Internal mammary artery (IMA) grafts were introduced by Green [22] in 1972; however, several years elapsed until they were fully accepted as standard procedures [23]. They were found to have several advantages, above all a significantly lower tendency for graft disease [22–25]. Indeed, the IMA has long been known to be one of the few arteries rarely becoming atherosclerotic. In addition, their biological behavior, especially also with regard to nitric oxide production differs markedly from veins [26]. In addition, they also need only one anastomosis and this between arteries.

In performing control angiograms after graft operations, IMA grafts must be included [27] even if their intubation is sometimes technically more

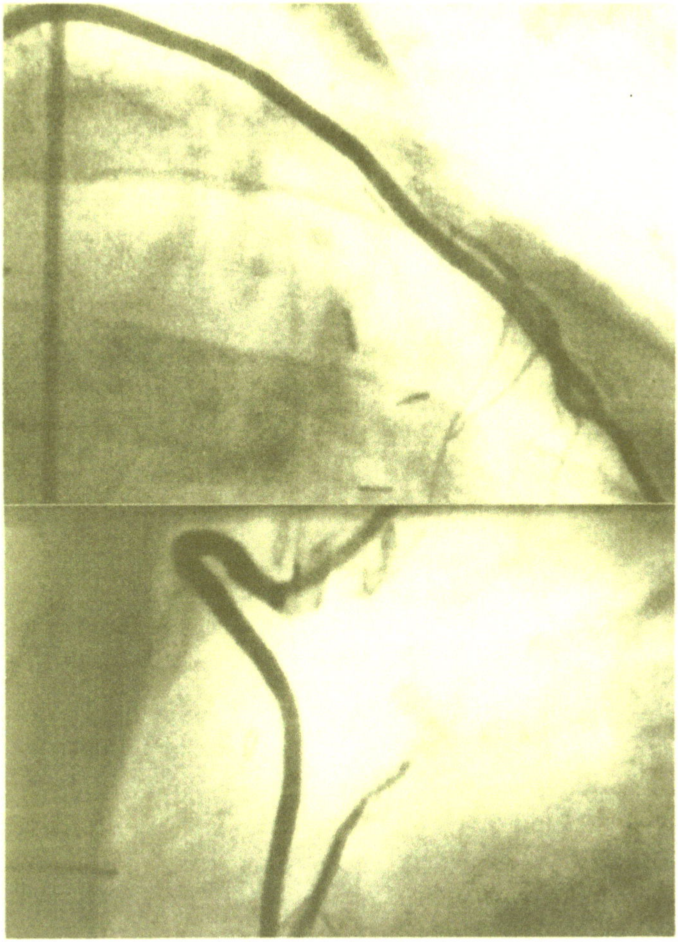

Fig. 6. Free arterial graft to the proximal LAD branch in RAO (*above*) and LAO (*below*) projection. The graft was taken from the right internal mammary artery. Note the smooth contours of the graft also at the anastomotic site

difficult (Fig. 10). Great care should be taken to perform strictly selective injections by fixing the catheter tip in the ostium of the internal mammary artery; subselective injections into the subclavian arteries often provide insufficient images, not visualizing well enough the anastomosis.

As to be expected, most of the abnormalities of IMA grafts are at the site of the anastomosis to the distal artery, most often the LAD [28]. Special angulations might be necessary to demonstrate these localized narrowings. IMA occlusions are rare and usually due either to an inadequately small size of the artery [29] or to technical failures, for example, insufficient tying off of side branches, leading to a steal phenomenon [30, 31] (Fig. 11). More

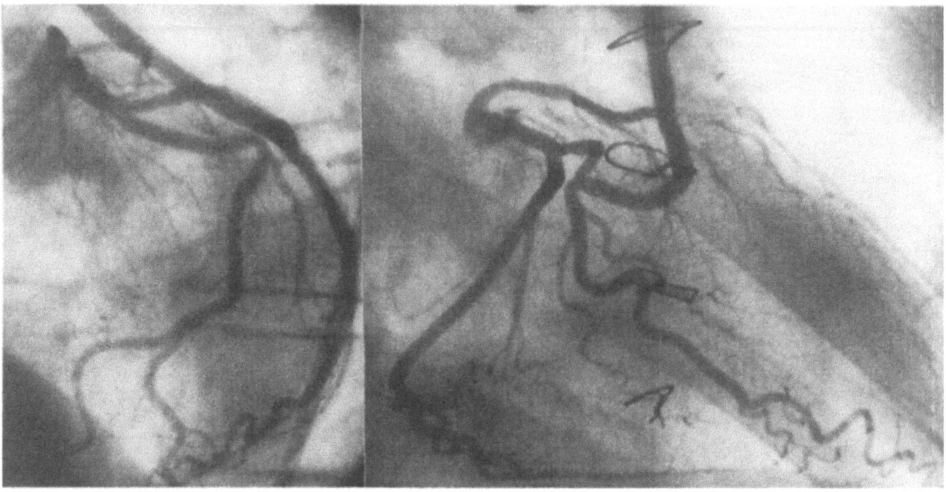

Fig. 7. Vein bypass graft to the first posterolateral branch of the left circumflex artery with an end to side anastomosis. *Left*, in LAO; *right*, in RAO projection. There is excellent retrograde filling to the main stem of the LCX and of a short intermediate branch. There is antegrade filling of the entire AV and right posterior descending branch, originating in this case from the LCX (balanced distribution type). All visualized branches have smooth contours

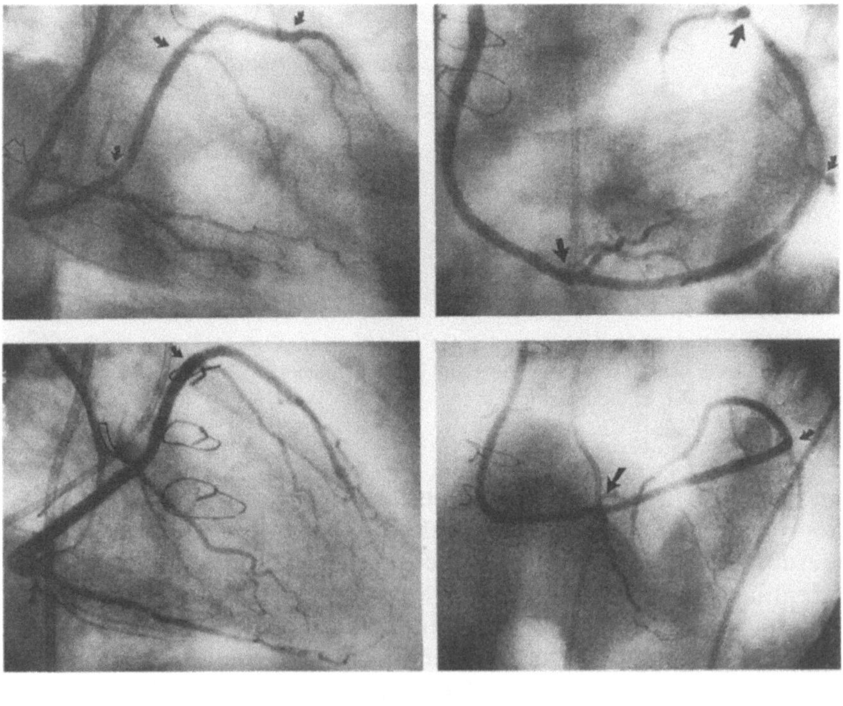

Fig. 8. Typical example of a snake graft taking its origin from the right lateral wall of the aorta, reaching with its first anastomosis (side to side) the RCA at the crux cordis (*upper left panel, open arrow*); the second anastomosis reaches the second posterolateral branch (*lower left panel, open arrow*), the third anastomosis (side to side) the first posterolateral branch, and the fourth anastomosis (end to side) the proximal portion of the left anterior descending branch. *Upper left and below*, two RAO projections in slightly different angles; *upper right and below*, two LAO projections in planar (*above*) and craniocaudal views

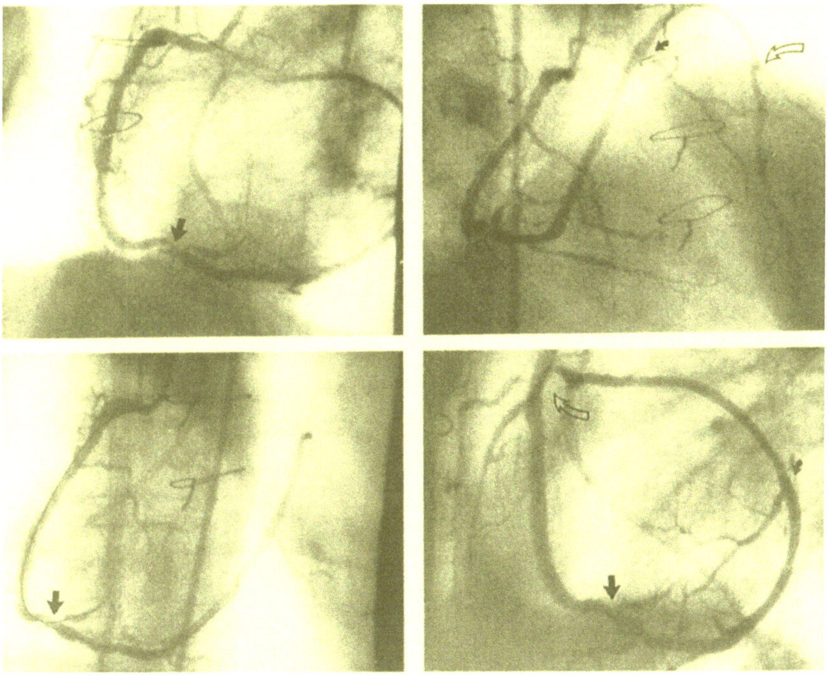

Fig. 9. Typical snake graft failure; there is a high-grade stenosis at the first anastomosis to the RCA, at the crux cordis (*dark arrow, upper and lower left panels*). The snake graft passes then to the left circumflex branch (*dark arrow, right upper and lower panels*) and from there to the LAD (*open arrows*). The high-grade stenosis at the RCA anastomosis was successfully dilated applying the double wire technique (*lower left panel*)

recently, also free grafts gathered from various arteries, for example, the gastroepiploic artery or the right internal mammary artery (Fig. 6) were successfully applied.

Graft Abnormalities: Physiological Changes of Graft Diameters

The wall of vein bypass grafts is capable of considerable adaptation. This concerns especially the intima, but also the media of the artery. Hence, during the first months vein grafts undergo considerable narrowing over their entire length without losing their smooth contours; this is due to wall thickening resulting from newly formed fibrous tissue or from vascular smooth muscle cell proliferation induced by the high pressure [17, 32–34]. This early decrease in luminal diameter, not induced by atherosclerosis, amounts to approximately 30% and is best seen in large grafts [17, 32,

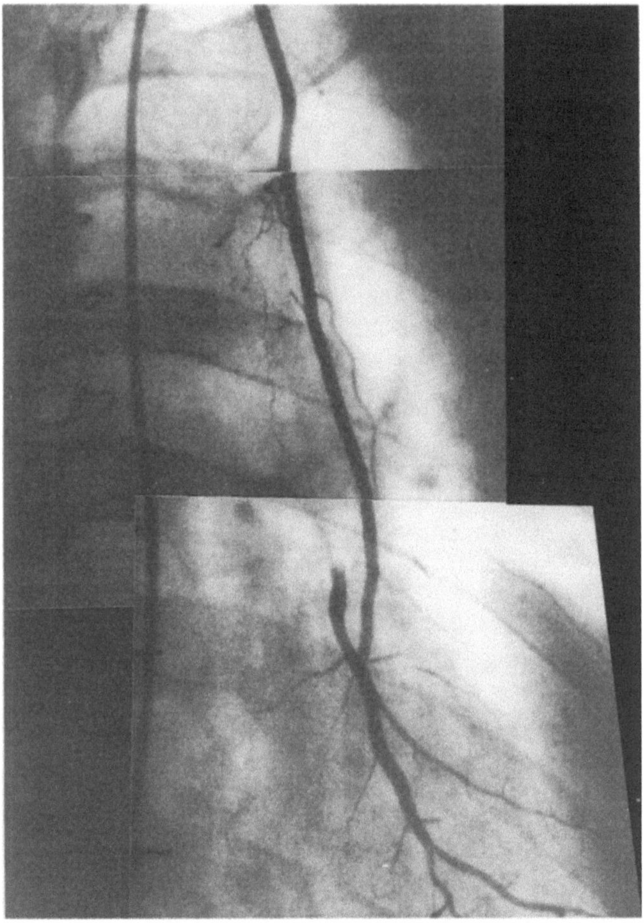

Fig. 10. Left internal mammary artery graft to the first posterolateral branch of the LCX artery (composite view). The LIMA is selectively intubated at its origin from the left subclavian artery; it is anastomosed with the proximal segment of the occluded PLA stenosis.

34–37]. It is important to note that proliferating changes of the venous wall do not suppress vasomotion; graft function and coronary flow are not impaired, as this luminal "narrowing" is accompanied by an increasè in blood flow velocity [2].

Vein grafts not only reduce their size over time, but under certain circumstances are also able to increase in luminal diameter [18, 38]; the latter occurs either acutely due to a sudden drop in vasomotor tone, such as after administration of nitrates [26] or dipyridamol or chronically through active growth [18]. Such circumferential growth, i.e., luminal widening of vein grafts can be observed when graft flow is permanently high. This is the case when flow to a myocardial area adjacent to the one perfused by the

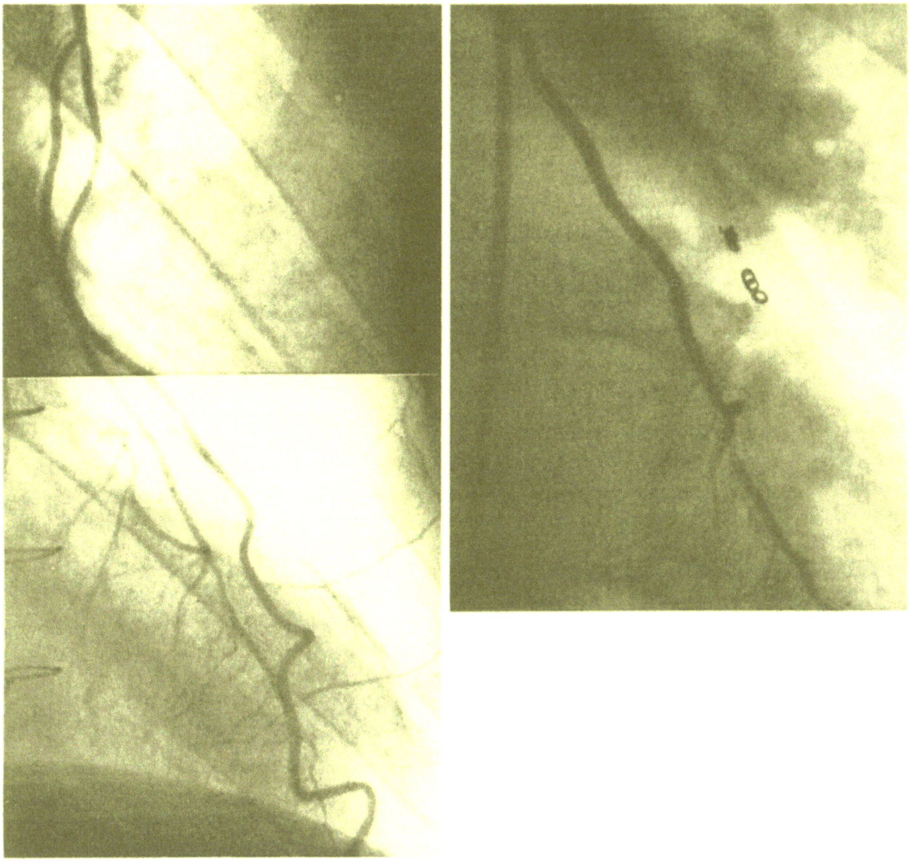

Fig. 11. IMA graft with steal phenomenon. There were two parallel running branches of the internal mammary artery; only one of them, the smaller, was anastomosed to the LAD branch (*left*); the larger was not tied off. This led to a classic steal phenomenon with severe angina pectoris. Therefore, 6 months later the unconnected branch was obliterated by selective injection of special plastic beads (*right*) [30]. From then on the patient remained free of angina

graft ceases due to occlusion of the related artery, and collaterals originating from an artery perfused by a vein graft now provide the additional flow (Fig. 12). In this situation the increased flow demand provides a strong stimulus for the production of angiotropic hormones in the graft wall resulting in circumferential graft growth leading to widening of the graft lumen [8, 33].

Typical for all physiological alterations of the graft wall is the angiographic smooth aspect of the luminal contour, which involves the entire length of the vein. In these cases the venous wall, not visualized by angiography, is either symmetrically thickened, and the internal circumferences and the lumen are reduced, or the site of the wall is increased in its entire circumference, and the lumen is widened. In both situations the silhouette is

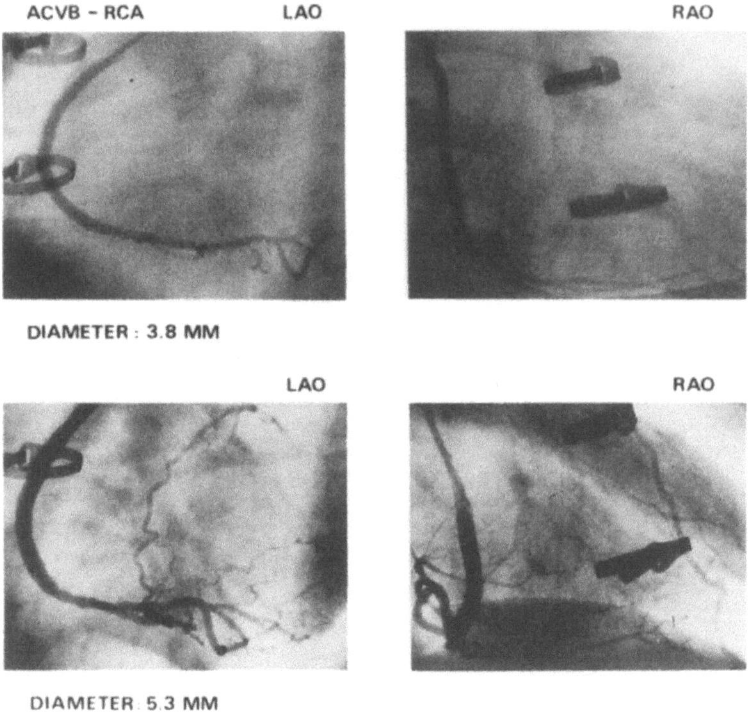

Fig. 12. Late postoperative increase of the size (diameter) of an RCA graft. On top the RCA graft 25 months after implantation in LAO (*left*) and RAO projection (*right*). *Below*, second angiogram 112 months postoperatively, 87 months after the first postoperative angiogram. This angiogram was performed after occlusion of the left anterior descending branch which is now perfused in a retrograde manner via septal branches from the right posterior descending branch. Note the increase in graft diameter from 3.8 to 5.3 mm in the presence of a marked increase in resting flow (from [18])

still smooth. As these changes are often subtle (changes in diameter less than 0.5 mm), they are observed mainly when angiograms performed at different intervals are compared, and luminal diameter changes are assessed by a computer-assisted system allowing accurate measurements and contour recognition [2, 4, 35, 39].

Atherosclerotic Changes of Grafts

Patency Rate

Approximately 10%–15% of grafts occlude at an early stage within the first hours or days postoperatively [4]. The reasons for early graft closure are multiple: a prominent cause is small graft size functioning as increased resistance leads to low flow, i.e., impaired runoff due to an inadequate relation between graft size and artery diameter. Diameters of arteries to be bypassed are between approximately 1 and 2.5 mm. Immediate postoperative flow values in grafts vary between 20 and 200 ml [1, 20, 40]. Early postoperative coronary flow, however, often is not representative for normal graft flow as there are several limiting factors [15, 16]; these include the quality of grafts which depends among other factors on the handling of the vein prior to insertion, the size of the distal and proximal anastomosis, the peripheral runoff, i.e., the presence of atherosclerosis beyond the distal anastomosis, the size of the artery, and the vitality of the perfused myocardial area. In addition, the postoperative course and the antithrombotic regimen are important factors for graft patency; initial high graft flow and constant rigorous antithrombotic and antiatherosclerotic measures contribute to a high patency rate [41–43].

Several studies reveal a long-term patency rate of approximately 60%–80% after 5 and of approximately 55%–70% after 10 years, i.e., an occlusion rate of approximately 2%–3% per year [1, 4, 19, 33, 43–47]. In contrast, the rate of diseased grafts often with clinically silent lesions, amounts to approximately 20% per year [48] and hence is markedly higher than the closure rate. Unfortunately, there are only few studies in the literature describing the natural attrition rate of grafts, i.e., the natural progression of graft atherosclerosis [45], which includes both the appearance of new, asymptomatic, low-grade and symptomatic preexisting high-grade lesions as well as graft occlusions. Noninvasive studies such as exercise tests and digital angiographic studies (see below) can reveal only symptomatic graft stenoses and occlusions; prospective studies of graft angiograms performed at regular intervals, independent of clinical indications, are still lacking. Hence, in spite of the large number of operations, very little is known on the natural evolution of graft disease [41] and the influences of risk factors [42, 49].

Late occlusions of grafts are usually due to new plaque formation and rupture of the fibrous cap followed by thrombotic occlusion, a similar process as in atherosclerosis of native coronary arteries [50]. Most often grafts are occluded directly at the origin of the aortic root. This, however, in many cases probably represents retrograde growth of the thrombus within the graft, starting at a distal occlusion site. In this situation, intubation is hardly possible as often only a small "nose" in the aortic wall can be visualized; often is the occlusion directly located at the inner surface of the aortic wall. The extent to which progression of graft atherosclerosis is influenced by the handling of grafts at the time of implantation is still debated [51]. Graft closure due to atherosclerosis in patients receiving adequate protective, prophylactive treatment usually does not occur before at least 5 years as the evolution of atherosclerotic lesions in most cases is rather slow [2]. It depends on the level of risk factors, especially hypercholesterolemia, smoking, and hypertension [38, 42, 43]. There are, however, also sex differences [47];

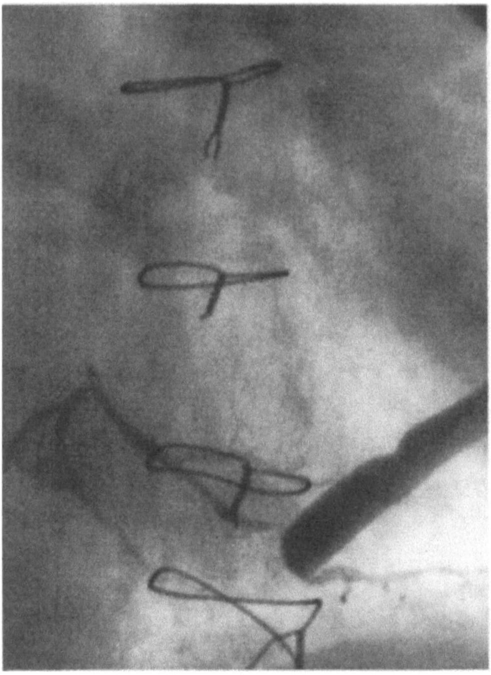

Fig. 13. Vein graft anastomosis to the second posterolateral branch of the LCX artery (RAO 30°). There is a clear mismatch between the size of the vein graft and the anastomosed artery; a high-grade stenosis is seen proximally to the anastomotic site. The vein graft shows a short, low-degree plaque

grafts in women – with the smaller size of coronary arteries – are usually smaller than those in men and therefore have a higher tendency for early occlusion [47, 52].

Morphology of Graft Alterations

As in atherosclerosis of coronary arteries, atherosclerosis in grafts at the beginning is localized, however, later becomes diffuse, depending on the age of the graft and risk factors inducing progression. Localized vein graft narrowings can be observed both at the anastomotic sites and over the entire length of the graft body.

Narrowing of Anastomoses

In contrast to atherosclerosis of coronary arteries vein grafts often demonstrate early narrowings at the anastomotic site. These anastomotic nar-

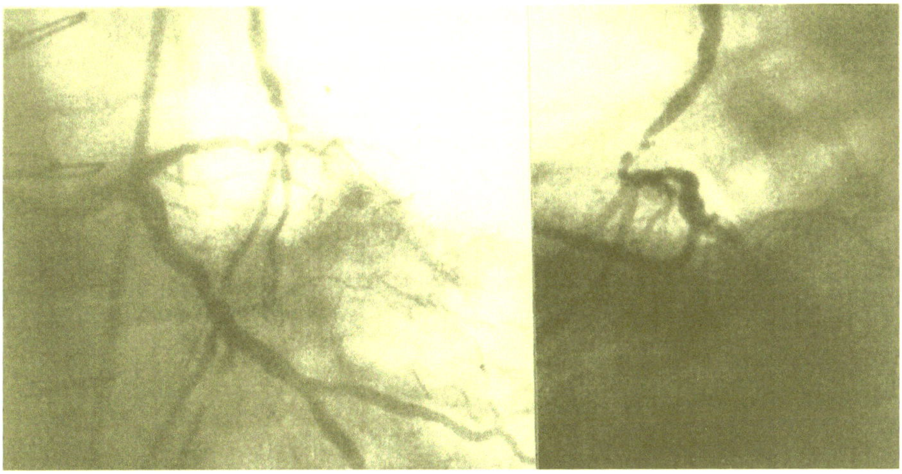

Fig. 14. Severe narrowing in the distal portion of an LAD graft, directly at the peripheral anastomosis. The graft was still patent but filling mainly in retrograde fashion when contrast material was injected into the native artery. Note the severely altered LAD segment from which also the first major septal branches originate. On the left RAO projection, on the right caudocranial LAO projection

rowings are frequently due to technical inadequacies occurring in connection with the implantation of the graft; some of its causes are large differences between the diameter of the vein and artery (Fig. 13), abnormal insertion angles, and extensive disease within the arterial wall at the site of anastomosis (Fig. 14). In addition, narrow anastomotic sites with increased resistance to flow and rough edges causing turbulence often lead to platelet accumulation and rapid development of atherosclerosis, further reducing the anastomotic lumen. In order to accurately visualize these narrowings, and especially to estimate or assess the size of the stenosis, special angulations and projections are often necessary; these narrowings proved to be short (1–2 mm), often with a septum-like aspect or an eccentric location with regard to the circumference of the vessel wall. The majority of these narrowings occur at the distal anastomotic site (Fig. 15); narrowings of the proximal, the aortic anastomoses are less frequent and usually easier to demonstrate (Fig. 16).

Stenoses Within the Graft Body Areas

With increasing age of the vein graft (8–10 years) new atherosclerotic lesions are observed with increasing frequency (see above). Morphologically they do not differ from those observed in native coronary arteries. They often are short, of a few millimetres long (1–5 mm; Fig. 17), sometimes of a typically

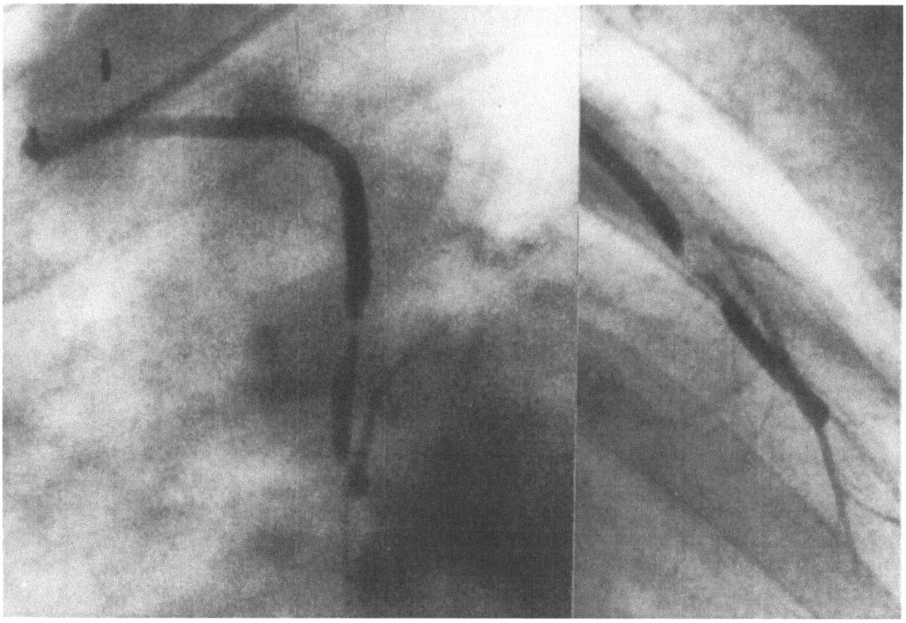

Fig. 15. High-grade concentric stenosis of the body and of the peripheral anastomotic site of an LAD graft; the peripheral stenosis is visible only in the RAO projection (*left*), not in the LAO projection of approx. 30° (*right*), which demonstrates mainly the eccentric stenosis of the graft body

complicated nature (Fig. 18), with slitlike incisions or aneurysmatic widening often containing thrombotic material (Fig. 19); many lesions are eccentrically located, but concentric lesions (Fig. 20), sometimes arranged in a row like a chain of pearls can often also be observed (Fig. 22); these are often of a low degree (<50% diameter stenosis) and therefore remain clinically silent. When graft stenoses lead to symptoms, to stable, exercise-induced angina, or to silent ischemia, they usually are of a relatively high degree (diameter stenosis of ≥80%) and are often more severe than symptomatic stenoses in native coronary arteries. This might be due to the lack of exercise induced increase in alphatone in veins [53, 54]; in native coronary arteries this leads

Fig. 16. High-grade stenosis at the proximal anastomotic site of a sequential graft to the first diagonal and the middle portion of the LAD branch. The stenosis is directly at the origin of the graft from the aortic root and is followed by a poststenotic aneurysmatic dilatation

Fig. 17. High-grade, eccentric and complicated stenosis in the middle of an LAD graft; the complex nature of the stenosis is best visualized in the *middle panel*, where an island of contrast medium surrounded by a contrast-free area can be observed. The stenosis was successfully dilated as shown in the lowest panel

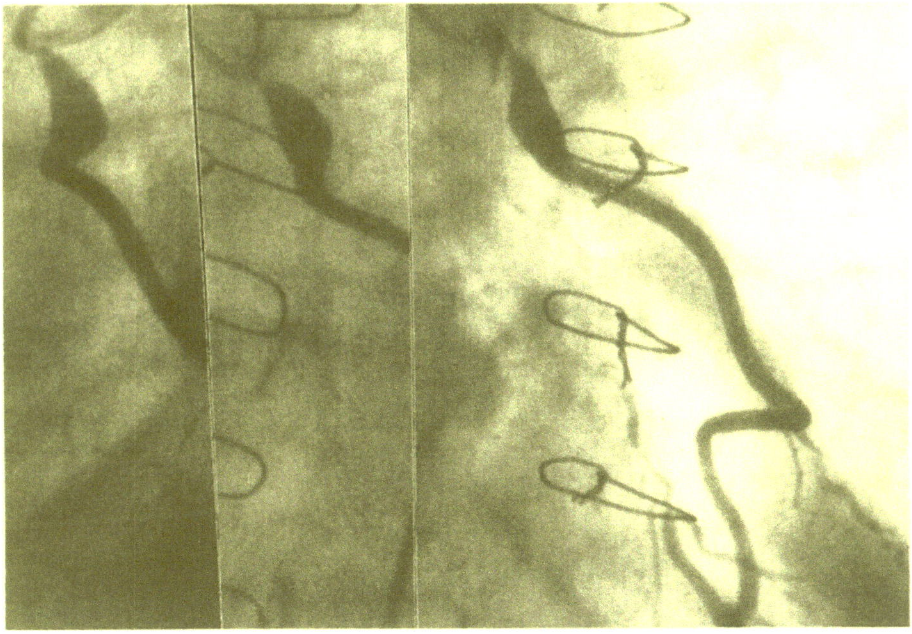

Fig. 16

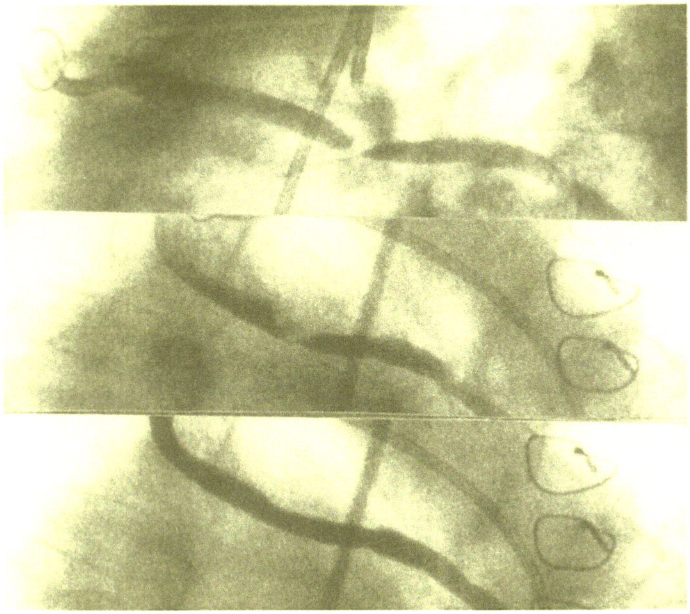

Fig. 17

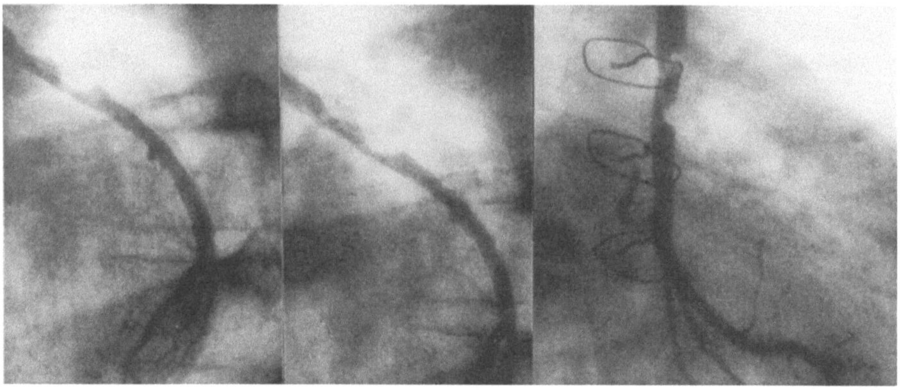

Fig. 18. High-grade stenosis in the middle portion of a graft to the first posterolateral branch of the left circumflex artery. The stenosis is eccentric and of complex nature as best shown on the frames in the *middle* (LAO) and *right* panels (mild RAO projection). There are several niches free of contrast medium, surrounding a small area filled with contrast medium, typical for a ruptured plaque (see: right panel)

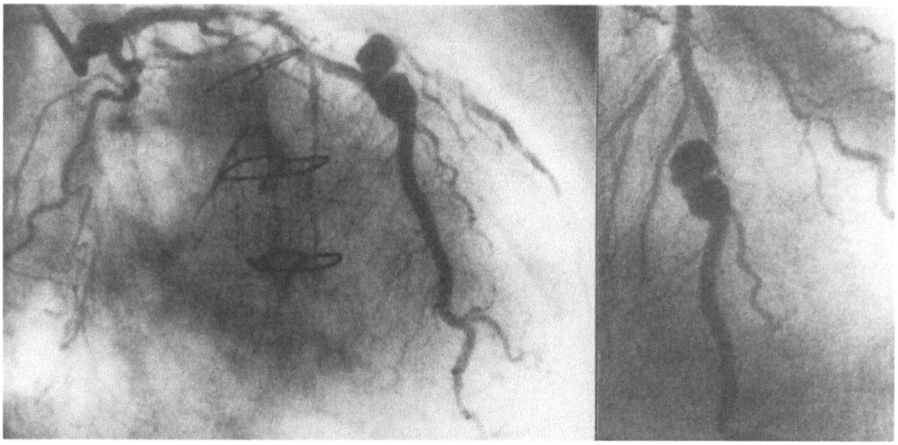

Fig. 19. Aneurysmatic dilatation of an occluded LAD graft; only the distal portion of the graft, directly above the distal anastomosis is filled by contrast medium; it demonstrates an irregular structure with a slitlike insertion. The LAD shows a long, high-grade concentric stenosis beginning after the first diagonal branch and including the first septal branch. RAO projection (*left*) and craniocaudal LAO projection (*right*)

to additional functional narrowing in eccentric stenoses during exercise, further reducing the lumen at the stenotic site and inducing ischemia even with relatively low-grade stenoses. As vasomotor tone is markedly reduced or even absent in veins [26], only high-grade stenoses become symptomatic. In some veins, in addition to atherosclerotic lesions, platelet thrombi

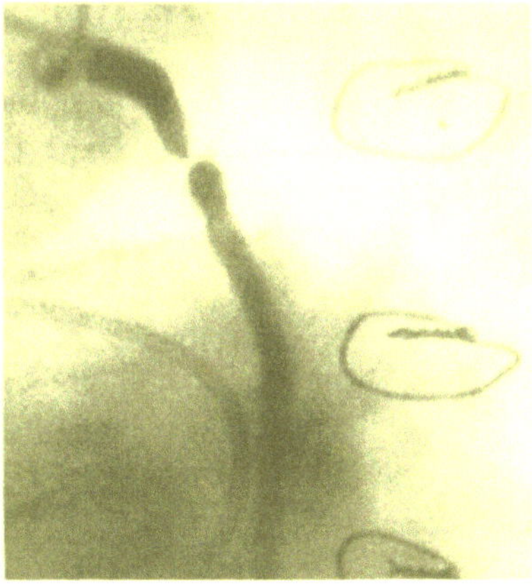

Fig. 20. High-grade, concentric stenosis of an LAD graft (PA projection)

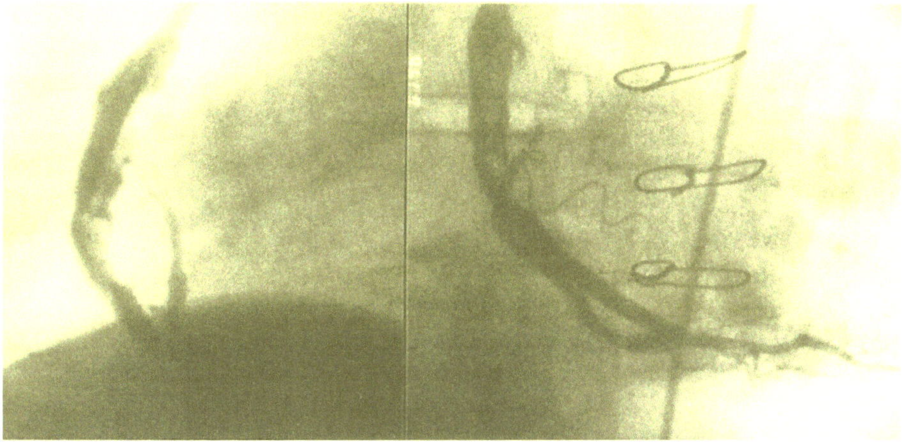

Fig. 21. Diffusely diseased graft to the RCA partially with aneurysmatic dilatation and filled with thrombotic material. This is recognized as islands with poor or no contrast, surrounded by zones of intensive contrast. From the still unstenosed distal anastomosis, there is good ante- and retrograde filling of the distal RCA

adhering to areas of diseased endothelium can further reduce the lumen and lead to early symptoms (Fig. 21).

As with stenoses in native coronary arteries, also the exact visualization of graft stenoses usually depends on a combination of several projections. Optimal projections are necessary to demonstrate the minimal stenotic diameter, the exact location and length of the stenosis, its relation to the vessel circumference (eccentric or concentric), and to provide exact morphologic description with regard to their complexity, i.e., the quality of the plaque and the presence of thrombi. Especially for vein grafts the search for

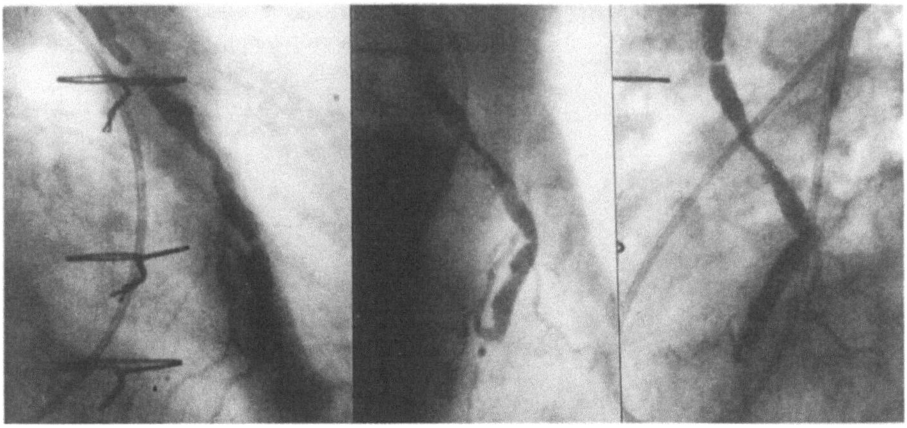

Fig. 22. Diffusely diseased LAD graft. All three projections (mild RAO, craniocaudal RAO, and LAO) show irregular contours along the entire length of the graft, even including the distal anastomosis; in addition there is a short, approx. 1-mm-long circular incisionlike constriction in the upper portion

thrombi adhering to the wall or to complicated plaques with rough edges is of great clinical importance.

Diffuse Graft Disease

Extensive progression of coronary artery disease often leads to diffuse graft alterations including the entire length of its body and also frequently its peripheral anastomosis (Fig. 22); sometimes thrombi are attached at various sites, probably due to spotty loss of endothelial surface, leaving islands of free collagen. Such grafts have a high tendency to progress rapidly towards total thrombotic occlusion, the thrombus forming either from the proximal part to the distal region or, on the other hand, leaving only a short proximal or distal segment still patent.

Technical Aspects of Graft Intubation

Fluoroscopic and angiographic times should be kept as short as possible. For this reason, the special catheters devised to intubate bypass as well as IMA grafts, with special curvatures on the tip of the catheter should be used to guarantee a minimal duration of fluoroscopy. The time of angiography should also be kept as short as possible by using biplane systems and the lowest possible X-ray doses. This is absolutely mandatory as many of these patients undergo repeated angiography within a short interval of a few months and years and therefore receive a relatively high cumulative radiation dose. These considerations should, however, not influence the quest for optimal visualization of grafts and stenoses, allowing the necessary clinical decisions with great reliability.

Indications for Graft Angiography

Clinical Indications

The preservation of graft integrity over a long period of time is of extreme clinical importance [55, 56]; therefore early recognition of graft failure is important; we recommend, at our institution, control angiography early after implantation, i.e., within the first 6–12 months. This is of special importance as low-grade stenoses (diameter stenosis <50%) cannot be detected by noninvasive techniques such as exercise or nuclear tests [2]; furthermore, even highgrade stenoses (diameter stenosis ≥70%), leading to ischemic episodes often remain clinically silent [57]. Immediate graft angiography is mandatory when ischemic symptoms (typical stable or unstable angina) recur and/or new signs of silent or symptomatic ischemia are observed in noninvasive tests (exercise ECG, stress thallium scintigraphy). This is of special importance as graft PTCA has become a true alternative to reoperation when performed early after the development of plaques. The sooner the stenotic graft undergoes PTCA, the greater is the chance for successful dilatation, i.e., long-term opening. Once a graft is occluded, chances for successful reopening by PTCA (not followed by early reocclusion) are much lower than in stenosed grafts [58]. Finally, it should be stressed that in the presence of new anginal pain after a symptom-free interval, especially of several years it is impossible to differentiate by noninvasive means whether the culprit stenosis is localized in a graft or in a native coronary artery. Progression of coronary artery disease takes place both in native coronary arteries and in vein grafts, even in successfully implanted ones. The success of secondary preventive measures (PTCA of a graft or of a native artery or reoperation) depends on the early detection of such new, clinically relevant plaques.

Angiographic Indications

Considering the fact that approximately 50% of grafts show considerable changes after 5–8 years, and that in the majority of cases progression of CAD in grafts remains clinically silent over a long time, routine graft angiography after an interval of approximately 5 to 8 years is recommendable, even in the absence of ischemic symptoms or of positive noninvasive tests, especially in patients with multivessel disease, where the results of noninvasive tests might be equivocal. This not only has prognostic implications but often also therapeutic consequences (graft-PTCA, or reoperation).

Early reangiography, within the first year after operation is recommended for special types of vein grafts, such as vein grafts with multiple anastomoses, sequential grafts, and especially snake grafts, grafts with special anastomotic sites and those grafts where special arteries were applied, for example, free arterial grafts (free IMA, gastroepiploic artery) (Fig. 6). In addition, early angiography is recommended especially in institutions starting bypass surgery, where local experience on early and late patency is still lacking and should be followed for reasons of clinical management. Indications for reangiography depend to a great deal on knowledge of the local situation. This includes also controls of IMA grafts, where initially anastomotic problems might occur. The long-term high patency rate of IMA grafts (see above) does not render early control worthwhile in experienced centers.

Noninvasive Angiographic Techniques to Visualize Bypass Grafts

Today, two non-invasive techniques are available that allow visualization of grafts by peripheral intravenous injection of contrast medium: digital subtraction angiography (DSA) [59] and computer tomography (CT) [60, 61]. Both techniques, however, range far below angiography with regard to their sensitivity of image acquisition. The information is rather crude when compared to angiography and at best can be used to decide on further invasive tests. Whereas DSA in special situations can still be helpful, especially in cases where it is able to demonstrate the entire length of the graft, CT is outmoded, as it represents only a very small portion of the graft in cross-section [60, 61]. It is therefore not discussed here.

Digital Subtraction Angiography (DSA)

The quality of DSA is limited by the amount of contrast medium (only two or three injections), the timing for optimal contrast filling of the graft, and the search for the best projection. There is an overlap of contrast medium in the aortic root with the proximal portion of the grafts, i.e., with the proximal implantation site and also an overlap with the cardiac silhouette. This requires special projections which often cannot be achieved due to the limitation in the amount of contrast material to be administered.

In optimal situations (Fig. 23) DSA is able to demonstrate large portions of the graft body. Comparisons with coronary angiography [59] confirm its ability to visualize isolated stenoses or occlusions well enough to serve as basis for clinical decisions. Difficulties arise in the simultaneous demonstration of both the proximal and the distal anastomoses. Hence, the indications

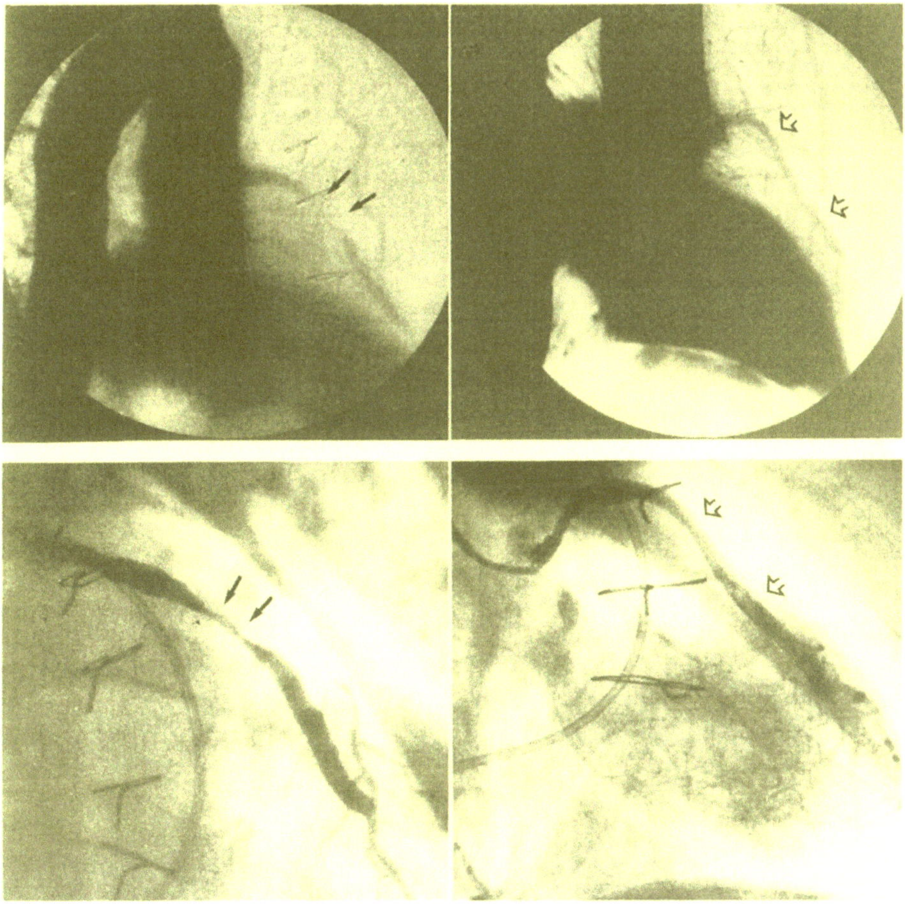

Fig. 23. Noninvasive demonstration of a diseased graft by DSA. Contrast material was infused intravenously and pictures were taken in RAO projection during systole (*upper left*) and during diastole (*upper right*). *Below*, selective injection of contrast material into the same vein graft to the LAD in two RAO projections. There is a long high-grade stenosis in the middle of the graft body, seen both by DSA and by selective contrast injection

for DSA of grafts have been considerably reduced in recent years. Today they concentrate on the differentiation between graft patency versus closure but do not attempt an exact visualization of high-grade stenoses, i.e., the assessment of the degree of stenosis.

Conclusions

At present and probably for a considerable time in the future, conventional angiography will remain the only reliable technique visualizing vein and

IMA grafts well enough to allow clinically relevant judgment on the extent and management of graft disease. Indications for graft angiography should be handled liberally as the best chances to restore and maintain graft patency are still early interventions. Only optimal graft visualization allows the necessary clinical conclusions and decisions. Angiography must be based on ample knowledge of graft anatomy and topography and in many cases exact knowledge of the surgical procedure is necessary before angiography. Graft angiography should combine a maximum of information with the shortest procedure possible as often relatively long fluoroscopic and angiographic times, i.e., radiation exposures, are required. Therefore, biplane angiography and, if possible, even digital image acquisition – to enhance contrast – are of great advantage, optimizing the visualization of minute details such as the recognition of platelet thrombi. Complete graft angiography should include visualization not only of the various vein and/or IMA grafts but also of the native coronary arteries, as in the presence of graft disease or failure decisions on future management depend on knowledge of the entire coronary system.

References

1. Lichtlen PR (1990) Koronarangiographie und Koronarchirurgie. In: Lichtlen PR (ed) Beiträge zur Kardiologie. Perimed, Erlangen, pp 537–582
2. Lichtlen PR, Nikutta P, Jost S et al. (1992) Anatomical progression of coronary artery disease in humans as seen by prospective, repeated, quantitated coronary angiography. Relation to clinical events and risk factors. Circulation 86:828–838
3. Freudenberg H, Lichtlen PR (1981) Limitations of intravital coronary angiography. A comparison with postmortem results in 87 cases. Circulation 63/64 [Suppl IV]:238 (abstract)
4. Lichtlen PR (1981) Koronarchirurgie. In: Krayenbühl HP, Kübler W (eds) Kardiologie in Klinik und Praxis, vol II. Thieme, Stuttgart, pp 43.1–43.22
5. Ambrose JA, Tannenbaum MA, Alexopoulos D et al. (1988) Angiographic progression of coronary artery disease and the development of myocardial infarction. J Am Coll Cardiol 12:56–62
6. Little WC, Constantinescu M, Applegate RJ et al. (1988) Can coronary angiography predict the site of a subsequent myocardial infarction in patients with mild-to-moderate coronary artery disease? Circulation 78:1157–1166
7. Ross R (1986) The pathogenesis of atherosclerosis – an update. N Engl J Med 314:488–499
8. Haudenschild CC (1990) Pathogenesis of atherosclerosis: state of the art. Cardiovasc Drugs Ther 4 [Suppl V]:993–1004
9. Steinberg D, Parthasarathy S, Carew T, Khoo JC, Witztum JL (1989) Beyond cholesterol: modifications of low-density lipoprotein that increase its atherogeneity. N Engl J Med 320:915–924
10. Faggiotto A, Ross R, Herker L (1984) Studies on hypercholesterolemia in the non-human primate. I. Changes that lead to fatty streak formation. Arteriosclerosis 4:323–340
11. Glagov S, Weisenberg E, Zarins C, Stankunavicius R, Kolettis GJ (1987) Compensatory enlargement of human atherosclerotic coronary arteries. N Engl J Med 316:1371–1375
12. Liebson PR, Klein LW (1992) Intravascular ultrasound in coronary atherosclerosis: a new approach to clinical assessment. Am Heart J 123:1643–1660

13. Fitzgerald PJ, St Goar FG, Conolly AJ et al. (1992) Intravascular ultrasound imaging of coronary arteries. Is three layer the norm? Circulation 86:154–158
14. Tobis JM, Mallery J, Mahon D et al. (1991) Intravascular ultrasound imaging of human coronary arteries in vivo. Analysis of tissue characteristics with comparison to in vitro histologic specimen. Circulation 83:913–926
15. Gibson CM, Saffian RD (1992) Limitations of cineangiography; impact of new technologies for image processing and quantitation. Trends Cardiovasc Med 2:156–160
16. Hermiller JB, Kusma JT, Spero LA, Fortin DF, Harding MB, Bashore TM (1992) Quantitative and qualitative coronary angiographic analysis: review of methods, utility and limitations. Cathet Cardiovasc Diagn 25:110–131
17. Campeau L, Enjalbert M, Lespérance J (1983) Atherosclerosis and late closure of aortocoronary vein bypass grafts: sequential angiographic study at 2 weeks, 1 year, 5–7 years and 10–12 years after surgery. Circulation 68 [Suppl II]:1–7
18. Herrmann G, Simon R, Amende I, Frank G, Borst HG, Lichtlen PR (1987) Late increase in luminal diameter of aorto-coronary venous bypass grafts associated with an increase in the vascular region under supply. J Am Coll Cardiol 10:10–16
19. Lawrie GM, Lie JT et al. (1976) Vein graft patency and intimal proliferation after aortocoronary bypass: early and long-term angiopathologic correlations. Am J Cardiol 38:856–861
20. Lichtlen P, Moccetti T, Halter J, Schönbeck M, Senning A (1972) Postoperative evaluation of myocardial blood flow in aorto-to-coronary vein bypass grafts using the Xenon-residue-detection technique. Circulation 46:445–455
21. Meester K, Veldkamp R, Tijssen JGP et al. (1991) Clinical outcome of single vessel sequential grafts in coronary bypass operations at 10 years follow-up. Eur J Cardiothorac Surg 101:1076–1081
22. Green GE (1972) Internal mammary artery for coronary artery anastomosis. 3 year experience with 165 patients. Ann Thorac Surg 14:260
23. Loop FD, Little BW, Cosgrove DM (1986) Influence of the internal mammary artery graft in 10 year survival and other cardiac event. N Engl J Med 314:1–6
24. Grondin CM, Campeau L, Lespérance J, Enjalbert M, Bourassa MG (1984) Comparison of late changes in internal mammary artery and saphenous vein grafts in two consecutive series of patients 10 years after operation. Circulation 70 [Suppl I]:208–212
25. Lytle BM, Loop FD, Cosgrove DM (1985) Long-term (5–12 years) serial studies of internal mammary artery and saphenous vein coronary bypass graft. J Thorac Cardiovasc Surg 89:248–258
26. Lüscher TF, Diederich D, Siebenmann R, Lehmann K et al. (1988) Difference between endothelium-dependent relaxation in arterial and in venous coronary bypass grafts. N Engl J Med 319:462–467
27. Kuttler H, Hauenstein KH, Kameda T, Wenz W, Schlosser V (1988) Significance of early angiographic follow-up after internal artery anastomosis in coronary surgery. Thorac Cardiovasc Surg 36:96–99
28. Dincer B, Barner HB (1983) The "occluded" internal mammary artery graft: restoration of patency after apparent occlusion associated with progression of coronary disease. J Thorac Cardiovasc Surg 85:318–320
29. Grondin CM, Lespérance J, Bourassa MB, Campeau L (1975) Coronary artery grafting with the saphenous vein or internal mammary artery. Comparison of late results in 2 consecutive series of patients. Ann Thorac Surg 20:605–618
30. Schmid C, Heublein B, Reichelt S, Borst HG (1990) Steal phenomenon caused by a parallel branch of the internal mammary artery. Ann Thorac Surg 50:463–464
31. Pelias AJ, del Rossi AJ (1985) A case of postoperative internal mammary steal. J Thorac Cardiovasc Surg 90:794–796
32. Stolte M (1977) Postmortale Untersuchungen nach Revaskularisations-Operation. Thoraxchirurgie 25:181

33. Herrmann G, Simon R, Haverich A, Lichtlen PR, Borst HG (1986) Langzeitergebnisse aortokoronarer Venenbypasschirurgie. Z Kardiol 75; [Suppl 1]:68 (abstr.)
34. Vlodaver Z, Edwards JE (1971) Pathologic changes in aorto-coronary arterial saphenous vein grafts. Circulation 44:719
35. Lichtlen P (1974) The aorto to coronary vein bypass graft: postoperative clinical and functional evaluation. J Cardiovasc Surg 15:163
36. Sheldon WC (1978) Effect of bypass graft surgery on survival; a 6–10 year follow-up study of 741 patients. Cleve Clin Q J Med 45:166
37. Buis B, Endlich B, Arntzenius AC (1975) A technique for measuring the diameter of coronary arteries and venous bypass grafts from 70 mm spot films. In: Lichtlen PR (ed) Coronary angiography and angina pectoris. Thieme, Stuttgart, p 265
38. Lawrie GM, Weilbacher DE, Henry PD (1990) Endothelium-dependent relaxation in human saphenous vein grafts. Eur J Cardiothorac Surg 100:612–620
39. Reiber JHC, Serruys PW, Kooijman CJ et al. (1985) Assessment of short-, medium-, and long-term variations in arterial dimensions from computer-assisted quantitation of coronary cineangiograms. Circulation 71:280–288
40. Liese W, Leitz K, Borst HG, Lichtlen P (1977) Patency-Rate im Früh- und Folgestadium des aorto-koronaren Venenbypass in Abhängigkeit vom Venentransplantat und intraoperativen Fluss. Schweiz Med Wochenschr 107:1581–1584
41. Neville RF, Sidway AN, Foegh ML (1992) The molecular biology of vein graft atherosclerosis and myointimal hyperplasia. Curr Opin Cardiol 7:930–938
42. Campeau L, Enjalbert M, Lespérance J et al. (1984) The relationship of risk factors to the development of atherosclerosis in saphenous vein bypass grafts and the progression of disease in the native circulation: a study 10 years after aorto-coronary bypass surgery. N Engl J Med 311:1329–1332
43. Johnson WD, Brenowitz JB, Kasper KL (1989) Factors influencing long-term (10 years to 15 years) survival after a successful coronary artery bypass operation. Ann Thorac Surg 48:19–25
44. Lawrie CM, Morris GS, Earle N (1991) Long-term results of coronary bypass surgery. Ann Surg 213:377–387
45. Holman WL (1992) Long-term results of coronary artery bypass grafting. Curr Opin Cardiol 7:990–996
46. Sergeant P, Lesafre E, Flameng W, Suy R, Blackstone E (1991) The return of clinically evident ischemia after coronary bypass grafting. Eur J Cardiothorac Surg 5:447–457
47. Sheldon WC (1978) Factors influencing patency of coronary bypass grafts. Cleve Clin Q J Med 45:109
48. Gottlieb SO, Brinker JA, Mellits ED et al. (1989) Effect of nifedipine on the development of coronary bypass graft stenoses in high-risk patients: a randomized, double-blind, placebo-controlled trial. Circulation 80 [Suppl]:II-228 (abstract)
49. Cox JL, Chiasson DA, Gotlieb AI (1991) Stranger in a strange land: the pathogenesis of saphenous vein graft stenosis with emphasis on structural and functional differences between veins and arteries. Prog Cardiovasc Dis 34:45–68
50. Davies MJ (1990) A macro and micro view of coronary vascular insult in ischemic heart disease. Circulation 82 [Suppl II]:38–46
51. Quist WC, Haudenschild CC, LoGefro FW (1992) Qualitative microscopy of implanted vein grafts: effects of graft integrity of morphologic fate. Eur J Cardiothorac Surg 103:671–677
52. Sheldon WC, Rincon D, Effler DB, Proudfit WL, Sones FM (1973) Vein graft surgery for coronary artery disease. Survival and angiographic results in 1000 patients. Circulation 47/48:III-184
53. Feigl O (1987) The paradox of adrenergic coronary vasoconstriction. Circulation 76: 737–745
54. Gage JE, Hess OM, Murakami T, Ritter M, Grimm J, Krayenbühl HP (1986) Coronary artery stenosis vasoconstriction during dynamic exercise in patients with classical angina pectoris: reversibility by nitroglycerin. Circulation 73:865–876

55. Brown G, Cuningham RA, DeRouen T et al. (1985) Improved graft patency in patients treated with platelet-inhibiting therapy after coronary bypass surgery. Circulation 72: 138–146
56. Angelini GD (1992) Saphenous vein graft failure: etiologic considerations and strategies for prevention. Curr Opin Cardiol 7:939–944
57. Hausmann D, Nikutta P, Hartwig CA, Daniel WG, Lichtlen PR (1987) ST-segment analysis in the 24-h Holter ECG in patients with stable angina pectoris and proven coronary artery disease. Z Kardiol 76:554–562
58. Jost S, Gulba D, Eckert S, Simon R, Amende I, Lichtlen P (1990) Angiographischer und klinischer Verlauf nach PTCA von aortokoronaren Venenbypass (ACVB)-Grafts. Z Kardiol 79 [Suppl]:1–20 (abstract)
59. Luska G, Hendrickx PH, Kuhl A, Lichtlen P (1985) Peripher-venöse digitale Subtraktionsangiographie (DAS) zur Kontrolle von aorto-koronaren Venenbypass-Grafts (ACVB). Fortschr Röntgenstr 142:35–40
60. Daniel WG, Döring W, Stender H, Lichtlen P (1983) Value and limitation of computed tomography in assessing aorto-coronary bypass graft patency. Circulation 67:983–987
61. Guthaner EF, Robert EW, Aldermann EL, Wexler L (1979) Long-term serial angiographic studies after coronary artery bypass surgery. Circulation 60:250–259

Left Ventricular Function: Systolic and Diastolic Alterations

H.P. Krayenbuehl†, M. Jakob, and O.M. Hess

Introduction

Assessment of the effect of coronary artery bypass surgery on left ventricular performance must consider a variety of factors. These include patient selection, extent of revascularization, intraoperative myocardial preservation techniques, perioperative infarction, graft patency, runoff of the peripheral vascular bed, ventricular loading conditions, and drug therapy. The timing of the evaluation is important because left ventricular function changes rapidly throughout the early postoperative recovery period, and during the first 3 months after surgery the heart remains under enhanced chronotopic and inotropic stimulation by excess circulation of catecholamines [1]. It is only thereafter that a more "intrinsic" left ventricular function reflecting the overall result of surgery can be determined.

Left Ventricular Function in the Immediate Postoperative Period After Coronary Artery Bypass Grafting

Despite modern intraoperative preservation techniques the myocardium is exposed to some degree of ischemic-hypoxic injury during surgery. Thus when reperfusion is reestablished, left ventricular function does not recover at once, but recovery may go through a phase of left ventricular functional depression or "stunning" [2, 3]. Using equilibrium-gated blood pool scintigraphy, Roberts et al. [4] found that in 90% of patients undergoing coronary bypass surgery left ventricular ejection fraction was significantly depressed 2 h postoperatively. At 24 h ejection fraction had again reached the preoperative value, and 7 days postoperatively ejection fraction exceeded the presurgical value. In patients studied by echocardiography significant postoperative reduction of systolic septal thickening was observed which was thought to be responsible, at least in part, for transient paradoxical septal motion [5]. In some patients spontaneous recovery of ejection fraction may require up to 48 h [6], and rarely inotropic support and ventricular assist are necessary to bridge the phase of dysfunction of the severely stunned myocardium [7]. Thus, in the early postoperative period depression of left ventricular ejection fraction is much more likely due to reversible myocardial stunning than to ongoing severe ischemia or infarction consequent to acute graft failure.

Resting Left Ventricular Systolic Function at Follow-Up After Coronary Bypass Surgery

Global Left Ventricular Function

Systolic ejection fraction is the most convenient measure to assess global left ventricular function. Many studies have evaluated ejection fraction using contrast or radionuclide ventriculography. We have pooled the data of various studies from which paired pre-/postoperative values for ejection fraction were available (Tables 1–3). It is realized, however, that single-plane contrast ventriculography as carried out in the 1970s might be suboptimal for the assessment of left ventricular ejection fraction and volumes in the presence of regional wall motion abnormalities, and that the limit of normality of ejection fraction varies widely, being as low as 45% in some studies with radionuclide ventriculography [8, 9].

The overall data including patients with patent and occluded grafts [8, 10–16] or with unknown graft status [5, 17, 18] have shown no postoperative change in ejection fraction (Table 1). The results did not differ whether restudies were carried out early (<3 months) or late (up to 13 months) postoperatively. Only one of the individual studies (Table 1) showed a significant change in postoperative ejection fraction [11]. In this particular cohort patients with occluded grafts (10 of 14 cases) predominated and hence were likely to be responsible for the postoperatively depressed left ventricular ejection fraction.

More relevant than overall data is the analysis of postoperative left ventricular function according to whether bypasses are patent or nonfunctioning (occluded or severely stenosed). Table 2 presents results of follow-up studies in patients whose bypasses were patent [9, 10, 12, 16, 19–31]. The pooled data show an increase in ejection fraction from 60% to 66% ($p < 0.005$), a decrease in left ventricular end-diastolic volume index from 87 to 81 ml/m^2 ($p < 0.01$) and an increase in heart rate from 78 to 90 bpm ($p < 0.001$). Left ventricular end-diastolic pressure decreased slightly but significantly from 14 to 11 mmHg ($p < 0.001$). Despite the general trend of an improvement of postoperative ejection fraction there were some differences among the individual studies because of clinical variables and timing. The results of most studies in patients with stable, albeit in part severe angina [10, 20, 24, 26, 29, 30] and/or a preoperative ejection fraction exceeding 61% [12, 21, 22, 28, 31] showed few changes in resting ejection

Table 1. Global left ventricular systolic function at rest before and after coronary artery bypass surgery (overall findings)

Reference	Technique	Restudy postoperative	*n*	EF (%) Before	EF (%) After	Comments
Hammermeister [10]	Angio ap/lat	4 months	40	53	50 (NS)	Disabling angina
Apstein [11]	Angio spl	9 months	14	62	54 ($p < 0.01$)	Stable angina
Righetti [5]	Radionuc	10 months	20	63	62 (NS)	Chronic CAD
Wolf [12]	Angio bipl	13 months	37	65	64 (NS)	Stable angina
Kent [8]	Radionuc	6 months	19	51	55 (NS)	Stable angina
Hellman [13]	Radionuc	10–14 days	36	66	68 (NS)	Chronic CAD
Freeman [17]	Radionuc	5.3 months	21	56	54 (NS)	Stable angina
Lim [14]	Radionuc	3 months	9	54	55 (NS)	Refractory angina, MI
			11	67	68 (NS)	Refractory angina
Kronenberg [15]	Radionuc	5.8 months	36	57	53	Chronic stable angina
Taylor [18]	Radionuc	1.5 months	56	65	64 (NS)	Chronic stable angina
Melandri [16]	Angio spl	9 months	77	58	61 (NS)	Chronic CAD
Mean				60	59	
				NS		

n, Number of observations; EF, left ventricular ejection fraction; ap/lat, anteroposterior and lateral biplane angiography; spl, single plane; bipl, biplane; Radionuc, radionuclide angiography; NS, not significant; CAD, coronary artery disease; MI, myocardial infarction.

Table 2. Global left ventricular systolic function before and after coronary artery bypass surgery (patients with patent grafts)

Reference	Technique	Restudy postoperative	n	EF (%) Before	EF (%) After	EDVI (ml/m^2) Before	EDVI (ml/m^2) After	LVEDP (mmHg) Before	LVEDP (mmHg) After	HR (bpm) Before	HR (bpm) After	Comments
Rees [19]	Angio spl	3 months	8	61	72 ($p < 0.05$)	95	86	11.8	8.2	80	89	Angina at minimal effort
Arbogast [20]	Angio spl	12 months	20	No change		No change						Severe angina
Chatterjee [21]	Angio spl	14 days	6	78	80 (NS)	85	86	8	7	67	86	No asynergy
			12	45	44	114	97	15	10	76	90	Asynergy without MI } 8 preinfarction angina, 10 chronic angina
			7	44	59 ($p < 0.05$)	106	108	17	10	85	99	Asynergy with MI
Bolooki [22]	Angio spl	4.5 months	7	68	81 (NS)			16.1	13.0	81	80	Preinfarction angina
			14	71	66 (NS)			13.5	11.9	84	87	Chronic angina
Hamby [23]	Angio spl	2–4 weeks	33	68	71 (NS)	66	64	11	9	81	96	BPLAD 17/33 UA
			47	60	69 ($p < 0.001$)	68	64	13	10	80	95	2 BP 17/47 UA
			10	61	71 ($p < 0.001$)	71	61	12	9	84	100	3 BP 4/10 UA
Hammermeister [10]	Angio ap/lat	4 months	28	54	52 (NS)	82	76			73	86	Disabling angina
Shepherd [24]	Angio spl	5 months	10	54	53 (NS)	76	69	13	14	77	85	Disabling angina
Chatterjee [25]	Angio spl	0.5–6 months	7	51	71 ($p < 0.001$)	72	69	11.3	9.2	73	89	5/7 UA
Chesebro [26]	Angio bipl	14 months	30	No change		No change		No change				Stable angina
Wolf [12]	Angio bipl	3 months	11	74	71 (NS)	74	80	8	11			Stable angina, no asynergy
			11	53	65 ($p < 0.05$)	92	81					Stable angina, with asynergy
Zir [27]	Angio spl	17 months	16	49	57 ($p < 0.01$)							Asynergy, 20/51 UA
Bussmann [28]	Angio spl	5 weeks	6	68	68 (NS)			21.3	15.5	78	94	Chronic angina
Hirzel [29]	Angio bipl	5.4 months	15	56	62 (NS)	108	89	17	13	81	92	Stable angina
Carroll [30]	Angio bipl	7.7 months	24	57	59 (NS)	114	108	23	17	67	75	Stable angina
Melandri [16]	Angio spl	9 months	50	58	64 ($p < 0.005$)							Chronic CAD
Dilsizian [9]	Radionuc	6–8 months	16	56	61 ($p < 0.025$)							Chronic stable angina, asynergy
Gibson [31]	Angio spl	6–695 days	27	69	68 (NS)							Chronic CAD
Mean				60	66	87	81	14.1	11.2	78	90	
				$p < 0.005$		$p < 0.001$		$p < 0.001$		$p < 0.001$		

EDVI, Left ventricular end-diastolic volume index, LVEDP, left ventricular end-diastolic pressure; HR, heart rate; BP, bypass; LAD, left anterior descending coronary artery; UA, unstable angina. Other abbreviations are as in Table 1. The p values of EF (in parentheses) refer to the statistics in the individual publications; the p values of the pooled data were obtained by the paired t test

Table 3. Global left ventricular systolic function before and after coronary artery bypass surgery (patients with occluded or severely stenosed grafts)

Reference	Technique	Restudy postoperative	*n*	EF (%)		EDVI (ml/m^2)		LVEDP (mmHg)		HR (bpm)		Comments
				Before	After	Before	After	Before	After	Before	After	
Rees [19]	Angio spl	3 months	6	59	50 (NS)	95	100	15.0	16.3	77	84	Resting angina
Arbogast [20]	Angio spl	12 months	19	Decrease		Increase						Severe angina
Shepherd [24]	Angio spl	5 months	12	59	49 ($p < 0.05$)	74	77	12	16	81	92	Disabling angina
Barry [33]	Angio spl	12 months	5	71	59							Chronic angina
Chesebro [26]	Angio bipl	14 months	22	No change								Stable angina
Apstein [11]	Angio spl	9 months	10	59	49 ($p < 0.01$)							Stable angina
Wolf [12]	Angio bipl	13 months	11	67	57 ($p < 0.025$)	84	86					Stable angina
Hirzel [29]	Angio bipl	5.4 months	37	61	59 (NS)	105	97	16	14	69	79	Stable angina
Dilsizian [9]	radionuc	6–8 months	4	59	58 (NS)							Chronic stable angina
Mean				62	54	90	90	14.3	15.4	76	85	
				$p < 0.005$								

Abbreviations as in Tables 1 and 2.

fraction postoperatively. In contrast, patients with acute preinfarction syndrome or unstable angina [21, 23, 25] and/or resting asynergy [9, 12, 27] elicited in most instances a marked postoperative improvement of ejection fraction. This increase in ejection fraction has been related to the correction of a state of chronic ischemia associated with hibernating myocardium the function of which is reestablished upon restoration of coronary flow [9, 32]. Finally it should be realized that in patients restudied early, i.e., less than 3 months postoperatively [21, 23, 25] ejection fraction might be abnormally high due to ongoing increased adrenergic stimulation [1].

A somewhat different picture as to postoperative resting ejection fraction is obtained when patients with occluded or severely stenosed grafts are evaluated separately (Table 3) [9, 11, 12, 19, 20, 24, 26, 29, 33]. Based on pooled data from seven studies ejection fraction decreased from 62 to 54% ($p < 0.005$) whereby a significant decrease was present in three of six individual studies. Too few data are available to evaluate the effect of nonfunctioning grafts on left ventricular end-diastolic volume and pressure.

Regional Left Ventricular Function

Several studies [9, 12, 23, 24, 27, 34, 35] have analyzed regional wall motion after coronary bypass surgery (Table 4). In regions supplied by patent grafts preoperative hypokinetic wall motion improved or became normal after surgery in a large percentage but not in all instances. Failure of resting hypokinetic regions to improve was found to be related to myocardial infarction or to a graft flow <60 ml/min [26]. Differentiation as to whether a preoperatively hypokinetic segment will improve its function after revascularization might be obtained from its reaction to an inotropic intervention or an acute reduction in preload and myocardial oxygen consumption. Improvement in function of an asynergic region after postextrasystolic potentiation [36, 37] or nitroglycerin [38, 39] generally heralds an improvement in postoperative regional wall motion.

Graft patency is not always associated with improved or at least unchanged postoperative regional wall motion. Shepherd et al. [24] have reported deterioration of wall motion (episode of postoperative infarction?) in 9 of 28 segments of ten patients supplied by patent grafts. This impairment of regional function however, was, not accompanied by a decrease in ejection fraction probably due to compensatory hyperfunction of other parts of the ventricular myocardium. Postoperative hyperfunction may also occur in grafted segments when an infarct has occurred elsewhere [26].

Regional contractile function in the perfusion territory of occluded grafts has been found to be decreased or at best unchanged with respect to the preoperative performance (Table 4). Chesebro et al. [26] using peak rate of systolic wall thickening to assess regional myocardial function in segments without preoperative infarction observed a consistent decrease of this velocity

Table 4. Systolic regional wall motion at rest before and after coronary bypass surgery

Reference	Technique	Restudy postoperative	Patent grafts (before/after)		Occluded grafts (before/after)	
			Improvement	Deterioration	Improvement	Deterioration
Bourassa [34]	Angio spl	12–18 months	71% of hypokin. sgm			37% of normal or hypokin. sgm
Hamby [23]	Angio spl	2–4 weeks	94% of sgm with asynergy			
Shepherd [24]	Angio spl	5 months	21% of sgm	32% of sgm	0%	36% of sgm
Wolf [12]	Angio bipl	13 months	Asynergic sgm: % short. 12 → 36% Normokin. sgm: % short. 41 → 43%			% short. 43 → 37%
Zir [27]	Angio spl	17 months	Asynergic sgm		No change	
Brundage [35]	Radionuc	8.5 months	66% of hypokin. sgm		Hypokin. sgm: 90% with persisting hypokinesis	
Dilsizian [9]	Radionuc	6–8 months	65% of preop ischemic sgm		7% of preop ischemic sgm	

Hypokin, Hypokinetic; sgm, segment; % short, percentage segmental shortening; normokin, normokinetic. Other abbreviations as in Table 1.

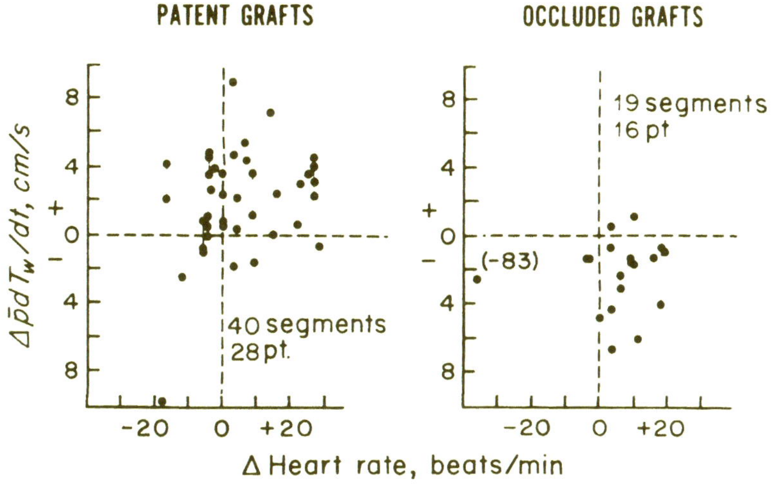

Fig. 1. Changes in peak rate of systolic wall thickening ($\Delta p/dT_w/dt$; postoperative minus preoperative) versus change in heart rate (postoperative minus preoperative) in segments without myocardial infarction supplied by patent grafts (*left panel*) and in segments without preoperative infarction supplied by occluded grafts (*right panel*). In the patients with patent grafts peak rate of systolic wall thickening was consistently higher at the postoperative than at the preoperative study irrespective of the change in heart rate. In the patients with occluded grafts peak rate of systolic wall thickening decreased after surgery although heart rate increased postoperatively. (From Chesebro et al. [26], reproduced with permission of the American Society for Clinical Investigation)

measure when grafts were occluded (Fig. 1). With patent grafts peak rate of systolic wall thickening increased in most instances compared to the preoperative value. Irrespective of the resting function no contractile reserve appears to exist in the supply regions of occluded grafts because in postextrasystolic beats augmentation of segmental motion is absent [37]. Rarely an increase in regional wall motion occurs despite occluded grafts probably via improved blood supply through collaterals from patent grafts in adjacent areas [40].

Left Ventricular Systolic Function During Exercise After Coronary Bypass Surgery

Left ventricular function during exercise has been assessed by standard hemodynamic parameters [33, 41–44] and indices of ejection performance determined by contrast [28–30] or radionuclide [8, 9, 13–15] ventriculography.

Standard hemodynamic parameters are variable during exercise in patients with patent and occluded grafts. Rutherford et al. [41] and Campeau et al. [42] found a similar left ventricular end-diastolic pressure and stroke work index during exercise in groups of patients with patent and occluded grafts. Among patients with patent grafts only those with preoperative hypokinesis and not those with preoperative normal left ventricular contraction or akinesis showed postoperative hemodynamic improvement during exercise consisting of a significant fall in left ventricular end-diastolic pressure and increase in stroke work index [42]. Vliestra et al. [43] reevaluated 31 patients with an abnormal preoperative hemodynamic exercise response 17 months after bypass surgery. A group of 11 patients with complete revascularization differed significantly from another group of 20 patients with incomplete revascularization in that postoperative reaction to exercise was improved. This improvement consisted in a lower left ventricular end-diastolic pressure and a higher stroke work index at the postoperative than at the preoperative exercise study. In contrast, only 5 out of the 20 patients with incomplete revascularization had an improved left ventricular functional response during exercise according to the above criteria. Thus, although specific groups of patients may have different response patterns of standard hemodynamic measures during exercise after bypass surgery, these parameters have a too low sensitivity and specificity to allow a fiducial assessment of the revascularization status in individual patients.

When ischemia occurs during exercise, de novo regional hypokinesis or accentuation of preexisting wall motion abnormalities associated with a fall in ejection fraction has been consistently documented by angiographic [28–30] and radionuclide ventriculography [8, 9, 13–15, 17, 18]. Following successful revascularization exercise left ventricular shortening dynamics were significantly improved compared with preoperative exercise data [8, 9, 13–15, 17, 18, 28–30]. Some [13, 15, 17, 18, 30] but not all studies [8, 9, 14, 29] have also shown a significant increase in ejection fraction from rest to exercise following surgery. In this context it should be pointed out that an adequate comparison of pre- and postoperative exercise studies requires stress tests at matched loads [15]. In patients with occluded grafts [9, 13, 28] or incomplete revascularization [29] the ejection fraction decreases with exercise, and its absolute value during exercise is similar to the exercise ejection fraction at the preoperative evaluation (Figs. 2, 3). Thus, the assessment of ejection dynamics during exercise is a powerful tool for the diagnosis of eventual postoperative stress-induced ischemia and hence the state of revascularization.

Left Ventricular Diastolic Function After Coronary Bypass Surgery

Left ventricular diastole encompasses three distinct phases, namely isovolumic relaxation, the early rapid filling period, and the period of passive diastolic filling which is terminated by atrial systole [45]. In coronary heart

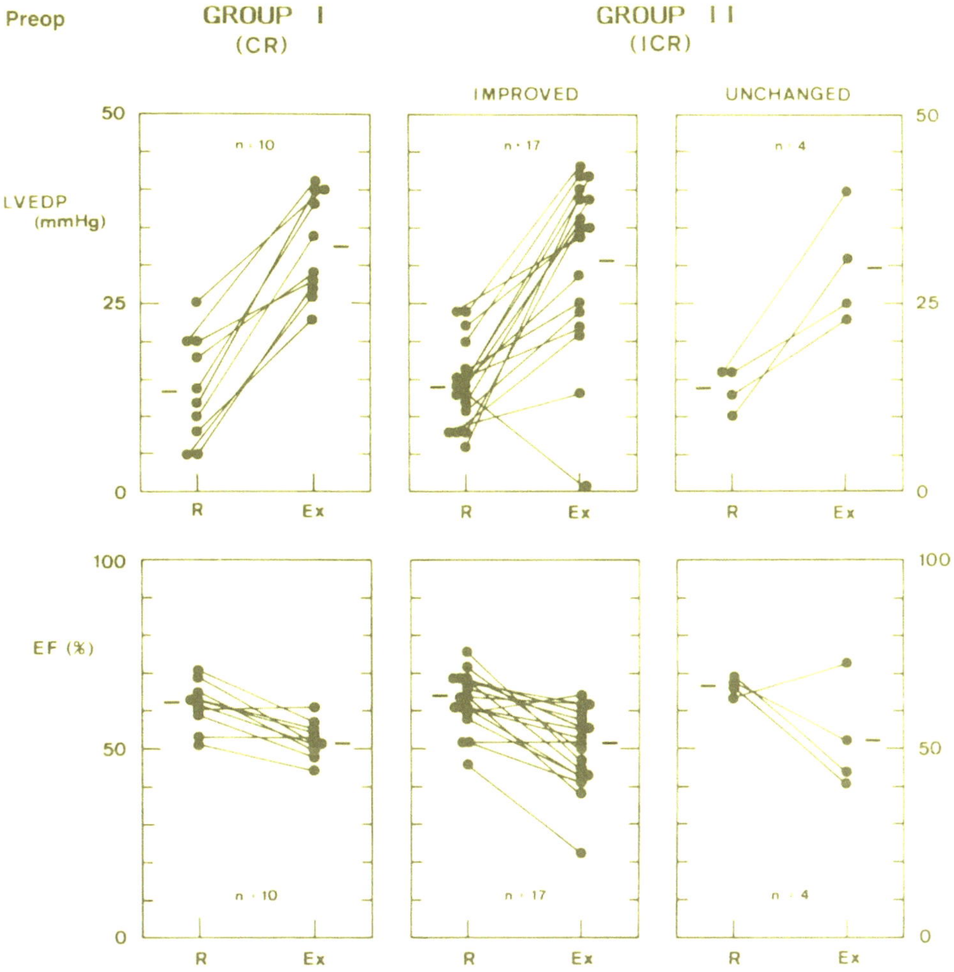

Fig. 2. Preoperative left ventricular end-diastolic pressure (*LVEDP*) and ejection fraction (*EF*) at rest (*R*) and during bicycle ergometry (*Ex*) in patients with coronary artery disease without infarction. Group I includes patients with subsequently complete revascularization; in group II are those with subsequently incomplete revascularization. Among the group II patients 17 patients had an improved revascularization index according to Levine et al. [51]; in 4 patients this index was unchanged postoperatively. Ex induced a sizeable increase in LVEDP and decrease of EF of similar extent in the three groups. *Horizontal bars*, mean values; CR, complete revascularization; *ICR*, incomplete revascularization; *n*, number of observations. (From Hirzel et al. [29], reproduced with permission of the publisher)

disease all three phases may undergo functional derangements which can be assessed by the time constant of left ventricular pressure decay, the peak rate of early rapid filling, and the steepness of the passive left ventricular diastolic pressure-volume relationship, respectively. Thus, the proper hemodynamic assessment of left ventricular relaxation and passive diastolic

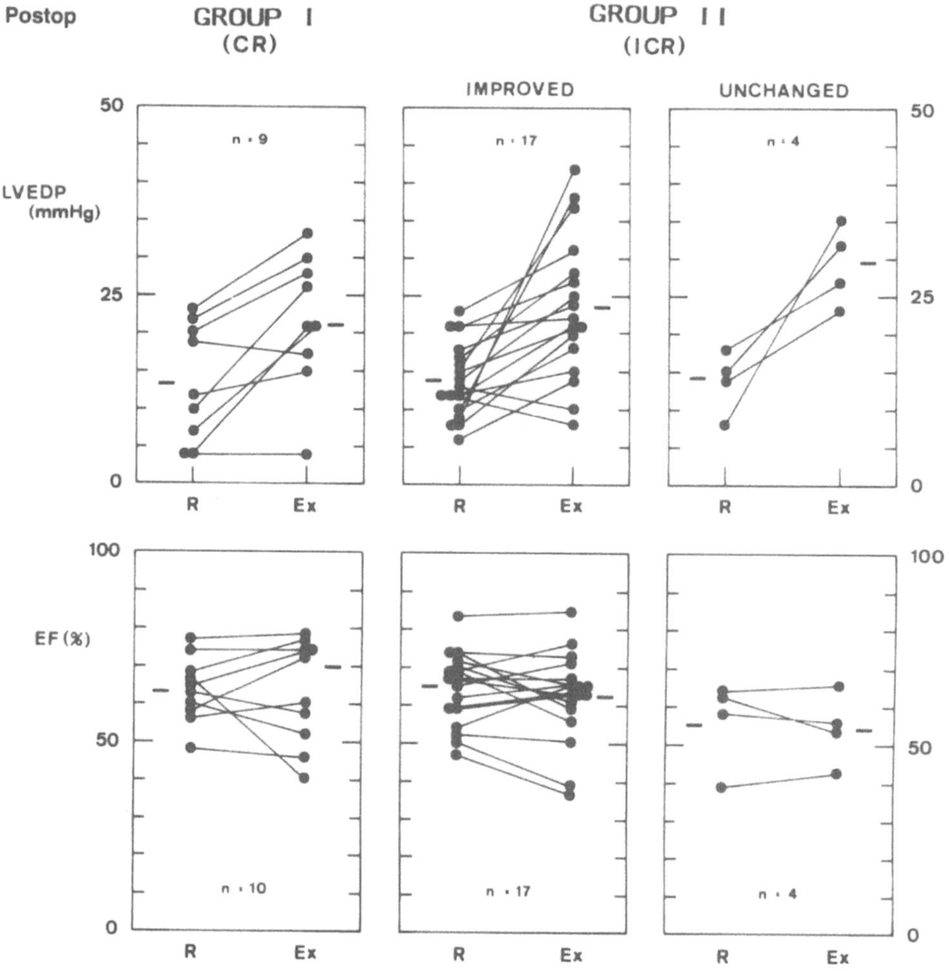

Fig. 3. Postoperative left ventricular end-diastolic pressure (*LVEDP*) and ejection fraction (*EF*) at rest (*R*) and during bicycle ergometry (*Ex*) in the same three patient groups as depicted in Fig. 2. In the patients with complete revascularization (*CR*) and improved vascularization LVEDP during Ex is lower than at the preoperative study. In the patients with unchanged vascularization after surgery LVEDP increases to the same value as at the preoperative study. In the completely revascularized patients (group I) and in the patients with improved vascularization EF during Ex was higher at the postoperative than at the preoperative study. In the patients with unchanged vascularization exercise EF was unchanged. (From Hirzel et al. [29], reproduced with permission of the publisher)

function requires invasive measurements whereas peak filling velocity (in cm/sec) and rate (ml/sec) can be determined by Doppler echocardiography and magnetic resonance imaging. It must, however, be pointed out that the isolated assessment of early filling dynamics gives an incomplete and sometimes misleading picture of left ventricular "diastolic function" because early rapid filling is determined by a variety of factors such as elastic recoil, speed of relaxation, atrial driving pressure, and left ventricular passive chamber compliance [46]. Some of these factors have antagonistic effects on the magnitude of early diastolic filling velocity and rate. For instance, increased atrial driving pressure may "normalize" reduced early rapid filling consequent to loss of elastic recoil (high end-systolic volume) and/or decreased rate of relaxation. Thus, caution is mandatory in using the popular Doppler echocardiographic diastolic velocity measurements to evaluate left ventricular "diastolic function."

There are only few data available concerning the various aspects of left ventricular diastolic function after coronary bypass surgery [30, 31, 47]. Especially, information on the effect of graft failure on diastolic function is lacking. In patients with patent grafts restudied 7.7 months after surgery we have found at rest no change in the time constant of left ventricular pressure decay, peak early filling rate, or diastolic pressure-volume relationship [30]. Similarly, Gibson et al. [31] and Lawson et al. [47], using angiography and Doppler echocardiography, respectively, observed no change in early diastolic filling dynamics after bypass surgery. During postoperative exercise the workload which was matched to the preoperative

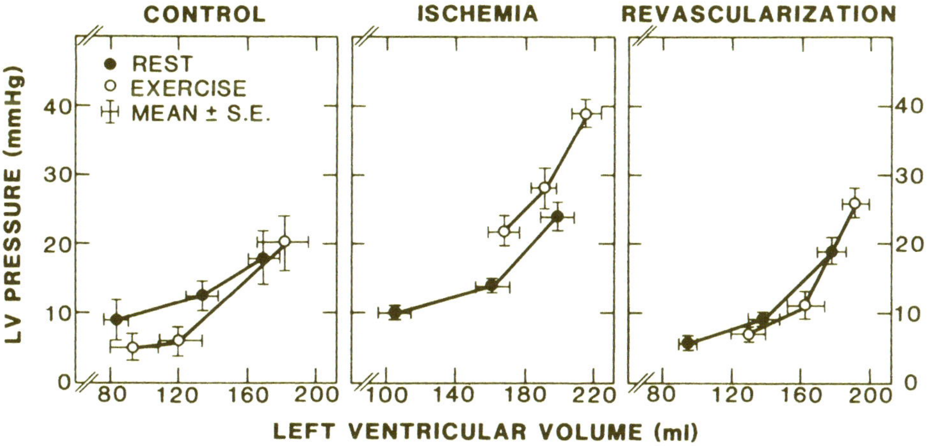

Fig. 4. Resting and exercise diastolic pressure-volume relationships in controls, preoperative patients with exercise-induced ischemia, and after revascularization. Coordinates of pressure are averages at three diastolic points: the early diastolic pressure nadir, mid-diastole and end-diastole. *Left*, the control group had a downward shift in the early diastolic pressure-volume relationship; *middle*, during preoperative exercise an upward shift developed; *right*, the preoperative upward shift was reversed by revascularization. Despite the lack of ischemia left ventricular end-diastolic pressure was significantly elevated during postoperative exercise. Moreover, there was no early diastolic pressure reduction during exercise as in the controls. Hence, despite full revascularization there remain some minute abnormalities of the passive diastolic pressure-volume relationship. (From Carroll et al. [30], reproduced with permission of the American Heart Association)

level there were, however, significant improvements in left ventricular diastolic function [30]; the time constant of left ventricular pressure decay decreased from 37 to 30 ms ($p < 0.01$), peak early filling rate increased from 950 to 1260 ml/s ($p < 0.01$), the lowest early diastolic left ventricular pressure decreased from 21 to 6 mmHg ($p < 0.001$), and the left ventricular end-diastolic pressure from 37 to 25 mmHg ($p < 0.001$). The preoperatively observed upward shift of the left ventricular diastolic pressure-volume curve during exercise was reversed by revascularization (Fig. 4). Nevertheless, there remained some minute alterations of diastolic function mainly concerning the pressure decay and the passive diastolic pressure-volume relationship in this optimally revascularized group of patients when compared to the exercise dynamics of controls. These diastolic abnormalities manifested during exercise were not due to acute ischemia because systolic regional wall motion disorders were absent. They are likely to reflect increased amounts of interstitial fibrosis and myocardial hypertrophy which were observed in transmural left ventricular biopsies of patients with coronary artery disease but fully preserved left ventricular contractile function at rest [48].

The knowledge of these diastolic functional abnormalities in patients with patent grafts is important when ischemia-induced diastolic functional derangements related to graft occlusion or progression of coronary artery disease are to be properly assessed.

Left Ventricular Function in Candidates for Coronary Reoperation

Some 50% of reoperations are carried out for graft failure, 20%–30% primarily for progression of native coronary artery disease, and the remainder for incomplete initial revascularization. Although the impact of left ventricular dysfunction on the risk of reoperation has not been formally established one might infer from the results of the first operations in CASS [49] that there is increasing operative mortality with increasing left ventricular dysfunction. Thus, it is of great practical importance to what extent left ventricular function is altered in postoperative patients who are candidates for reoperation [50]. Because the consequences of graft failure in these symptomatic patients might not necessarily be comparable to those of graft blockage or stenoses occasionally detected in postoperative patients recatheterized for routine purposes, we have evaluated left ventricular function in 22 patients who underwent reoperation for vein graft failure and had both the invasive study prior to the initial bypass grafting and that in view of repeat surgery at the Division of Cardiology of the Medical Policlinic of the University Hospital in Zurich between 1977 and 1989.

Demographic and hemodynamic data of these patients are given in Table 5. All were men and their functional limitation according to the NYHA class was similar prior to the first and the second coronary bypass

Table 5. Demographics and left ventricular systolic function in 22 patients reoperated for vein graft failure

	Age (years)	NYHA class	VI	EF (%)	EDVI (ml/m^2)	LVEDP (mmHg)	HR (bpm)
Cath prior to initial CABG	54	2.8	−2.1	58	99	10.6	79
Cath prior to repeat surgery	58	2.8	−2.0	51	103	13.5	69
p		NS	NS	<0.05	NS	NS	<0.01

Cath, Catheterization; CABG, coronary artery bypass grafting; VI, vascularization index. Other abbreviations as in Tables 1 and 2. The *p* values were obtained by the paired *t* test; NS, not significant.

operation. Only vein grafts were used at the initial surgery. On average only 1.3 of 3.4 placed grafts per patient were functioning prior to repeat surgery and the vascularization index according to Levine et al. [51], which takes into account the state of the native arteries, and that of the grafts was reduced to a similar extent at both catheterizations. There was an interval of 44 months between the two invasive studies.

Similarly to the pooled data of the literature in patients with nonfunctioning grafts (Table 3), ejection fraction was decreased in the 22 patients who were reoperated on for vein graft failure (Table 5). The reduction in ejection fraction occurred essentially in a subgroup of 7 patients (group 1) who had suffered a clinical myocardial infarction during the time span from the initial surgery to the second catheterization (decrease from 65% to 49%; Fig. 5). In the other 15 patients (group 2) ejection fraction remained stable (55% at the first and 52% at the second catheterization). Interestingly, the vascularization index prior to repeat surgery did not differ in the two subgroups (−1.7 in group 1 and −2.2 in group 2) although graft patency was less in group 1 (0.6 of 3.1 per patient, 19%) than in group 2 (1.4 of 3.5 per patient, 40%).

Thus, the experience at our hospital demonstrates that the patients reoperated for vein graft failure are those whose ejection fraction was essentially unchanged (in two-thirds) or had moderately decreased consequent to an intercurrent myocardial infarction (in one-third).

Summary

Depression of left ventricular systolic function in the early postoperative period is seldom the consequence of acute graft failure but is much more likely due to reversible myocardial stunning consequent to some degree of intraoperative ischemic-hypoxic injury.

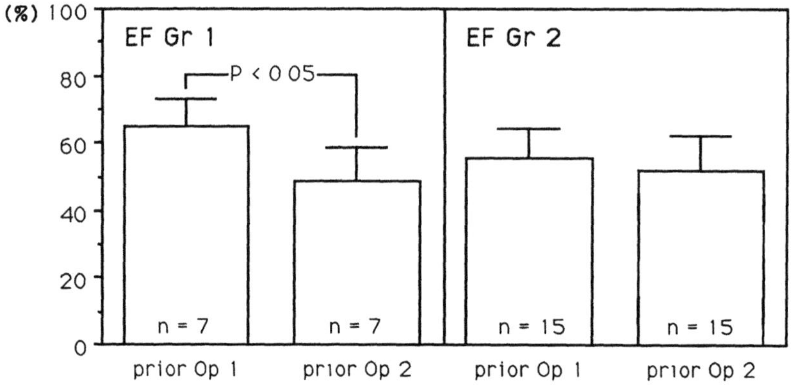

Fig. 5. Left ventricular ejection fraction (*EF*) prior to the initial coronary operation (*Op 1*) and prior to repeat surgery due to vein graft failure. In a subgroup of 7 patients (*Gr 1*) who had suffered a clinical myocardial infarction during the time span from the initial surgery to the second catheterization EF decreased significantly whereas in 15 patients (*Gr 2*) without an event of infarction ejection fraction remained essentially unchanged. *Bars*, mean values ±1 SD

With bypasses patent at follow-up investigations, resting left ventricular systolic function was found to change little if preoperative ejection fraction exceeded 60%. In contrast, patients with acute preinfarction syndrome or unstable angina and resting asynergy elicit in most instances a marked postoperative improvement of ejection fraction. With nonfunctioning grafts at follow-up resting ejection fraction decreased significantly in 50% of the reported studies.

With grafts patent, exercise regional left ventricular shortening dynamics and ejection fraction improve compared with preoperative exercise data. In patients with occluded grafts or incomplete revascularization the ejection fraction decreases during exercise, and its absolute value is similar to the preoperative exercise ejection fraction.

Left ventricular diastolic function remains unchanged at rest after successful revascularization. During exercise, however, significant improvements were noted, such as a decrease in the time constant of left ventricular pressure decay, an increase in the early peak filling rate, and a decrease in the early diastolic and end-diastolic left ventricular pressure. No data on follow-up diastolic function in patients with occluded grafts are available.

In our experience patients recruited for reoperation due to vein graft failure are those whose ejection fraction was unchanged or had only moderately decreased consequent to an intercurrent myocardial infarction.

References

1. Boudoulas H, Lewis RP, Vasko JS, Karayannacos PE, Beaver BM (1976) Left ventricular function and adrenergic hyperactivity before and after saphenous vein bypass. Circulation 53:802–806
2. Braunwald E, Kloner RA (1982) The stunned myocardium: prolonged, postischemic ventricular dysfunction. Circulation 66:1146–1149
3. Braunwald E (1991) Stunning of the myocardium. Cardiovasc Drugs Ther 5:849–852
4. Roberts AJ, Spies SM, Sanders JH, Moran JM, Wilkinson CJ, Lichtenthal PR, White RL, Michaelis LL (1981) Serial assessment of left ventricular performance following coronary artery bypass grafting. J Thorac Cardiovasc Surg 81:69–84
5. Righetti A, Crawford MH, O'Rourke RA, Schelbert H, Daily PO, Ross J Jr (1977) Interventricular septal motion and left ventricular function after coronary bypass surgery. Am J Cardiol 39:372–377
6. Breisblatt WM, Stein KL, Wolfe CJ, Follansbee WP, Capozzi J, Armitage JM, Hardesty RL (1990) Acute myocardial dysfunction and recovery: a common occurrence after coronary bypass surgery. J Am Coll Cardiol 15:1261–1269
7. Ballantyne CM, Verani MS, Short HD, Hyatt C, Noon GP (1987) Delayed recovery of severely "stunned" myocardium with the support of a left ventricular assist device after coronary artery bypass graft surgery. J Am Coll Cardiol 10:710–712
8. Kent KM, Borer JS, Green MV, Bacharach SL, McIntosh CL, Conkle DM, Epstein SE (1978) Effects of coronary artery bypass on global and regional left ventricular function during exercise. N Engl J Med 298:1434–1439
9. Dilsizian V, Bonow RO, Cannon RO III, Tracy CM, Vitale DF, McIntosh CL, Clark RE, Bacharach SL, Green MV (1988) The effect of coronary artery bypass grafting on left ventricular systolic function at rest: evidence for preoperative subclinical myocardial ischemia. Am J Cardiol 61:1248–1254
10. Hammermeister KE, Kennedy JW, Hamilton GW, Stewart DK, Gould KL, Lipscomb K, Murray JA (1974) Aortocoronary saphenous-vein bypass. Failure of successful grafting to improve resting left ventricular function in chronic angina. N Engl J Med 290:186–192
11. Apstein CS, Kline SA, Levin DC, Baltaxe HA, Killip T (1977) Left ventricular performance and graft patency after coronary artery-saphenous vein bypass surgery: early and late follow-up. Am Heart J 93: 547–555
12. Wolf NM, Kreulen TH, Bove AA, McDonough MT, Kessler KM, Strong M, LeMole G, Spann JF (1978) Left ventricular function following coronary bypass surgery. Circulation 58:63–70
13. Hellman CK, Kamath ML, Schmidt DH, Anholm J, Blau F, Johnson WD (1980) Improvement in left ventricular function after myocardial revascularization. J Thorac Cardiovasc Surg 79:645–655
14. Lim YL, Kalff V, Kelly MJ, Mason PJ, Currie PJ, Harper RW, Anderson ST, Federman J, Stirling GR, Pitt A (1982) Radionuclide angiographic assessment of global and segmental left ventricular function at rest and during exercise after coronary artery bypass surgery. Circulation 66:972–979
15. Kronenberg MW, Pederson RW, Harston WE, Born ML, Bender HW Jr, Friesinger GC (1983) Left ventricular performance after coronary artery bypass surgery. Prediction of functional benefit. Ann Intern Med 99:305–313
16. Melandri G, Maresta A, Contrafatto I, Tartagni F, Magnani B (1987) Effects of coronary artery revascularization and perioperative myocardial infarction on left ventricular wall motion. Int J Cardiol 15:47–54
17. Freeman MR, Gray RJ, Berman DS, Maddahi J, Raymond MJ, Forrester JS, Matloff JM (1981) Improvement in global and segmental left ventricular function after coronary bypass surgery. Circulation 64 [Suppl II]:34–39

18. Taylor NC, Barber RW, Crossland P, English TA, Wraight EP, Petch MC (1983) Effects of coronary artery bypass grafting on left ventricular function assessed by multiple gated ventricular scintigraphy. Br Heart J 50:149–156
19. Rees G, Bristow JD, Kremkau EL, Green GS, Herr RH, Griswold HE, Starr A (1971) Influence of aortocoronary bypass surgery on left ventricular performance. N Engl J Med 284:1116–1120
20. Arbogast R, Solignac A, Bourassa MG (1973) Influence of aortocoronary saphenous vein bypass surgery on left ventricular volumes and ejection fraction. Am J Med 54:290–296
21. Chatterjee K, Swan HJC, Parmley WW, Sustaita H, Marcus HS, Matloff J (1973) Influence of direct myocardial revascularization on left ventricular asynergy and function in patients with coronary heart disease. Circulation 47:276–286
22. Bolooki H, Mallon S, Ghahramani A, Sommer E, Vargas A, Slavin D, Kaiser GA (1973) Objective assessment of the effects of aorto-coronary bypass operation on cardiac function. J Thorac Cardiovasc Surg 66:916–933
23. Hamby RI, Tabrah F, Aintablian A, Hartstein ML, Wisoff BG (1974) Left ventricular hemodynamics and contractile pattern after aortocoronary bypass surgery. Am Heart J 88:149–159
24. Shepherd RL, Itscoitz SB, Glancy DL, Stinson EB, Reis RL, Olinger GN, Clark CE, Epstein SE (1974) Deterioration of myocardial function following aortocoronary bypass operation. Circulation 49:467–475
25. Chatterjee K, Matloff JM, Swan HJC, Ganz W, Kaushik VS, Magnusson P, Henis MM, Forrester JS (1975) Abnormal regional metabolism and mechanical function in patients with ischemic heart disease: improvement after successful regional revascularization by aortocoronary bypass. Circulation 52:390–399
26. Chesebro JH, Ritman EL, Frye RL, Smith HC, Connolly DC, Rutherford BD, Davis GD, Danielson GK, Pluth JR, Barnhorst DA, Wallace RB (1976) Videometric analysis of regional left ventricular function before and after aortocoronary artery bypass surgery: correlation of peak rate of myocardial wall thickening with late postoperative graft flows. J Clin Invest 58:1339–1347
27. Zir LM, Dinsmore R, Vexeridis M, Singh JB, Harthorne JW, Daggett WM (1979) Effects of coronary bypass grafting on resting left ventricular contraction in patients studies 1 to 2 years after operation. Am J Cardiol 44:601–606
28. Bussmann WD, Mayer V, Kober G, Kaltenbach M (1979) Ventricular function at rest, during leg raising and physical exercise before and after aortocoronary bypass surgery. Am J Cardiol 43:488–493
29. Hirzel HO, Wegmüller R, Grimm J, Krayenbuehl HP (1982) Die Funktion des linken Ventrikels bei Patienten mit koronarer Herzkrankheit vor und nach aorto-koronarer Bypass-Operation in Ruhe und unter fahrradergometrischer Belastung. Herz 7:63–75
30. Carroll JD, Hess OM, Hirzel HO, Turina M, Krayenbuehl HP (1985) Left ventricular systolic and diastolic function in coronary artery disease: effects of revascularization on exercise-induced ischemia. Circulation 72:119–129
31. Gibson DG, Greenbaum RA, Pridie RB, Yacoub MH (1988) Correction of left ventricular asynchrony by coronary artery surgery. Br Heart J 59:304–308
32. Braunwald E, Rutherford JD (1986) Reversible ischemic left ventricular dysfunction: evidence for the "hibernating myocardium." J Am Coll Cardiol 8:1467–1470
33. Barry WH, Pfeifer JF, Lipton MJ, Tilkian AG, Hultgren HN (1976) Effects of coronary artery bypass grafting on resting and exercise hemodynamics in patients with stable angina pectoris: a prospective randomized study. Am J Cardiol 37:823–829
34. Bourassa MG, Lespérance J, Campeau L, Saltiel J (1972) Fate of left ventricular contraction following aortocoronary venous grafts. Early and late postoperative modifications. Circulation 46:724–730
35. Brundage BH, Massie BM, Botvinick EH (1984) Improved regional ventricular function after successful surgical revascularization. J Am Coll Cardiol 3:902–908

36. Popio KA, Gorlin R, Bechtel D, Levine JA (1977) Postextrasystolic potentiation as a predictor of potential myocardial viability: preoperative analyses compared with studies after coronary bypass surgery. Am J Cardiol 39:944–953
37. Cooper MW, Lutherer LO, Stanton MW, Lust RM Jr (1986) Postextrasystolic potentiation: Regional wall motion before and after revascularization. Am Heart J 111:334–339
38. Helfant RH, Pine R, Meister SG, Feldman MS, Trout RG, Banka VS (1974) Nitroglycerin to unmask reversible asynergy: correlations with post coronary bypass ventriculography. Circulation 50:108–113
39. Chesebro JH, Ritman EL, Frye RL, Smith HC, Rutherford BD, Fulton RE, Pluth JR, Barnhorst DA (1978) Regional myocardial wall thickening response to nitroglycerin. A predictor of myocardial response to aortocoronary bypass surgery. J Clin Invest 57:952–957
40. Kolibash AJ, Goodenow JS, Bush CA, Tetalman MR, Lewis RP (1979) Improvement of myocardial perfusion and left ventricular function after coronary artery bypass grafting in patients with unstable angina. Circulation 59:66–74
41. Rutherford BD, Gau GT, Danielson GK, Pluth JR, Davis GD, Wallace RB, Frye RL (1972) Left ventricular haemodynamics before and soon after saphenous vein bypass graft operation for angina pectoris. Br Heart J 34:1156–1162
42. Campeau L, Elias G, Esplugas E, Lespérance J, Bourassa MG, Grondin CM (1974) Left ventricular performance during exercise before and one year after aortocoronary bypass surgery for angina pectoris. Circulation 50 [Suppl II]:103–110
43. Vliestra RE, Chesebro JH, Frye RL, Wallace RB (1981) Improvement of left ventricular exercise hemodynamic function after aorto-coronary artery bypass grafting. J Thorac Cardiovasc Surg 81:85–91
44. Chesebro JH, Ritman EL, Frye RL, Smith HC, Vliestra RE, Pluth JR (1982) Left ventricular performance before and after aortocoronary bypass surgery. Circulation 65 [Suppl II]:98–105
45. Brutsaert DL, Rademakers FE, Sys SU (1984) Triple control of relaxation: implications in cardiac disease. Circulation 69:190–196
46. Carroll JD, Hess OM, Hirzel HO, Krayenbuehl HP (1983) Dynamics of left ventricular filling at rest and during exercise. Circulation 68:59–67
47. Lawson WE, Seifert F, Anagnostopoulos C, Hills DJ, Swinford RD, Cohn PF (1988) Effect of coronary artery bypass grafting on left ventricular diastolic function. Am J Cardiol 61:283–287
48. Hess OM, Schneider J, Nonogi H, Carroll JD, Schneider K, Turina M, Krayenbuehl HP (1988) Myocardial structure in patients with exercise-induced ischemia. Circulation 77:967–977
49. Myers WO, Davis K, Foster ED, Maynard C, Kaiser GC (1985) Surgical survival in the Coronary Artery Surgery Study (CASS) registry. Ann Thorac Surg 40:245–260
50. Egloff L, Studer M, Rothlin M, Hess OM, Turina M, Senning Å (1984) Koronare Reoperation – ja oder nein? Schweiz Med Wochenschr 114:1123–1126
51. Levine JA, Bechtel DJ, Cohn PF, Herman MV, Gorlin R, Cohn LH, Collins JJ Jr (1975) Ventricular function before and after direct revascularization surgery. Circulation 51: 1071–1078

Biological Characteristics and Coronary Bypass Grafts

Endothelium and Vascular Smooth Muscle Function of Coronary Bypass Grafts

T.F. Lüscher, Z. Yang, and B.S. Oemar

Introduction

The current surgical technique to treat patients with coronary artery disease is the implantation of autologous blood vessels into the aorta and distal to an obstructing lesion into the coronary circulation. Although this therapeutic approach does not prevent progression of the atherosclerotic process in the coronary circulation, it does provide appropriate blood flow if the blood vessels remain open and able to adapt their blood flow to the requirements of the coronary circulation. The function and patency of coronary bypass grafts is influenced by (a) the runoff into the coronary vascular bed supplied by the graft, (b) blood-borne factors (i.e., platelets, coagulation factors, cardiovascular risk factors), and (c) biological properties of the bypass vessel itself. Recently, it became obvious that biological properties of blood vessels very considerably depend on their anatomical origin, native physiological role, and size [1]. In addition, clinical experience with a number of coronary bypass vessels has supported the notion that biological properties of grafts are a crucial determinant of their function and patency [2]. Of particular importance are the antithrombotic properties of bypass vessel, their ability to adapt to the requirements of the coronary circulation, and their propensity to develop proliferative atherosclerotic changes after implantation.

Coronary Bypass Vessels

A number of blood vessels has been used for coronary bypass grafting, in particular the saphenous vein [3], veins of the upper limb, internal mammary artery [2], radial artery, right gastroepiploic artery [4, 5], and epigastric artery [6]. These blood vessels differ in their function and patency when used as coronary bypass grafts. Clinical studies have demonstrated that the internal mammary artery exhibits the highest patency rate, while in venous grafts occlusions commonly occur (see Loop, this volume; [2, 3]) particularly in the absence of antithrombotic drugs and in patients with cardiovascular risk factors. While the radial artery exhibits unsatisfactory results, newer arterial bypass vessels such as the right gastroepiploic artery and epigastric artery appear promising (see Suma, this volume; [4–6]). However, particularly with the right gastroepiploic artery, postoperative spasm can represent a clinical problem.

The different behavior of various bypass vessels as grafts must be related to different biological properties of the blood vessel wall, as differences in function and patency persist even when different types of bypass vessels are compared within the same patient or those supplying the same coronary vascular bed (i.e., left anterior descending coronary artery; [2]). This chapter updates a previously published review [7] and discusses the vascular biology of different coronary bypass vessels and the implications of these differences for their antithrombotic properties, physiological regulation, and propensity to develop proliferative changes.

The Role of the Endothelium

The endothelium plays a regulatory role as an activator and inactivator of circulating and local hormones, as a source regulating coagulation and platelet function, and a regulator of vascular tone and growth (see [1]).

The activity of *angiotensin-converting enzyme* (ACE) or kininase II which converts angiotensin I into a more potent vasoconstrictor peptide angiotensin II and inactivates bradykinin is more pronounced in the saphenous vein as compared to the internal mammary artery [8]. Hence, inhibition of the enzyme by ACE inhibitors augments endothelium-dependent relaxations to bradykinin and inhibits angiotensin I induced vasoconstrictions in the vein but not in the artery.

The *endothelial L-arginine pathway* is an important local regulator of platelet vessel wall interaction and vascular tone (Fig. 1) [9–11]. Indeed, nitric oxide which is formed from L-arginine is both a potent vasodilator and inhibitor of platelet adhesion and aggregation [12, 13]. Nitric oxide activates soluble guanylyl cyclase in vascular smooth muscle [14] and platelets and thereby reduces intracellular levels of calcium; this then mediates relaxation and platelet inhibition, respectively. The formation of nitric oxide in response to receptor-operated agonists is much less pronounced in the saphenous vein (even in preparations without endothelial damage; see below) than in the internal mammary artery (Fig. 2) [11, 15, 16], while the gastroepiploic artery exhibits similar endothelial function in response to acetylcholine, histamine, and substance P as the internal mammary artery (Fig. 3) [17]. All bypass vessels relax effectively in response to nitrovasodilators, indicating that their vascular smooth muscle is capable of forming cGMP [17]. Indeed, in the gastroepiploic artery the cGMP accumulated after stimulation with nitrovasodilators exceeds that of other bypass vessels [18].

In addition to relaxing factors, endothelial cells also release contracting factors (see [1]). No evidence for production of endothelium-derived con-

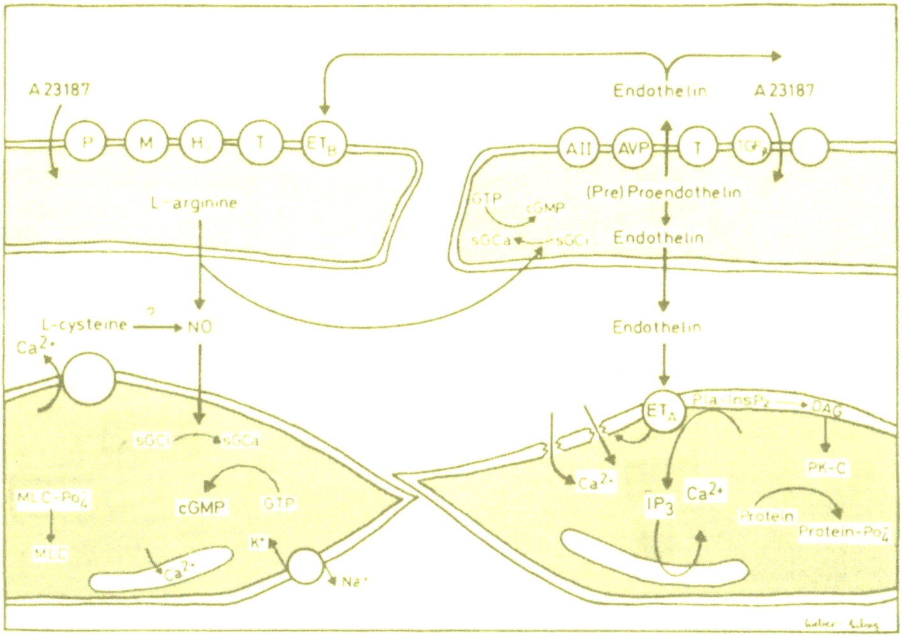

Fig. 1. Production of endothelium-derived nitric oxide (*NO*) and endothelin (*ET*) in the blood vessel wall. NO activates soluble guanylyl cyclase (sGC_i) which increases cyclic GMP. cGMP decreases intracellular Ca^{2+} and causes relaxation. NO increase cGMP in endothelial cells where it inhibits the production of ET. ET activates the vascular smooth muscle receptor (*open circle*; ET_A) mediating contraction via activation of Ca^{2+} channels, phospholipase C, inositol trisphosphate (IP_3), and diacyglycerol (*DAG*). ET also activates endothelial receptors (ET_B) linked to the formation of NO and prostacyclin. *AII*, Angiotensin II; *AVP*, arginine vasopressin; H_I, histaminergic receptor; *M*, muscarinic receptor; *MLC*, myosin light chain; *P*, substance P; *PK-C*, protein kinase C; *T*, thrombin receptor; TGF-β, transforming growth factor beta. (Modified from Luscher [76])

tracting factor in human arteries has been shown so far. By contrast, the endothelial cells of saphenous vein can release endothelium-derived contracting factors such as thromboxane A_2 in response to acetylcholine and prostaglandin H_2 in response to histamine [11]; both prostaglandins cause contraction and platelet activation.

Of particular interest for graft function is the fact, that the production of nitric oxide is stimulated by platelet-derived products such as adenosine diphosphate and triphosphate in the mammary artery, but not in the saphenous vein (even in veins in which the presence of functional endothelium has been previously confirmed by a relaxation to bradykinin [19]). Hence, mammary artery grafts exhibit endothelium-dependent relaxations and inhibition of platelet function at sites where platelets are activated (Fig. 4) [19]; this tends to flush away and disaggregate evolving platelet clots, while in the saphenous vein this important protective mechanism is not well

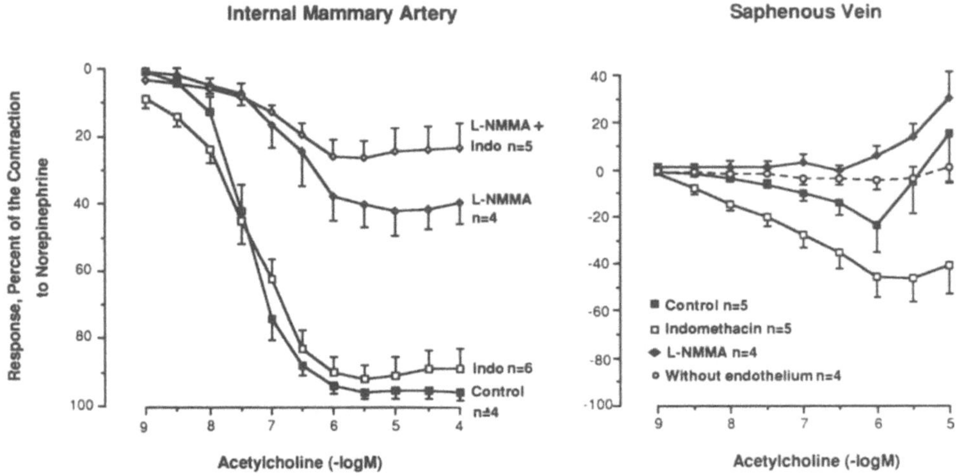

Fig. 2. The endothelial L-arginine pathway in human arterial and venous coronary bypass vessels. In the internal mammary artery acetylcholine causes full relaxation, which is unaffected by indomethacin but blunted by the inhibitor of nitric oxide formation L-N^G-monomethyl arginine (*L-NMMA*; *left panel*). In the saphenous vein the relaxations to acetylcholine are less pronounced, augmented by indomethacin and also prevented by L-NMMA (*right panel*). (Modified from Yang et al. [11])

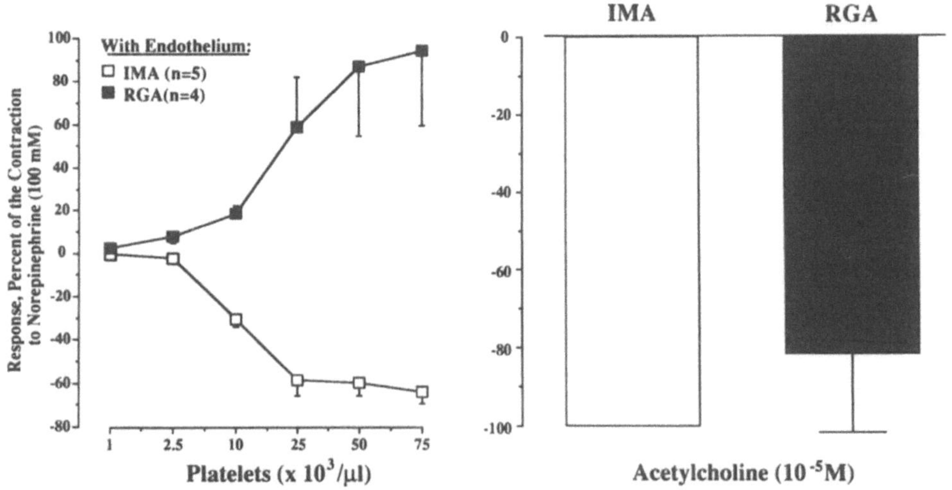

Fig. 3. Endothelium-dependent responses to platelets (*left panel*) and acetylcholine (*right panel*) in the internal mammary artery (*IMA*) and right gastroepiploic artery (*RGA*). While acetylcholine evokes comparable vascular relaxation in the two bypass vessels, platelets cause endothelium-dependent relaxations in the IMA but only contractions in the RGA. (Modified from Li et al. [20])

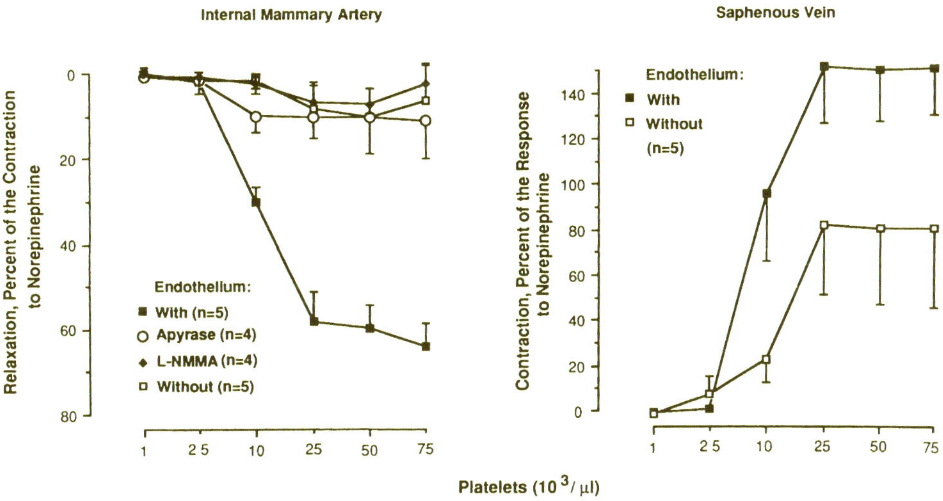

Fig. 4. Effects of aggregating platelets in the human internal mammary artery (*left*) and saphenous vein (*right*). While in the artery, platelets cause potent endothelium-dependent relaxations prevented by apyrase (to breakdown ATP and ADP) or L-N^G-monomethyl arginine (*L-NMMA*), platelets evoke potent and strong contractions facilitated by the endothelium in the vein. (Modified from Yang et al. [19])

developed (Fig. 5). Similar to the saphenous vein, the gastroepiploic artery exhibits marked contractions in response to aggregating platelets (Fig. 3) [20].

In addition, hormones such as bradykinin, histamine, and substance P are potent stimulators of nitric oxide production in mammary and gastroepiploic arteries, while the response particularly to histamine is less pronounced in the saphenous vein [11, 15–19]. Shear stress exerted by the circulating blood also stimulates the formation of nitric oxide (see [1]) and mediates flow-dependent vasodilation for instance during exercise. Internal mammary artery grafts but not saphenous vein grafts dilate in vivo during atrial pacing [21]. Thus, nitric oxide importantly contributes to the ability of arterial bypass vessels to respond to the flow requirements of the myocardium.

Prostacyclin is another endothelial mediator which is released in greater amounts in the mammary artery than in the saphenous vein [22]. Nitric oxide and prostacyclin potentiate each others action at the level of platelets, and hence both mediators contribute to antithrombotic properties of the endothelium [13]. Little is known about *tissue plasminogen activator* formed in coronary bypass vessels, another important endothelial mediator which helps to dissolve evolving blood clots.

Endothelin is a new 21 amino acid peptide produced and released by endothelial cells (Fig. 1) [23]. The peptide exhibits potent vasoconstrictor

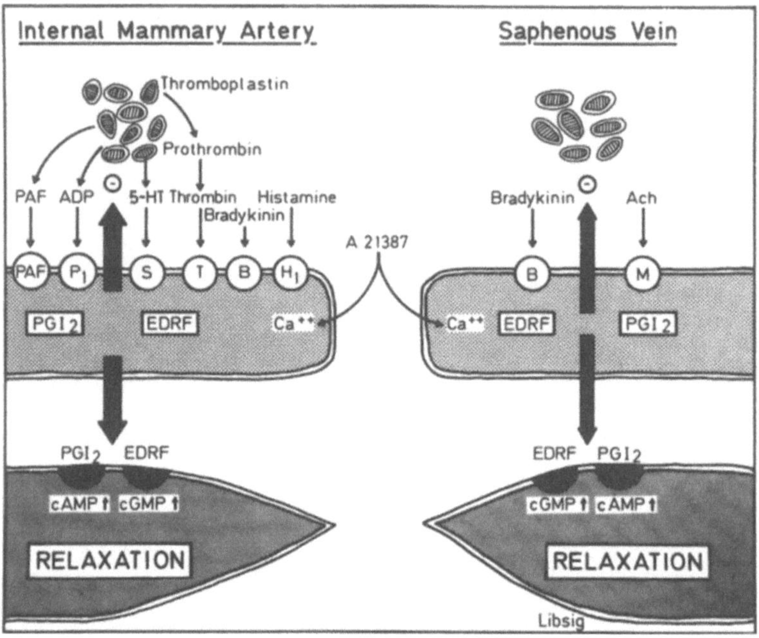

Fig. 5. Platelet vessel wall interaction in arterial (*left*) and venous coronary bypass grafts (*right*). In the internal mammary artery, platelets activate purinergic (P_l) and thrombin receptors (T) linked to the formation of endothellal-derived relaxing factor or nitric oxide. This mechanism leads to vasodilation and inhibition of platelet function and thereby plays an important protective role to maintain local graft blood flow and patency. In contrast in the vein, this pathway is less developed, and the contractile effects of thromboxane A_2 ($T\chi A_2$) and serotonin (*5-HT*, 5-hydroxytryptamine) predominate. *ADP*, Adenosine diphosphate; *Ach*, acetylcholine; *cGMP*, cyclic 3′5′-guanosine monophosphate; S_2, $5HT_2$-serotonergic receptor; O, receptor

effects on vascular smooth muscle which exceed those of norepinephrine, angiotensin II, and serotonin in human bypass grafts [24]. In both the mammary artery and saphenous vein, endothelium-derived nitric oxide or nitrovasodilators but not Ca^{2+} antagonists effectively inhibit endothelin-induced contractions [24, 25]. The amount of endothelin formed in coronary bypass vessels remains to be determined, but thrombin, angiotensin II and transforming growth factor beta (TGF-β; released from platelets) may stimulate the production of this potent peptide (Fig. 1; [23, 26]).

Endothelial cells are also a source of *growth inhibitors and activactors* (Fig. 6) [27, 28]. Important growth inhibitors secreted by endothelial cells are heparin and heparan sulfates, TGF-β_1 (which under certain conditions also may have proliferative properties; see below) and possibly also nitric oxide and prostacyclin [29–31]. Nitric oxide and prostacyclin may both have direct inhibitory effects on vascular smooth muscle proliferation via a formation of cGMP and cAMP, respectively, at least under certain con-

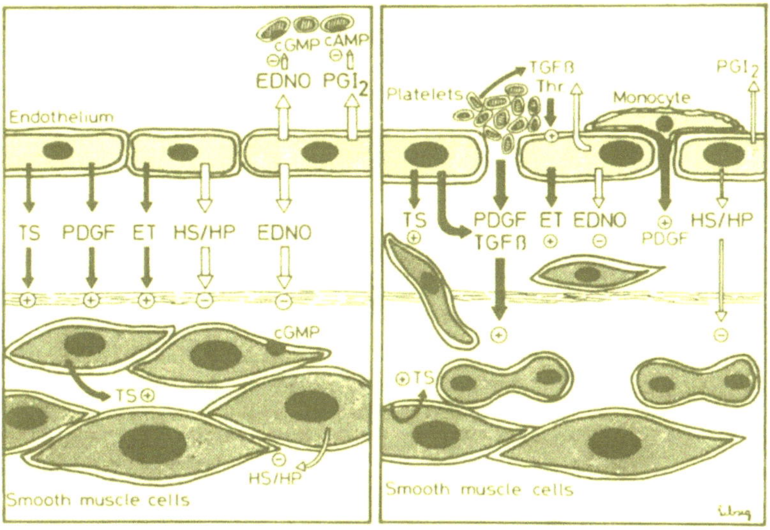

Fig. 6. Putative regulation of proliferative responses in the blood vessel wall. While under normal conditions, inhibitory stimuli (⊖) prevent vascular smooth muscle cell from modulating their phenotype, migrating, and proliferating (*left panel*), the latter responses predominate in the atherosclerotic blood vessel wall. ⊕, Stimulation; ⊖, inhibition; *HS/HP*, heparan sulfate/heparin; *Thr*, thrombin; *TS*, thrombospondin. (From Lüscher [7], by permission)

ditions; in addition, the antithrombotic properties of both mediators may be important. Indeed, deactivation of adhering and aggregating platelets may prevent or reduce the release of platelet-derived growth factor (PDGF) and other mediators and thereby limit the concentration of these potent proliferative substances within the blood vessel wall.

On the other hand, endothelial cells at least under certain conditions can produce growth factors, in particular PDGF and TGF-β (Fig. 6) [27–29]. TGF-β_1 stimulates proliferation of vascular smooth muscle cells at low concentrations, but is a potent antiproliferative substance at higher concentrations [29]. The effects of endothelin on proliferative responses of cells in culture are controversial; in vascular smooth muscle endothelin appears to exert no consistent proliferative effects on its own but may facilitate responses of other growth factors.

Vascular Smooth Muscle Cells

Vascular smooth muscle cells are the most important component of the media. They are primary regulators of vascular tone. In addition, vascular smooth muscle cells can change their phenotype (i.e., phenotypic modulation), secrete substances, migrate, and proliferate, an important process in atherosclerosis.

Contractile properties of coronary bypass vessels are determined by the number of receptors on the vascular smooth muscle cell membrane, their signal transduction pathway, the size of the blood vessels, the thickness of the media, and its histological composition. Indeed, muscular arteries such as the gastroepiploic artery exhibit marked contractile responses to all contractile agonists such as norepinephrine, serotonin, and potassium chloride [17, 32], while in elastic arteries such as the mammary artery the absolute increase in tension is less pronounced. The saphenous vein due to its size can exhibit marked contractile responses [15, 16].

The reactivity of the media to vasoconstrictor agents, however, is reduced by the endothelium through the basal release of nitric oxide [11] (see above). This basal release of nitric oxide is less pronounced in the saphenous vein than in the internal mammary artery and hence basal release of nitric oxide does reduce the effects of vasoconstrictor substances such as norepinephrine and serotonin in arterial bypass vessels but not in the saphenous vein [11, 16]. Endothelin, on the other hand, potentiates contractions of vascular smooth muscle to most vasoconstrictor agonists even at low and threshold concentrations in the mammary artery but not in the saphenous or mammary vein [33]. The mechanism involves an increased calcium sensitivity [33]. Thus, normally the endothelium protects vascular smooth cells of arterial grafts from vasoconstrictor substances; an increased formation of endothelin (for instance by thrombin or TGF-β released at sites of activated coagulation and platelets) may increase vascular tone and endanger graft blood flow.

Venous grafts exhibit marked *proliferative responses* as soon as they are implanted into the arterial circulation, leading to stenosis and eventually occlusion of the graft [2]; proliferation of vascular smooth muscle cells importantly contribute to this process [34]. Since in the mammary artery and also the gastroepiploic artery such changes are much less common, different biological properties of vascular smooth muscle cells of these arteries and the vein must be involved. Indeed, both arteries are almost free of atherosclerosis both as native vessels and after implantation in the coronary circulation [35–38]. This indicates that the smooth muscle cells of these arteries are less likely to dedifferentiate, migrate, and proliferate than those of the saphenous vein. Alternatively, more recent theories assume that there are two types of vascular smooth muscle cells in the media, one which is contractile and another which is dedifferentiated and able to proliferate and migrate [39]; under these conditions, one would suspect that the number of the latter type of vascular smooth muscle cells may be more prevalent in saphenous veins than in the mammary artery.

In the saphenous vein, vascular smooth muscle cell proliferation probably occurs in response to increases in transmural pressure and pulsatility [40] (Fig. 7; see "Chronic Changes After Implantation"). In addition, vascular

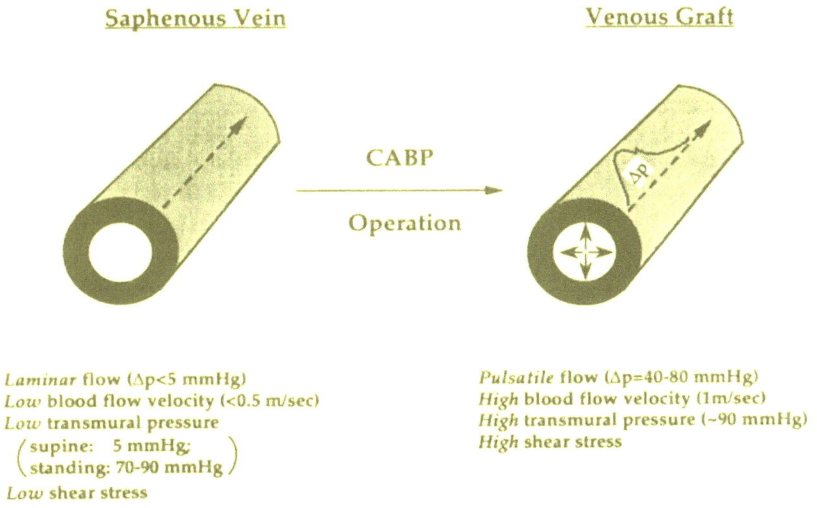

Fig. 7. Representation of hemodynamic changes occurring in the human saphenous vein after implantation in the coronary circulation during coronary artery bypass grafting (*CABG*)

injuries occurring during surgical preparation (see "Surgical Handling") leading to endothelial damage, and in turn local platelet activation and release of growth factors may make an important contribution. These events may be particularly important as recent clinical studies suggest that late vein graft stenoses are more dangerous (higher rate of death and cardiac events) than native coronary stenosis [41].

Surgical Handling

Surgical handling of coronary bypass vessels can profoundly affect their biological properties. Indeed, during *surgical preparation* endothelial damage occurs quite frequently, particularly in free grafts such as the saphenous vein and – if used as such – in the gastroepiploic or mammary artery [15, 42–48]. Endothelial denudation leads to platelet adhesion and aggregation and may contribute importantly to early graft occlusion [49]. In addition, adhering platelets release potent growth factors, in particular PDGF, which contribute to proliferative changes at sites of previous endothelial injury (Fig. 6).

The *pressurizing procedure* of grafts, which until recently was used frequently, also leads to extensive damage of the endothelium and (at higher pressure) the media. In many respects, the pressurizing procedure resembles angioplasty, and similar proliferative responses as those leading to restenosis may also be operative under these conditions, and hence this procedure should be avoided.

Although endothelial cells regrow within several days at sites of previous *mechanical endothelial injury*, their functional properties must not necessarily be normal after regeneration. Indeed, in the porcine coronary artery endothelial denudation is associated with specific dysfunctions of the regenerated endothelium, in particular with an impaired release of nitric oxide by platelet-derived serotonin, most likely due to a defective G_i protein associated with the serotonergic receptor [50].

Chronic Changes After Implantation

After implantation coronary bypass vessels are exposed to a different physiological environment with marked changes in blood flow velocities and diurnal changes in blood flow, transmural pressure, and pulsatility (particularly in the case of venous grafts; Fig. 7). In addition, at sites of vascular injury healing processes with marked migration and proliferation of vascular smooth muscle cells can occur (Fig. 6) [51]. Chronic vascular changes after implantation of coronary bypass vessels may relate to alterations of endothelial function and/or responses in vascular smooth muscle cells.

Endothelium-Dependent Vascular Responses. Compared to the saphenous vein studied before implantation, venous coronary bypass grafts develop somewhat more pronounced endothelium-dependent relaxations to acetylcholine, ADP, and thrombin after implantation, although the potency of these responses remains less pronounced than in arterial grafts [52]. Particularly at sites of mechanical injury (e.g., at the site of anastomoses) proliferative responses such as intimal hyperplasia develop. Intimal hyperplasia is associated with marked impairments of endothelium-dependent relaxations both in experimental animals and in humans [52–54]. In the rabbit reversed implantation of the jugular vein markedly reduces endothelium-dependent relaxation and a blunted reduction of cGMP in vascular smooth muscle [54].

Proliferative Processes. More insights into the biological mechanisms involved in proliferative responses, particularly within venous grafts after implantation, are crucial for the understanding and appropriate treatment of coronary bypass graft disease. Two intriguing observations help to elucidate this phenomenon. (a) The saphenous vein exhibits marked intimal hyperplasia and other proliferative changes only after implantation into the arterial side of the circulation. As under these conditions, most cardiovascular risk factors, particularly lipoproteins, circulating insulin, and glucose levels, remain the same, changes in hemodynamics such as pulsatile pressure, increased transmural pressure, increased shear forces due to increased flow velocities in the arterial circulation must contribute importantly (Fig. 7). Most likely, pulsatility represents the most important hemodynamic alteration to which saphenous veins are exposed to in the arterial circulation as pressure can also reach values of 70–80 mmHg during prolonged standing. (b) There are marked differences in the development of proliferative changes between venous and arterial conduits. This again suggests that different biological properties are crucially involved in venous bypass graft disease as the cells must respond differently to the same physiological environment.

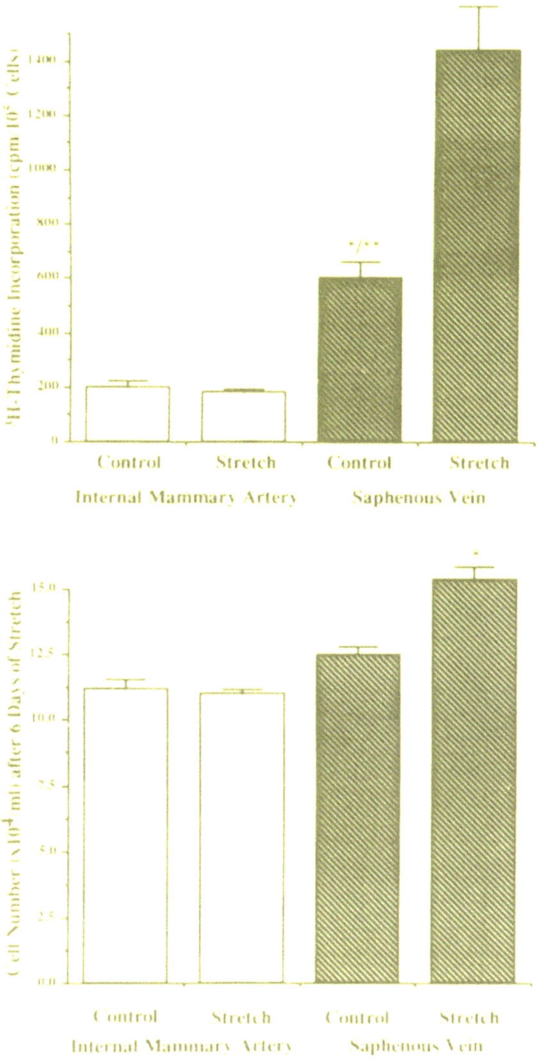

Fig. 8. Effects of pulsatile stretch on [^{3}H]thymidine incorporation (*top panel*) and cell replication (*lower panel*) of vascular smooth muscle cells in culture obtained from the human internal mammary artery (*open bars*) and saphenous vein (*hatched bars*). (From [40], by permission)

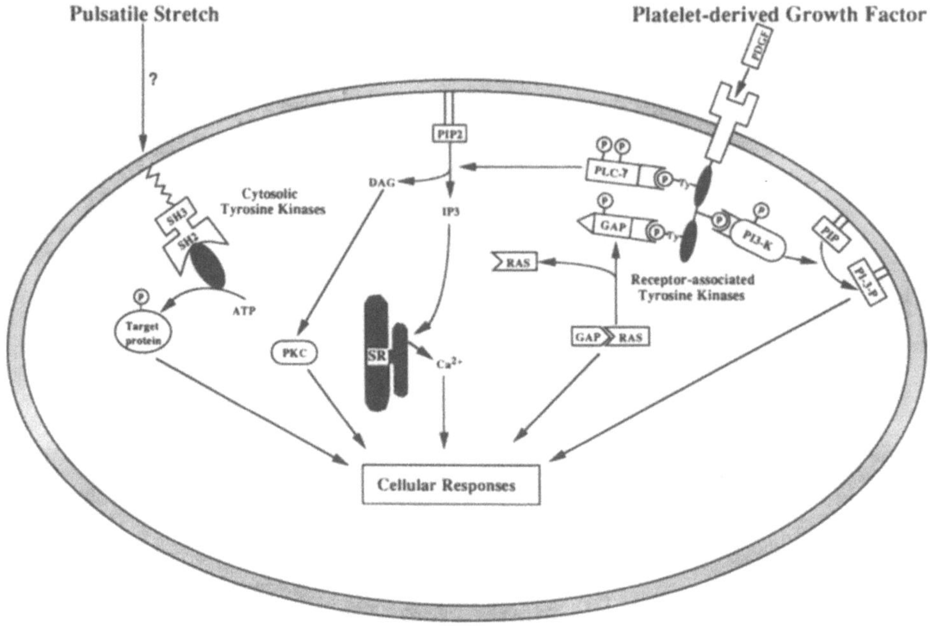

Fig. 9. Intracellular signal transduction pathway is activated by proliferative stimuli. Platelet-derived growth factor (*PDGF*) activates specific receptors. Autophosphorylation of these receptors by receptor-associated tyrosine kinases leads to activation of secondary pathways such as phospholipase C (*PLC-γ*), PI_3-*K* (phosphatidylinositide-3-kinase), and *GAP* (GTAse activating protein). Similar mechanisms may also be operative in response to pulsatile stretch, although the evidence so far is only indirect. *DAG*, diacylglycerol; IP_3, inositol triphosphate; *P*, phosphorus; *PIP*, phosphatidylinositol phosphate; PIP_2, phosphatidylinositol, 4,5-bisphosphate; *PKC*, protein kinase C; *RAS*, ras protein encoded by ras proto-oncogenes; *SH*, Src homology domain; *SR*, sarcoplasmatic reticulum

Changes in hemodynamics have been studied in vitro using pulsatile stretch exerted to vascular smooth muscle cells in culture. Interestingly, pulsatile stretch markedly increases [^{3}H]thymidine incorporation in venous vascular smooth muscle cells and also increase cell number (Fig. 8) [40] while the internal mammary artery smooth muscle cells remained markedly resistant to this mechanical stimulus. These experimental data strongly suggest that changes in pulsatility and possibly also pressure contribute importantly to venous bypass graft disease.

The mechanisms by which pulsatile stretch stimulates cell growth must involve tyrosine kinase activation, since the specific tyrosine kinase inhibitor genistein (Fig. 9) [55] is able to inhibit this response. The exact mechanisms (e.g., which tyrosine kinase is involved) remain to be investigated.

In addition, implantation of saphenous veins into the coronary circulation is almost always associated with endothelial damage (see above). At sites where endothelial damage occurs platelets adhere, and in turn several growth factors are released, such as PDGF and TGF-β_1 Interestingly, PDGF is a very potent mitogen in the human saphenous vein vascular smooth muscle cells with a half-maximal concentration in nanomolar range, while PDGF does not stimulate growth in human mammary artery vascular smooth muscle, although fetal calf serum is effective [55]. Most likely, these differences are related to a different expression of PDGF receptors and/or a different efficiency of the signal transduction pathways in vascular smooth muscle of the two blood vessels (Fig. 9) [55]. TGF-β_1, on the other hand, does not stimulate growth but rather markedly inhibits PDGF-induced and stretch-induced proliferation in the human saphenous vein [55].

Effects of Cardiovascular Risk Factors

Bypass graft function and patency is known to be negatively influenced by the presence of hypercholesteremia, diabetes, hypertension, and smoking. All cardiovascular risk factors impair endothelial function and affect that of vascular smooth muscle cells [1].

Hypertension, oxidized low-density lipoproteins, diabetes, and particularly atherosclerosis impair endothelium-dependent relaxations (see [1]). While in early stages a defective receptor-operated formation of nitric oxide due to insufficient mobilization and/or synthesis of intracellular L-arginine is responsible [56, 57], later stages of atherosclerosis are associated with a generalized impairment of endothelial function [58–62]. On the other hand, oxidized low-density lipoprotein and possibly also diabetes and atherosclerosis may increase the production of endothelin [63].

Furthermore, low-density lipoproteins can stimulate growth of human vascular smooth muscle cells in culture which may explain part of their atherosclerotic potential, since migration and proliferation of vascular smooth muscle cells play a dominant part in that process (Fig. 6) [64].

Effects of Cardiovascular Drugs

As an increased platelet vessel wall interaction has been implicated in vein graft dysfunction and occlusion, *platelet inhibitors* as well as coumarins have been extensively used. Aspirin prevents the formation of thromboxane A_2, but does not interfere with other platelet-derived mediators such as ADP, ATP, serotonin, and growth factors. To prevent platelet-induced contractions in the human mammary artery without endothelium or the saphenous vein, a combined blockade of type 2 serotonergic receptors (by ketanserin) and of the endoperoxide/thromboxane A_2 receptor (for instance, by SQ13080) is required [19]. The development of more potent platelet inhibitors such as monoclonal antibodies against the glycoprotein IIb/IIIa (which inhibit the final common pathway in the activation process of platelets) may provide new and more potent therapeutic tools in the prevention of vein graft occlusion. As the endothelium of the mammary artery has marked antithrombotic capacities, the use of antiplatelet drugs is less important in patients receiving arterial grafts, provided no major endothelial damage has occurred during implantation which would promote platelet activation.

Calcium antagonists such as nifedipine improve endothelial function [65] and not only appear to reduce the formation of new lesions in the coronary circulation [66] but also may be beneficial in reducing the complications of vein graft disease [67]. This antiproliferative effect of calcium antagonists may be related to inhibition of calcium entry [68] but may also involve other mechanisms such as inhibiton of tyrosine kinase and/or an interference of intracellular mechanisms mediating proliferation distal to this enzyme. In vascular smooth muscle cells in culture obtained from the human saphenous vein, verapamil markedly inhibits PDGF-stimulated smooth muscle cell growth but is unable to reduce proliferative responses stimulated by pulsatile stretch [55]. Preliminary experiments of our group suggest that the inhibition of PDGF-stimulated cell proliferation by verapamil is due to an interference of the calcium antagonist with postreceptor activation events because verapamil does not inhibit PDGF-induced receptor autophosphoration, which is a crucial step leading to cell proliferation (Fig. 9).

In the rat and rabbit, inhibition of ACE by *cilazapril* improves endothelial function [69] and prevents intimal hyperplasia after mechanical injury by a balloon catheter [70]. Although this therapeutic approach has proven inefficient in preventing restenosis in patients undergoing percutaneous transluminal coronary angioplasty, it remains possible that drugs of this class are effective in the prevention of intimal proliferation of venous grafts. Indeed, at least in the rat cilazapril inhibits wall thickening of the jugular vein implanted into the arterial circulation [71].

Certain *nitrovasodilators* such as 3-morpholino-sydnonimine (SIN-1; the active metabolite of molsidomine) have a spectrum of action resembling that of endothelium-derived nitric oxide [72]. It remains to be shown whether such nitric oxide donors are effective in preventing vein graft disease either through their ability to inhibit platelet activation, platelet-induced vasospasm, ischemia and/or vascular smooth muscle proliferation. Preliminary data of our group suggest that the nitric oxide donor SIN-1 has no significant antiproliferative effects in saphenous vein grafts, at least as judged from experiments performed in vascular smooth muscle cells in culture obtained from this blood vessel. Indeed, SIN-1 even at high concentrations does not prevent the [^{3}H]thymidine incorporation in venous vascular smooth muscle cells stimulated either by pulsatile stretch or PDGF [55].

Another approach to inhibit intimal thickening of venous graft is the use of *heparin*. In vitro study, heparin was found to strongly inhibit smooth muscle cell proliferation in culture [73]. In rabbit and rat vein graft models, heparin administrated intravenously inhibits the early but not late development of intima thickening [74, 75]. The effects of heparin on human vein graft intima thickening remain to be investigated.

Thus, three main biological factors importantly determine the pathogenesis of coronary bypass graft disease: (a) increased vasoconstrictor responses of the blood vessel wall to circulating hormones, (b) an increased platelet–vessel wall interaction, and (c) proliferation and migration of vascular smooth muscle cells. The endothelial cells from arterial bypass grafts release more relaxing factors (i.e., nitric oxide, prostacyclin) than venous bypass grafts. Furthermore, the endothelium of the saphenous vein produces contracting factors (i.e., cyclooxygenase-derived products PGH_2/TxA_2). These differences explain the increased platelet–vessel wall interaction in the saphenous vein. Moreover, smooth muscle cells from the saphenous vein, but not those from internal mammary artery proliferate in response to growth factors, i.e., PDGF, and mechanical forces such as pulsatile stretch. Hence, different biological properties of endothelial and smooth muscle cells of arterial and venous bypass vessels are most likely crucially involved in the development of coronary bypass graft disease, particularly in saphenous vein grafts. Based on these findings, cardiovascular drugs which protect endothelial function, inhibit platelet–vessel wall interaction and/or inhibit smooth muscle cell proliferation and migration would have the greatest clinical impact.

Acknowledgements. The authors would like to acknowledge the invaluable collaboration of Ludwig von Segesser, Erwin Bauer, Robert Siebenmann, Peter Stulz, and Marko Turina in this project. Further, we are indebted to Amanda de Sola Pinto and to Bernadette Weber-Libsig for their help in preparation of the manuscript. Original research reported in the manuscript was supported by grants from the Swiss National Research Foundation (no. 32-32541.91), Swiss Cardiology Foundation, Karl Mayer Foundation, Vaduz/Liechtenstein, Hartmann-Müller Foundation, and the Schweizerische Rentenanstalt.

References

1. Lüscher TF, Vanhoutte PM (1990) The endothelium modulator or cardiovascular function. CRC Press, Boca Raton, pp 1–215
2. Loop FD, Lytle BW, Cosgrove DM (1986) Influence of the internal mammary-artery graft on 10-year survival and other cardiac events. N Engl J Med 314:1–6
3. Lytle BW, Loop FD, Cosgrove DM, Ratliff NB, Easley K, Taylor PC (1985) Long-term (5 to 12 years) serial studies of internal mammary artery and saphenous vein coronary bypass grafts. J Thorac Cardiovasc Surg 89:248–258

4. Pym J, Brown PM, Charrette EJP, Parker JO, West RO (1987) Gastroepiploic-coronary anastomosis, a viable alternative bypass graft. J Thorac Cardiovasc Surg 94:256–259
5. Suma H, Fukumoto H, Takeuchi A (1987) Coronary artery bypass grafting by utilizing in situ right gastroepiploic artery: basic study and clinical application. Ann Thorac Surg 44:394–397
6. Puig LB, Ciongolli W, Cividanes VL, Dontos A, Kopel L, Bittencourt D, Assis VC, Jatente AD (1990) Inferior epigastric artery as a free graft for myocardial revascularization. J Thorac Cardiovasc Surg 99:251–255
7. Lüscher TF (1991) Vascular biology of coronary bypass grafts. Curr Opin Cardiol 6:868–876
8. Yang Z, Arnet U, von Segesser L, Siebenmann R, Turina M, Lüscher TF (1993) Different effects of angiotensin-converting enzyme inhibition in human arteries and veins. J Cardiovasc Pharmacol 22 (Suppl 5):S17–S22
9. Furchgott RF, Zawadzki JV (1980) The obligatory role of endothelial cells in the relaxation of arterial smooth muscle by acetylcholine. Nature 288:373–376
10. Palmer RMI, Ferrige AG, Moncada S (1987) Nitric oxide release accounts for the biological activity of endothelium-derived relaxing factor. Nature 327:524–526
11. Yang Z, von Segesser L, Bauer E, Stulz P, Turina M, Lüscher TF (1991) Different activation of endothelial L-arginine and cyclooxygenase pathway in human internal mammary artery and saphenous vein. Circ Res 68:52–60
12. Palmer RMJ, Ashtor DS, Moncada S (1988) Vascular endothelial cells synthesize nitric oxide from L-arginine. Nature 333:664–666
13. Radomski MW, Palmer RMJ, Moncada S (1987) The anti-aggregating properties of vascular endothelium: interactions between prostacyclin and nitric oxide. Br J Pharmacol 92:639–646
14. Rapoport RM, Murad F (1983) Agonist-induced endothelium-dependent relaxation in rat thoracic aorta may be mediated through cGMP. Circ Res 52:352–357
15. Lüscher TF, Diederich D, Siebenmann R, Lehmann K, Stulz P, von Segesser L, Yang Z, Turina M, Grädel G, Weber G, Bühler FR (1988) Difference between endothelium-dependent relaxations in arterial and in venous coronary bypass grafts. N Engl J Med 319:462–467
16. Yang Z, Diederich D, Schneider K, Siebenmann R, Stulz P, von Segesser L, Turina M, Bühler FR, Luscher TF (1989) Endothelium-derived relaxing factor and protection against contractions induced by histamine and serotonin in the human internal mammary artery and in the saphenous vein. Circulation 80:1041–1048
17. Yang Z, Siebenmann R, Studer M, Egloff L, Lüscher TF (1992) Similar endothelium-dependent relaxation, but enhanced contractility of the right gastroepiploic artery as compared to the internal mammary artery. J Thorac Cardiovasc Surg 104:459–464
18. O'Neil GS, Chester AH, Allen SP, Luu TN, Tadjkarimi S, Ridley P, Khagani A, Musumeci F, Yacoub MH (1991) Endothelial function of human gastroepiploic artery: implications for its use as a bypass graft. J Cardiovasc Surg 102:561–565
19. Yang Z, Stulz P, von Segesser L, Bauer E, Turina M, Lüscher TF (1991) Different interactions of platelets with arterial and venous coronary bypass vessels. Lancet 337: 939–943
20. Li X-N, Stulz P, Siebenmann PR, Yang Z, Luscher TF (1992) Different effects of activated platelets in the right gastroepiploic and internal mammary arteries. J Thorac Cardiovasc Surg 104:1294–1302
21. Hanet C, Schroeder E, Michel X, Gosyns J, Dion R, Verhelst R, Wijns W (1991) Flow-induced vasomotor response to tachycardia of the human internal mammary artery and saphenous vein grafts late following bypass surgery. Circulation 84 [Suppl III]:268–274
22. Subramanian VA, Hernandez Y, Rtack-Goldman K, Grabowski EF, Weksler BB (1986) Prostacyclin production by internal mammary artery as a factor in coronary artery bypass grafts. Surgery 100:376–383
23. Yanagisawa M, Kurihara H, Kimura S, Tomobe Y, Kobayashi M, Mitsui Y, Yazaki M, Goto K, Masaki T (1988) A novel potent vasoconstrictor peptide produced by vascular endothelial cells. Nature 332:411–415

24. Lüscher TF, Yang Z, Tschudi M et al. (1990) Interaction between endothelin-1 and endothelium-derived relaxing factor in human arteries and veins. Circ Res 66:1088–1094
25. Yang Z, Bauer E, von Segesser L, Stulz P, Turina M, Luscher TF (1990) Different mobilization of calcium in endothelin-1-induced contractions in human arteries and veins: effects of calcium antagonists. J Cardiovasc Pharmacol 16:654–660
26. Boulanger C, Lüscher TF (1990) Release of endothelin from the porcine aorta: inhibition by endothelium-derived nitric oxide. J Clin Invest 85:587–590
27. Lüscher TF (1990) Endothelial control of vascular tone and growth. Clin Exp Hypertens [A] A12(5):897–902
28. DiCorleto PE, Fox PL (1988) Growth factor production by endothelial cells. In: Una R (ed) Endothelial cells, vol 2. CRC Press, Boca Raton, pp 51–62
29. Battegay EJ, Raines EJ, Seifert RA, Bowen-Pope DF, Ross R (1990) TGF-beta induces bimodal proliferation of conneective tissue cells via complex control of an autocrine PDGF loop. Cell 63:515–524
30. Castellot JJ, Addonizio ML, Rosenberg RD, Karnovsky MJ (1981) Cultured endothelial cells produce a heparin-like inhibitor of smooth muscle cell growth. J Cell Biol 90:372
31. Garg UC, Hassid A (1989) Nitric oxide-generating vasodilators and 8-bromo-cyclic guanosine monophosphate inhibit mitogenesis and proliferation of cultured rat vascular smooth muscle cells. J Clin Invest 83:1774–1777
32. Dignan RJ, Zeh T, Dyke CM, Lee KF, Lutz HA, Ding M, Wechsler AS (1992) Reactivity of gastroepiploic and internal mammary arteries. Relevance to coronary artery bypass grafting. J Thorac Cardiovasc Surg 103:116–122
33. Yang Z, Richard V, von Segesser L, Bauer E, Stulz P, Turina M, Lüscher TF (1990) Threshold concentrations of endothelin-1 potentiate contractions to norepinephrine and serotonin in human arteries: a new mechanism of vasospasm? Circulation 82:188–195
34. Garratt KN, Edwards WD, Kaufmann UP, Vlietstra RE, Holmes DR (1991) Differential histopathology of primary atherosclerotic and restenotic lesions in coronary arteries and saphenous vein bypass grafts: analysis of tissue obtained from 73 patients by directional atherectomy. J Am Coll Cardiol 17:442–448
35. Singh RN (1983) Atherosclerosis and the internal mammary arteries. Cardiovasc Intervent Radiol 6:72–77
36. Shelton ME, Forman MB, Bajaj A, Virmani R, Bajaj A, Stoney WS, Atkison JB (1988) A comparison of morphologic and angiographic findings in long-term internal mammary artery and saphenous vein bypass grafts. J Am Coll Cardiol 20:297–307
37. Sisto T (1990) Atheriosclerosis in internal mammary and related arteries. Scand J Thorac Cardiovasc Surg 24:7–11
38. Suma H, Takanashi R (1990) Arteriosclerosis of the gastroepiploic and internal thoracic arteries. Ann Thorac Surg 50:413–416
39. Ross R (1986) The pathogenesis of atherosclerosis – an update. N Engl J Med 314:488–500
40. Predel HG, Yang Z, von Segesser L, Turina M, Bühler FR, Luscher TF (1992) Implications of pulsatile stretch on growth of saphenous vein and mammary artery smooth muscle. Lancet 340:878–879
41. Lytle BW, Loop FD, Taylor PC, Simpfendorfer C, Kramer JR, Ratliff NB, Goormastic M, Cosgrove DM, Schnauffer MJ (1992) Vein graft Disease: the clinical impact of stenoses in saphenous vein bypass grafts to coronary arteries. J Thorac Cardiovasc Surg 103:831–840
42. Lehmann KH, von Segesser L, Müller-Glauser W, Siebenmann R, Schneider K, Lüscher TF, Turina M (1989) Internal-mammary coronary artery grafts: is their superiority also due to a basically intact endothelium? Thorac Cardiovasc Surg 37:187–189
43. Quis WC, LoGerfo FW, Haudenschild CC (1988) Optimal preparation of vein grafts prevents the morphological changes of arterialization (abstract). Circulation 78 [Suppl II]:635
44. Angelini GD, Breckenridge IM, Psaila JV, Williams HM, Henderson AH, Newby C (1987) Preparation of human saphenous vein for coronary artery bypass grafting impairs its capacity to produce prostacyclin. Cardiovasc Res 21:28–33

45. Angelini GD, Christie MI, Bryan AJ, Lewis MJ (1989) Surgical preparation impairs release of endothelium-derived relaxing factor from human saphenous vein. Ann Thorac Surg 48:417–420
46. Lawrie GM, Weilbacher DE, Henry PD (1990) Endothelium-dependent relaxaton in human saphenous vein grafts: effects of preparation and clinicopathologic correlations. J Thorac Cardiovasc Surg 100:612–620
47. Lawrie GM (1990) Invited letter concerning: endothelial preservation in human saphenous veins. J Thorac Cardiovasc Surg 100:149–630
48. Barner HB, Fischer VW (1990) Invited letter concerning: endothelial preservation in human sapehnous veins. J Thorac Cardiovasc Surg 100:149–150
49. Angelini GD, Bryan AJ, Williams HMJ, Morgan R, Newby AC (1990) Distention promotes platelet and leukocyte adhesion and reduces short-term patency in pig arteriovenous bypass grafts. J Thorac Cardiovasc Surg 99:433–439
50. Shimokawa H, Flavahan NA, Vanhoutte PM (1989) Natural course of the impairment of endothelium-dependent relaxations after balloon endothelium-removal in porcine coronary arteries. Circ Res 65:740–753
51. Angelini GD, Bryan AJ, Williams HMJ, Soyombo AA, Williams A, Tovey J, Newby AC (1992) Time-course of medial and intimal thickening in pig venous arterial grafts: relationship to endothelial injury and cholesterol accumulation. J Thorac Cardiovasc Surg 103:1093
52. Ku DD, Caulfield JB, Kirklin JK (1991) Endothelium-dependent responses in long-term human coronary artery bypass grafts. Circulation 83:403–411
53. Miller VM, Reigel MM, Hollier LH, Vanhoutte PM (1987) Endothelium-dependent responses in autogenous femoral veins grafted into the arterial circulation of the dog. J Clin Invest 80:1350–1357
54. Komori K, Schini VB, Gloviczki P, Bourchier RG, Vanhoutte PM (1991) The impairment of endothelium-dependent relaxations in reversed vein grafts is associated with a reduced production of cyclic guanosine monophosphate. J Vasc Surg 14:67–75
55. Yang Z, Von Segesser L, Stulz P, Turina M, Lüscher TF (1992) Pulsatile stretch and platelet-derived growth factor (PDGF): important mechanisms for coronary venous bypass graft disease (abstract). Circulation 86:I-84
56. Kugiyama K, Kerns SA, Morrisett JD et al. (1990) Impairment of endothelium-dependent arterial relaxation by lysolecithin in modified low-density lipoproteins. Nature 344:160–162
57. Tanner FC, Noll G, Boulanger CM, Lüscher TF (1991) Oxidized native low density lipoproteins inhibit relaxations of porcine coronary arteries: role of scavenger receptor and endothelium-derived nitric oxide. Circulation 83:2012–2020
58. Shimokawa H, Vanhoutte PM (1989) Impaired endothelium-dependent relaxation to aggregating platelets and related vasoactive substances in porcine coronary arteries in hypercholesterolemia and in atherosclerosis. Circ Res 64:900–904
59. Bossaller C, Habib GB, Yamamoto H et al. (1987) Impaired muscarinic endothelium-dependent relaxation and cyclic guanosine 5′-monophosphate formation in atherosclerotic human coronary artery and rabbit aorta. J Clin Invest 79:170–174
60. Förstermann U, Mügge A, Alheid U, Haverich A, Frölich JC (1988) Selective attenuation of endothelium-mediated vasodilation in atherosclerotic human coronary arteries. Circ Res 62:185–190
61. Ludmer PL, Selwyn AP, Shook TL et al. (1986) Paradoxical vasoconstriction induced by acetylcholine in atherosclerotic coronary arteries. N Engl J Med 315:1046–1051
62. Gollino P, Piscione F, Willerson JT et al. (1991) Divergent effects of serotonin on coronary-artery dimensions and blood flow in patients with coronary atherosclerosis and control patients. N Engl J Med 324:641–648
63. Boulanger CM, Tanner FC, Hahn AWS, Buhler FR, Lüscher TF (1986) Oxidized low density lipoproteins induce mRNA expression and release of endothelin from human and porcine endothelium. Circ Res 58:305–309

64. Scott-Burden T, Resink TJ, Hahn AWA, Baur U, Box RG, Bühler FR (1989) Induction of growth-related metabolism in human vascular smooth muscle cells by low density lipoprotein. J Biol Chem 264:12582–12589
65. Habib JB, Bossaller C, Wells S, Williams C, Morrisett JD, Henry PD (1986) Preservation of endothelium-dependent vascular relaxation in cholesterol-fed rabbit by treatment with the calcium blocker PN 200-110. Circ Res 58:305–309
66. Lichtlen PR, Hugenholtz P, Rafflenbeul W, Jost S, Deckers JW (1991) Retardation of angiographic progression of coronary artery disease by nifedipine. Lancet 335:1109–1113
67. Seitelberger R, Zwölfer W, Huber S et al. (1991) Nifedipine reduces the incidence of myocardial infarction and transient ischemia in patients undergoing coronary bypass grafting. Circulation 83:460–468
68. Block LH, Emmons R, Vogt E, Sachinidis A, Vetter W (1989) Calcium blockers inhibit the action of recombinant platelet-derived growth factor in vascular smooth muscle cells. Proc Natl Acad Sci USA 86:2388–2392
69. Clozel M, Kuhn H, Hefti F (1990) Effects of angiotensin-converting enzyme inhibitors and of hydralazine on endothelial function in hypertensive rats. Hypertension 16:532–540
70. Powell JS, Clozel J-P, Müller RKM, Kuhn H, Hefti F, Hosang M, Baumgarner HR (1989) Inhibitors of angiotensin-converting enzyme prevent myointimal proliferation after vascular injury. Science 245:186–188
71. Roux SP, Clozel J-P, Kuhn H (1991) Cilazapril inhibits wall thickening of vein bypass graft in the rat. Hypertension 18 [Suppl II]:43–46
72. Lüscher TF, Richard V, Yang Z (1989) Interaction between endothelium-derived nitric oxide and SIN-1 in human and porcine blood vessels. J Cardiovasc Pharmacol 14 [Suppl 11]:76–80
73. Guyton JR, Rosenberg RD, Clowes AW, Karnovsky MJ (1980) Inhibition of rat arterial smooth muscle cell proliferation by heparin. In vivo studies with anticoagulant and non-anticoagulant heparin. Circ Res 46:625–634
74. Hirsch GM, Karnovsky MJ (1991) Inhibiton of vein graft intimal proliferative lesions in the rat by heparin. Am J Pathol 139:581–587.
75. Kohler TR, Kirkman T, Clowes AW (1989) Effects of heparin on adaptation of vein grafts to the arterial circulation. Arteriosclerosis 9:523–528
76. Lüscher TF (1991) Endothelin. J Cardiovasc Pharmacol 18 [Suppl 10]:15–22

Smooth Muscle Cell Proliferation Responses in Organ Cultures of Human Saphenous Vein

G.D. Angelini and A.C. Newby

Introduction

Occlusion of saphenous vein coronary artery bypass grafts remains a major limitation to the clinical benefits of the procedure, despite more than 25 years of experience [1]. Early occlusion rates can be minimized by optimizing techniques for surgical preparation [2] and anastomosis and by the use of perioperative and early post-operative antithrombotic therapy [3]. Unfortunately, no modification of technique or drug regime has been shown to reduce late vein graft occlusion [4]. This is known to result from excessive proliferation of vascular smooth muscle cells (VSMCs) and the superimposition of atheroma on the resulting thickened intima [5]. The relationship of intimal thickening to the conditions of implantation has been investigated in animal models. Briefly summarized, intimal thickening occurs only after implantation into a high-pressure (arterial) location and is not related to adventitial disruption [6, 7]. Qualitative and quantitative time course studies [8, 9] indicate also that intimal thickening occurs progressively long after the restoration of a morphologically intact endothelium and the termination of measurable platelet and leucocyte adhesion. These observations imply that intimal thickening is an intrinsic response of the vessel wall itself to the altered haemodynamics [10]. Understanding the mechanisms underlying this response may be helpful in developing strategies to reduce vein graft occlusion.

In pursuit of this objective, we have investigated whether intimal thickening occurs in segments of human saphenous vein maintained in culture. We argued that this experimental model would offer advantages over pathological studies in that the progression of intimal thickening could be studied in human tissue over a conveniently short period under controlled and reproducible conditions. Furthermore the impact of technical and pharmacological interventions could be evaluated by quantitative comparison using relatively small numbers of samples. Organ culture is also superior to isolated cell culture methods because it allows the investigation of interactions between VSMCs and their native extracellular matrix and with other vessel wall and blood cells, such as endothelium and monocyte/macrophages.

Establishment of the Model

Our first concern was to establish whether tissue viability can be maintained in organ culture and then to locate, identify and quantify any proliferating cells. Segments of human saphenous vein were cultured by adapting the method of Pedersen and Bowyer for rabbit aorta [11]. In their work they point to the importance of dehydration, mechanical trauma, vasospasm and coagulation as causes of endothelial disruption during vessel preparation. For this reason, in the initial studies [12] we collected vessels that had been subjected to a minimum of surgical dissection directly into HEPES-buffered tissue culture medium containing papaverine and heparin. Segments were immersed or maintained moist in this medium throughout the subsequent procedures. Vessel segments were immediately taken to the tissue culture laboratory, and as much as possible of the adventitia was removed with microvascular scissors, taking care not to stretch or compress the vessel. The vessels were then cut with the scissors longitudinally along their upper aspect, pinned out with minuten pins intimal surface uppermost onto set Sylgard silicone resin and then cut into 1-cm-long segments. The vessel segments were then transferred onto the surface of nylon mesh (to facilitate diffusion of nutrients) in petri dishes containing set Sylgard resin. Tissue culture was conducted for periods of up to 2 weeks in bicarbonate-buffered medium supplemented with 30% fetal bovine serum at 37°C under 95% air/5% CO_2. The medium was renewed every 2–3 days.

Viability

Based on previous acute experiments [13, 14], we chose measurements of adenosine triphosphate (ATP) concentration and the ratio of the concentrations of ATP and adenosine diphosphate (ADP) as the most sensitive markers of the viability of the predominant VSMCs. Indeed, we showed directly that removal of the endothelium, which constitutes a minor component of the total cell wall population, did not detectably affect these parameters [14]. DNA concentration was also measured as a marker of total cell density. For endothelial viability we used light and scanning electron microscopy in combination with morphometry. Prostacyclin production is a quantitative biochemical marker of the endothelial function in human saphenous vein [15], but it is affected by culturing itself and therefore could not be applied for these studies (A.A. Soyombo, G.D. Angelini, A.C. Newby, unpublished observations). Moreover, many of our patients had been receiving aspirin preoperatively, and we have shown that this greatly diminishes venous prostacyclin production [16].

Segments prepared for culture had more than 80% of the intimal surface covered with endothelium (Fig. 1a) and had values of ATP concentration

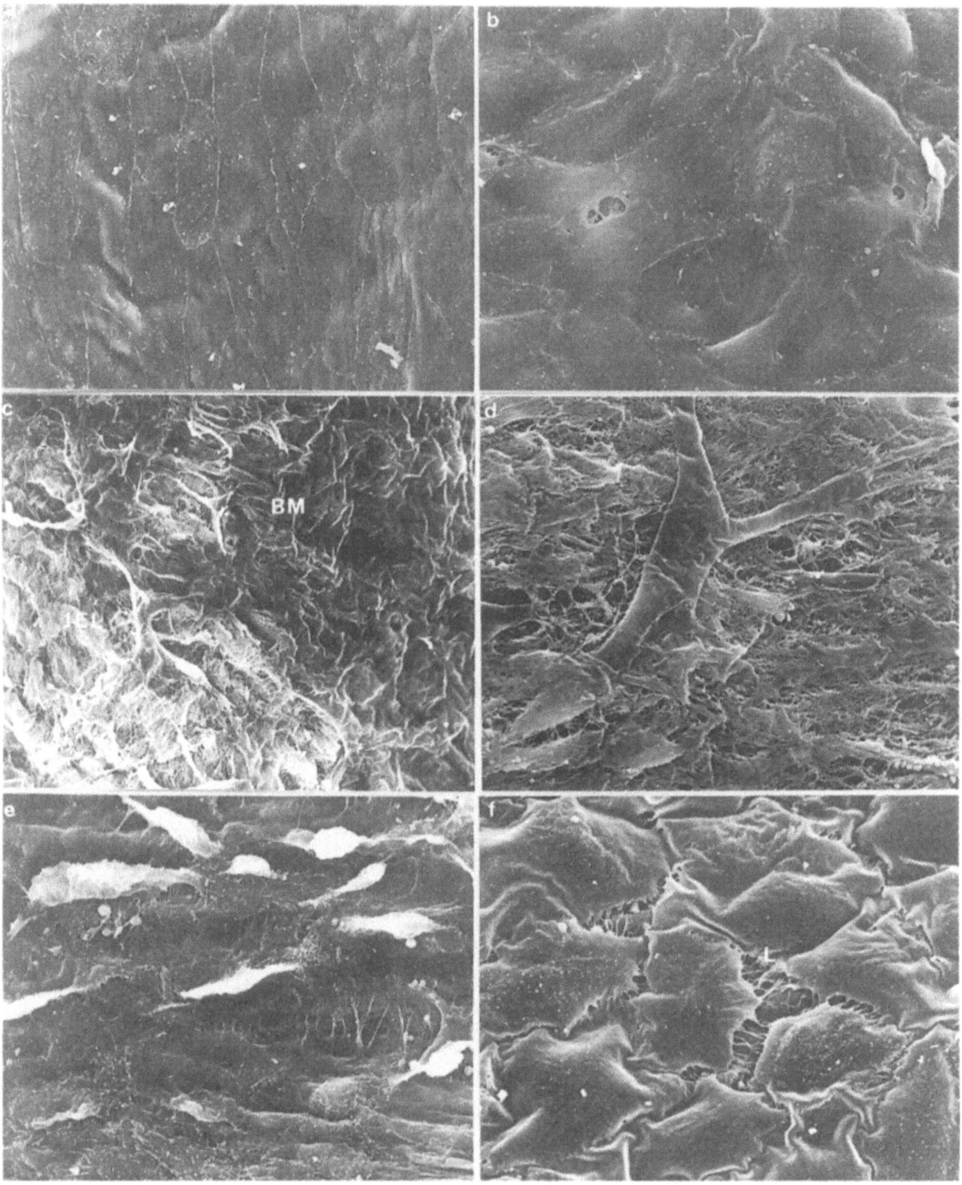

Fig. 1a–f. Scanning electron micrographs of the intimal surface of freshly isolated, de-endothelialized and surgically prepared veins before and after culturing. **a** Freshly isolated vein before culture. **b** Freshly isolated vein after 14 days in culture. **c** De-endothelialized vein before culture. Note the smooth basement membrane (*BM*) and the exposed filamentous internal elastic lamina. **d** De-endothelialized vein cultured for 14 days. **e** Surgically prepared vein before culture. Note the rolled-up appearance of endothelial cells with exposure of smooth basement membrane and deeper filamentous structures. **f** Surgically prepared vein after 14 days in culture. Note the presence of cuboid cells with fine projections. Initial magnification ×1000. (Reproduced from [24] with permission)

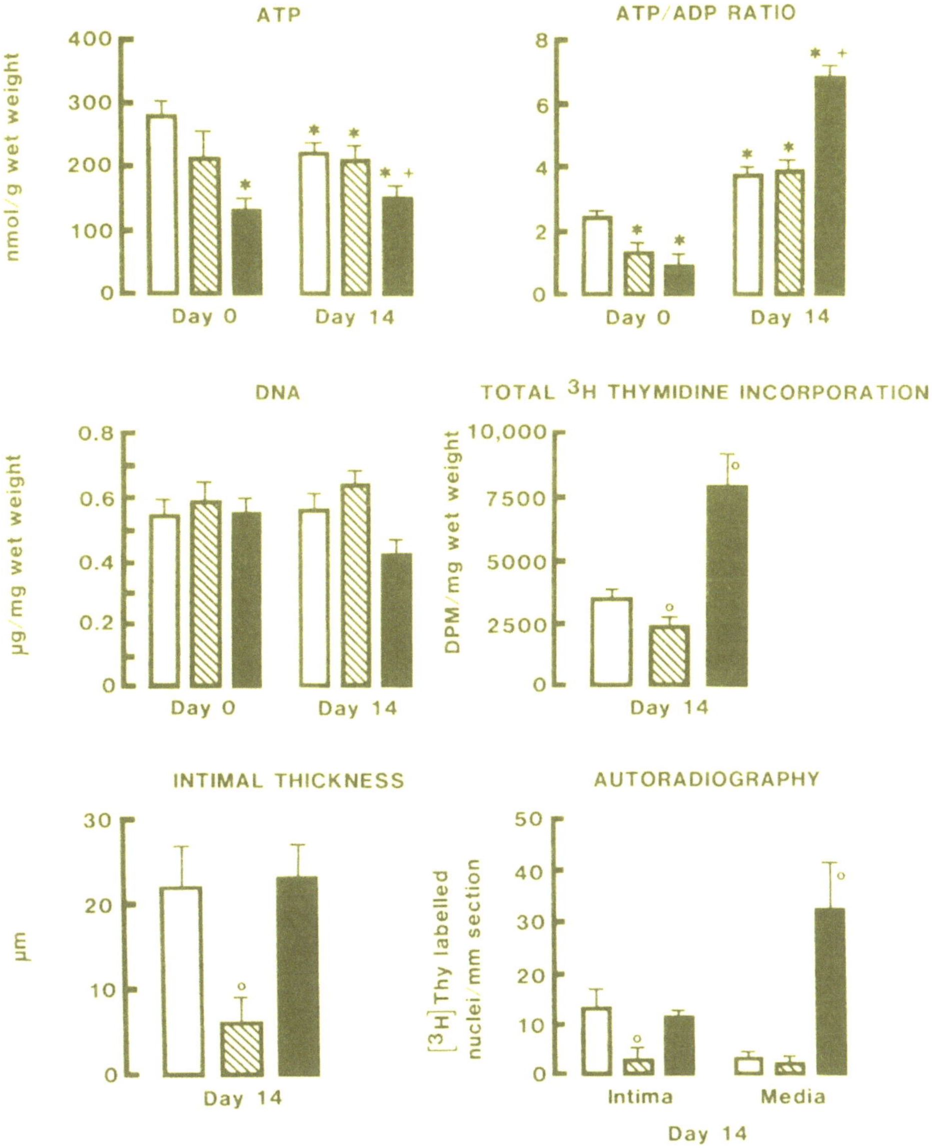

Fig. 2. Summary of biochemical and morphometric analyses of veins. *White bars*, freshly isolated; *hatched bars*, de-endothelialized; *black bars*, surgically prepared. *, $p < 0.05$ versus freshly isolated vein on day 0; +, $p < 0.05$ versus freshly isolated vein on day 14; 0, $p < 0.001$ versus freshly isolated vein

(Fig. 2) and ATP/ADP ratio (Fig. 2) similar to those in vessel segments taken for analysis immediately after removal from patients [14]. Culture of these vessels for 2 weeks led to a 20% fall in ATP concentration, suggesting that some loss of cell viability had occurred (Fig. 2). Endothelial coverage remained virtually complete throughout the culture period, although some separation of the cells and development of fine filamentous projections was noted (Fig. 1b). Thus the culture method of Pedersen and Bowyer [11] provided adequate VSMC and endothelial viability.

We have subsequently found that the presence of papaverine in the collecting medium is not essential. Furthermore, variation of the geometry of the culture system is possible. For example, we have been able to culture 6-mm punch biopsies either as described above or in wells lined with silicone grease so as to waterproof the adventitial surface [17]. Hence diffusion of nutrients and oxygen from the intimal side appears to be enough only to maintain viability. So far we have not performed prolonged culture in a fully defined culture medium, but viability can be maintained for to 24h in serum-free medium [18].

Cell Proliferation

Intimal thickening was investigated by morphometry of transverse histological sections stained either with haematoxylin and eosin, the elastic Van Gieson stain or a modified trichrome stain [19]. Cell proliferation was located and quantified in similar sections from veins that had been cultured with [^{3}H]thymidine and then subjected to autoradiography. VSMCs and endothelial cells were identified by immunocytochemistry with specific antibodies or by lectin binding [12].

Cultured veins showed progressive thickening of the intima in transverse sections (Fig. 3). The new intima that developed in culture was easily distinguished as an elastin-poor, mucopolysacharride-rich layer in appropriately stained preparations (Fig. 3). In sections where a distinct internal elastic lamina was visible, pre-existing intimal thickening could be identified as an elastin-rich layer (Fig. 3). This pre-existing intima was therefore clearly distinct from the intima that developed in culture. Interestingly, however, the amount of pre-existing intima was correlated with the development of neointima in culture (C.M. Holt, S.E. Francis, G.D. Angelini, unpublished observations). Intimal thickening was quantified by either a manual or computer-assisted method [19].

Cultured veins also showed a progressive incorporation of [^{3}H]thymidine when this was present throughout the culture period (Fig. 2). Manual counting of cells which incorporated thymidine showed that proliferating cells were virtually confined to the new intima (Fig. 4b). After 2 weeks in culture only approximately 50% of the new intimal cells had taken up thymidine [12], which implies that the remaining intimal cells arose by

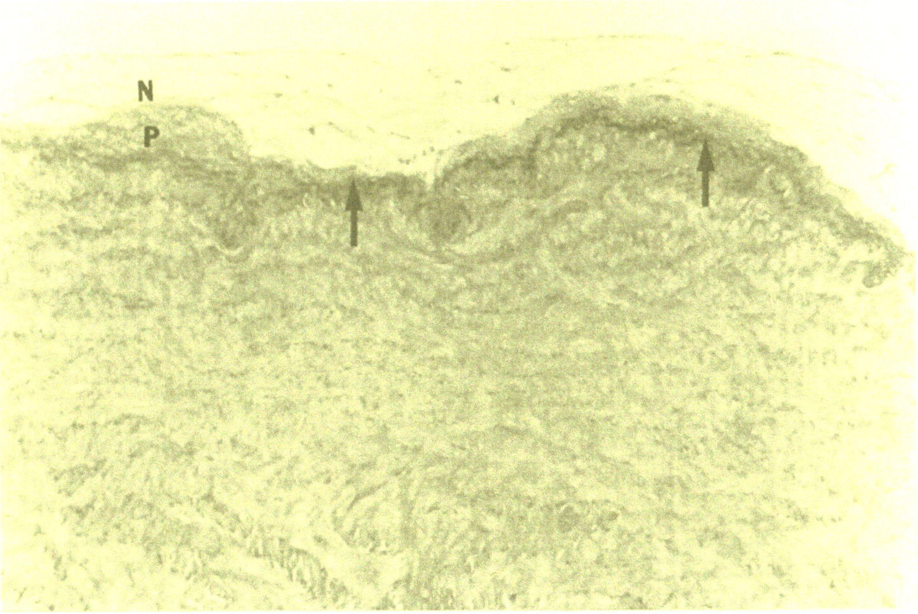

Fig. 3. Histological appearance of cultured vein. A transverse section (5 μm) of a freshly isolated vein cultured for 14 days. Note the internal elastic lamina (*arrows*) with pre-existing intima (*P*) and new intima (*N*). Initial magnification ×112

migration from the media or pre-existing intima. Interestingly, there was no corresponding zone of proliferating cells at the cut edges of the segments or at the adventitial surface. Thus VSMC proliferation was directed to the intima, despite the exposure of all vein surfaces to culture medium. This implies that the subendothelial microenvironment favours VSMC proliferation. Endothelial cell VSMC contact is unlikely to be necessary for this effect, however, because in pulse-labelled preparations proliferating cells are seen scattered throughout the neointima (A.A. Soyombo and A.C. Newby, unpublished observations).

Some discussion is warranted on the validity of the various ways in which intimal enlargement is quantified. Firstly, since the majority of the cells in the intima are smooth muscle cells (see below), ignoring the contribution of endothelial cells introduces only a small error, although these could be accounted for by the use of cell specific stains. In the intima, where the proportion of labelled cells is high, it is practicable to quantify proliferation in the conventional terms of a thymidine-labelling index. Absolute measures (i.e., cells/mm of intima) are superior, however, because they give an estimate of the amount of intima formation, whereas the thymidine index merely indicates the proportion of those cells that have undergone S phase. Since many intimal cells have arisen by migration and

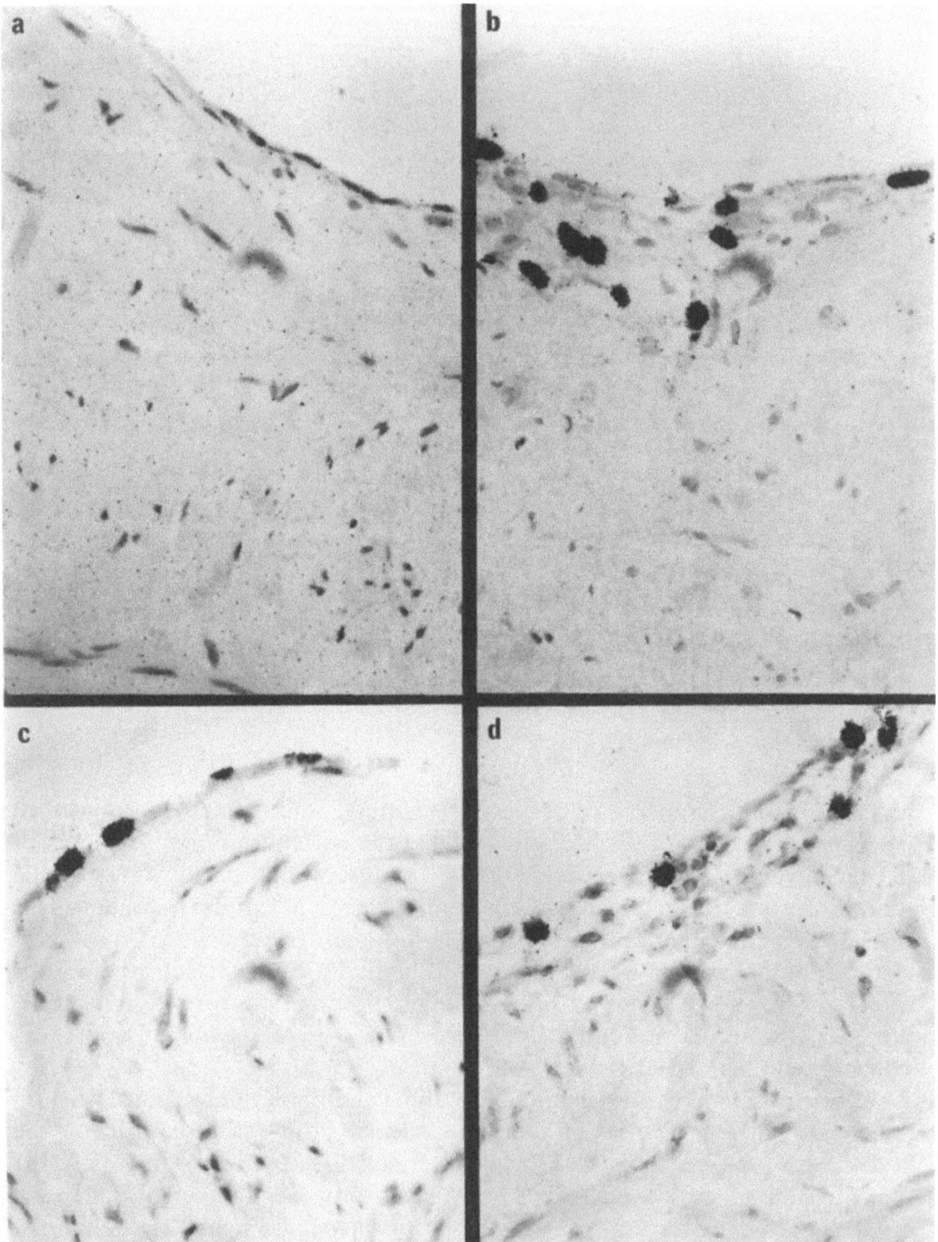
a
b
c
d

have not subsequently divided, an intervention that affects principally migration rather than proliferation of smooth muscle cells might increase the thymidine-labelling index despite decreasing the amount of intima formation. Thus measurement of thymidine index alone would be misleading. In the media, where the thymidine index is extremely low, data can be more readily accumulated from whole sections by counting only the labelled cells and relating this to the area in the section. This is valid because the density of total cells (from morphometry or from DNA measurements, e.g., Fig. 2) is fairly constant.

Identification of Intimal Cells

The majority of the intimal surface cells were identified as endothelial cells by staining with U. europaeus lectin [12] or with monoclonal antibodies (QB-end-10). A few of the intimal surface cells were identified as smooth muscle cells by staining with two different monoclonal antibodies for smooth muscle cell actin [12]. Some endothelial cells were seen penetrating into the neointima as capillary-like structures, but these constituted a relatively small component [12]. The majority of cells in the neointima were positively identified as smooth muscle cells [12]. This was in marked contrast to the adventitia where the majority of the cells (presumably fibroblasts) were not stained with antibodies to actin. Serial sectioning confirmed that the neointima consisted of a majority of smooth muscle whereas the minority of cells that were not stained were endothelial cells [12]. Thus there was no evidence that fibroblasts contributed significantly to intimal enlargement in this model, as is the case in vivo. Fibroblast proliferation was occasionally observed from the adventitial surface, but these cells grew as a monolayer on the nylon mesh and floor of the dishes.

Surgical Interventions

Response to injury mechanisms has been implicated on theoretical grounds in the intimal proliferation that occurs during atherogenesis, in vein grafts and after angioplasty [20]. These may, in part, involve loss of thrombo-

Fig. 4a–d. Autoradiograms of transverse sections. Transverse sections (5 μm) were subjected to autoradiography and counterstained with haematoxylin and eosin. **a** Freshly isolated vein cultured for 1 day only in the presence of [^{3}H]thymidine. Note the absence of silver-labelled nuclei. **b** Freshly isolated vein cultured for 14 days in the presence of [^{3}H]thymidine. Note the presence of silver-labelled cells in the intima. **c** De-endothelialized vein cultured for 14 days with [^{3}H]thymidine. Note the much fewer silver-labelled cells. **d** Surgically prepared vein cultured for 14 days in the presence of [^{3}H]thymidine. Note the silver-labelled cells in both the intimal and medial (*arrow*) layers. Initial magnification ×112 resistance of the endothelial surface with resulting platelet activation and growth factor release [21]. However, platelet-independent mechanisms are also well recognized from in vivo and in vitro experiments. For example, release of basic fibroblast growth factor from damaged VSMCs has recently been implicated in the proliferation of rat carotid artery cells after angioplasty [22]. Surgical preparation of saphenous vein is known to be a potential cause of injury to both endothelium and VSMC [23]. It was reasonable to ask, therefore, whether endothelial removal or the injury to the medial VSMC which occurs during surgical preparation has any influence on subsequent proliferative responses in organ culture.

Endothelial Removal

Endothelial removal from freshly-isolated vessels by gentle abrasion before culturing [24] had no effect on initial or final ATP or DNA concentration (Fig. 2). The ATP/ADP ratio was slightly decreased intially but recovered during culture (Fig. 2). Endothelial regrowth was not observed after culture, although a few intimal surface cells with VSMC morphology were present (Fig. 1d). Intimal thickness (Fig. 2) and the number of intimal thymidine-labelled cells (Fig. 2) were both reduced by approximately 75%. Interestingly, the thymidine-labelling index was not altered (data not shown), which implies that the major effect of endothelium was to encourage cells to migrate into the intima rather than to act as a source of growth factor. This is not surprising in the presence of 30% serum. The overall thymidine incorporation (Fig. 2) and the number of medial labelled cells (Fig. 2) were not affected by endothelial removal.

Routine Surgical Preparation

We [24] chose to compare freshly isolated veins obtained after the minimum of dissection with samples obtained from the same patients after routine surgical preparation and storage in blood. This has the ethical and practical advantage of making use of otherwise discarded material and is also representative of the clinical situation. Nevertheless, there is an inevitable variability in the amount of injury suffered by each surgically prepared segment.

Surgically prepared segments had a substantially lower endothelial coverage (Fig. 1e) and medial ATP concentration (Fig. 2) than paired freshly isolated segments, consistent with many previous observations (see above). After culturing the endothelial coverage (Fig. 1f) and ATP concentration (Fig. 2) appeared to recover towards the values obtained with cultured freshly isolated vessels. Interestingly, the DNA concentration tended to be lower in cultured surgically prepared veins (Fig. 2), consistent with necrosis of injured cells.

Intimal thickening (Fig. 2) was similar in cultured surgically prepared and freshly isolated vessels. In two subsequent independent series of experiments (A.A. Soyombo, A.C. Newby, C.M. Holt, S.E. Francis, G.D. Angelini, unpublished observations) surgical preparation tended to increase intimal thickness and the number of intimal labelled cells in parallel. Taken together, these data imply that surgical preparation had a tendency to increase intimal proliferation, but that this may have been close to maximal even in freshly isolated vessels given the presence of 30% serum in the cultures.

Overall incorporation of [^{3}H]thymidine was significantly greater in cultured surgically prepared vessels (Fig. 2). The effect was more pronounced in cultures continuously labelled with thymidine for 14 days than in cultures pulse-labelled for the last 24 h (A.A. Soyombo, A.C. Newby, unpublished observations). This implies that the greatest difference in thymidine incorporation was during the early days of culture. The number of thymidine-labelled cells in the medial layer was greatly increased by surgical preparation (Fig. 2); the difference was again greatest in the continuously labelled cultures where it amounted to more than ten fold [24]. These data showed that injury promoted the production of a factor that could stimulate VSMC proliferation over and above any effect of serum. The data reviewed above regarding endothelial removal make it unlikely that this resulted from endothelial injury. It is most likely, therefore, that this factor was derived from injured VSMC themselves.

Other Applications of the Model

Interaction with Blood Cells

Short-term (24-h) and long-term (up to 14 days) co-culture of human saphenous vein with human monocytes has been achieved [17, 25]. These experiments may help to clarify the mechanisms of acute interactions (e.g., cell adhesion) and longer term (e.g., growth regulation) controls.

Comparison with Other Human Conduits

Similar methods have been used to organ culture segments of human internal mammary [19], gastroepiploic and inferior epigastric arteries (T. Taylor, G.D. Angelini, unpublished observations). In general, some degree of intimal cell proliferation has been observed with all these vessels and appears to be partially endothelium dependent in mammary arteries [19] as well as saphenous veins. In a direct comparison (C.M. Holt, S.E. Francis, G.D. Angelini, unpublished observations), the degree of intimal thickening and medial cell proliferation in internal mammary artery was significantly less than in surgically prepared saphenous vein, which may help to explain their differing tendency for intimal proliferation when implanted as conduits. However, the difference in organ culture was not apparent in comparison to freshly isolated veins, which demonstrates a greater susceptibility of vein to surgical-preparative injury. Whether this underlies the different subsequent behaviour of the conduits remains to be investigated.

Normal and diseased human coronary artery segments obtained from the hearts of transplant recipients can also be subjected to organ culture [26]. These experiments offer for the first time the possibility of studying the dynamics of events underlying lesion formation. As a simple example, measurement of the thymidine incorporation after serum-free organ culture for 24 h give the first estimates of VSMC proliferation rates in atherosclerotic plaques [27].

Comparison with Nonhuman Vessels

Similar organ culture methods have been described for segments of rat, rabbit, and pig aorta [11, 28–30]. We have also established organ cultures of pig saphenous vein and vein grafts [18]. In the rabbit intimal proliferation is rarely observed [11] although both intimal and medial cell proliferation may be provoked by injury [30]. In the smaller rat aorta a greater tendency for cells to grow out from the cut edges was noted [28]. In the pig aorta selective intimal thickening occurred [29] and was endothelium-dependent [31], as in our experiments. The greater thickness of the pig aortic media apparently renders diffusion of substrates and oxygen difficult so that a necrotic core of VSMC is present in the cultures [29]. From our results we might expect that these necrosing cells provide a source of growth-stimulatory activity, but this has not been directly demonstrated. At present there are too few comparative data to conclude what factors (e.g., thickness of the internal elastic lamina, presence of pre-existing intima, age, state of development) might influence the degree of intimal thickening seen in these different vessels.

Pharmacological Interventions

The models that we have described are fully quantitative and so allow the stastistical evaluation of data obtained with putative inhibitors of intimal thickening. Given the underlying variability, approximately ten paired samples are neeed to test for a 50% reduction with 95% confidence of achieving $p < 0.05$. The advantages of using the organ culture over isolated cells is that the composite influences on proliferation, migration and matrix formation can also be investigated. Disadvantages are the cumbersome nature of the morphometric analyses and the limited availability of material, which almost preclude detailed concentration-response and time course experiments. The long culture period necessary to measure effects may either be an advantage or a disadvantage. Certainly, the action of highly unstable agents is difficult to study, but a cumulative effect of low concentrations of agents may be more readily observable in such a long-term organ culture.

Analogues of cAMP and cGMP, as well as the phosphodiesterase inhibitor isobutylmethylxanthine have been shown to inhibit intimal thickening in the model [32]. Conversely, heparin [33] and a prostaglandin analogue (T. Taylor, G.D. Angelini, unpublished observations) were ineffective. Too few data are presently available to determine whether the organ culture will prove an accurate predictor of effects of drugs in clinical trials.

What Has Been Learned so Far?

The first exciting finding of these organ culture experiments is that intimally directed VSMC proliferation occurs even in vessel segments totally immersed in culture medium. This implies that the vessel has an intrinsic polarity which determines the direction in which proliferation takes place. The most obvious structural polarity is the presence of endothelium on the intimal surface, and the effect of endothelial removal suggests that this is of major importance. The production of growth factors including PDGF and basic fibroblast growth factor has been described from endothelial cells [34], although it is not obvious why these should be effective in addition to serum. Establishment of a chemoattractant gradient of a growth factor such as PDGF might possibly be involved. Another possibility is secretion of matrix-degrading enzymes, since recent evidence suggests that these are essential for smooth muscle migration and proliferation [35]. Moreover, such enzymes are known to be secreted vectorially from the abluminal surface of endothelial cells [36]. The precise nature of the endothelium-derived proliferation factor or factors implicated in our studies and those of Gotlieb and co-workers [31] remains to be elucidated. It is tempting to speculate that such factors play some part in the pathogenesis of intimal proliferation in vein grafts and in arteries during atherosclerosis formation and after angioplasty.

The organ culture work similarly identifies proliferation factors produced during injury to VSMC. Such factors presumably also explain the association of medial injury with VSMC proliferation in experimental animal models [37, 38]. The nature of these factors is presently uncertain, but growth factors [22] or matrix-degrading enzymes are two attractive possibilities.

Work in the organ culture has confirmed suggestions from animal models that the presence of VSMC in the intima predisposes to further intimal proliferation. Whether this results from the selection of a highly proliferative subpopulation of cells or from differences in the regulation (e.g., by the extracellular matrix) is not clear.

Future Developments

The development of fully defined culture conditions will broaden the scope of the organ culture model for investigating growth factor production and growth regulation by cells intrinsic to the vessel wall. Preliminary results indicate that cell viability can be maintained during short-term serum-free culture of human [26] and pig vessels [18]. Moreover, both pig [18] and human [26] vascular tissues secrete growth factor activity detectable by bioassays. Further characterization of the nature and regulation of growth factor production in these vessels should shed light on the underlying mechanism of intimal proliferation in vein grafts and also in arterial pathologies. The preserved morphology in the organ culture allows also for co-localization studies of proliferating cells and cells producing growth-promoting activities. For example, messenger RNAs for PDGF A and B chains are co-localized by in situ hybridization with proliferating (i.e., intimal) but not quiescent (medial) VSMC in organ cultures of human saphenous vein (V. Thurston, A.C. Newby, unpublished observations).

Organ culture also offer a model for studying the long-term interactions between vessel wall cells, circulating cells and humoral pathogens such as lipoproteins. Initial studies indicate that circulating monocytes can inhibit VSMC proliferation in organ cultures [25] and this may be relevant to the attrition of the fibrous cap overlying advanced atherosclerotic plaques [39].

Implications for Late Vein Graft Patency

Our results so far imply that vein graft intimal thickening can be ameliorated by reducing surgical preparative injury. This can be achieved by avoiding overdistension by using a pressure-limiting device [40] or arterial pressure [23, 41] when checking the competence of side-branch ligatures. Endothelial disruption can be reduced by avoiding manipulation that leads to abrasion of the intimal surface [15]. Avoidance of injury was shown to improve early patency in pig model [2]. Conversely, distension of vein was shown to promote graft atherosclerosis by increasing cholesterol and lipoprotein deposition in grafts of hypercholesterolemic primates [42]. In the absence of a definitive clinical trial, organ culture studies add to the experimental evidence favouring the use of atraumatic methods of vein preparation.

Pharmacological intervention as well as optimal surgical technique will be needed to improve long-term patency. Only lipid-lowering therapy has been so far shown to decrease lesion formation in vein grafts [43]. Potent inhibitors of VSMC proliferation have not been available for clinical studies, however. The results of this study indicate that cAMP and cGMP pathways are possible therapeutic targets. While neither cAMP analogues nor isobutylmethylxanthine could be used in man, agents with similar actions are available for clinical studies. Stable analogues of prostacyclin and selective cAMP phosphodiesterase inhibitors (e.g., milrinone) have been shown to exert vasodilator effects [44], mediated by elevation of cAMP concentration in VSMC. Whether significant inhibition of VSMC proliferation in vein grafts can be achieved without excessive vasodilatation, or other side effects such as positive inotropy [44] remains to be established. Based on our data, nitrovasodilators or specific cGMP phosphodiesterase inhibitors may also be useful.

Organ culture represents a relatively new tool in the armoury of the cardiovascular researcher. As we have attempted to illustrate, it has some unique advantages for studying a progressive process, such as intimal thickening, in human material. Naturally, the results obtained give support to previous work with animal models and isolated cell cultures but, in addition, provide a greater emphasis on the cell-cell interactions that we believe lie at the heart of arterial pathologies. Inevitably with such a relatively new technique, we have generated many additional questions. However, endothelium-derived and injury-related proliferation factors have already been identified. Elucidating the nature of these factors is likely to shed light on the underlying mechanisms of intimal thickening. Twenty-five years of surgical experience have failed to solve the problems of late vein graft occlusion. It is our belief that a deeper understanding of the underlying cell biology is an essential pre-requisite to further progress.

Acknowledgements. Support by grants from the British Heart Foundation and the Heart Research Fund for Wales.

References

1. Grondin CM (1984) Late results of coronary artery grafting – is there a flag on the field? J Thorac Cardiovasc Surg 87:161–166
2. Angelini GD, Bryan AJ, Williams HMJ, Morgan R, Newby AC (1990) Distention promotes platelet and leukocyte adhesion and reduces short-term patency in pig arteriovenous bypass grafts. J Thorac Cardiovasc Surg 99:433–439
3. Fuster V, Chesebro JH (1985) Aorto-coronary artery vein graft disease: experimental and clinical approach for the understanding of the role of platelets and platelet inhibitors. Circulation 72 [Suppl V]:65–70
4. Angelini GD, Newby AC (1989) The future of saphenous vein as a coronary artery bypass conduit. Eur Heart J 10:273–280

5. Dilley RJ, McGeachie JK, Prendergast FJ (1988) A review of the histological changes in vein to artery grafts, with particular reference to intimal hyperplasia. Arch Surg 123: 691–696
6. Brody WR, Kosek JC, Angell WW (1972) Changes in vein grafts following aorto-coronary by-pass induced by pressure and ischaemia. J Thorac Cardiovasc Surg 64:847–854
7. Brody WR, Angell WW, Kosek JC (1972) Histologic fate of venous coronary artery bypass in dogs. Am J Pathol 66:111–130
8. Fonkalsrud EW, Sanchez M, Zerubavel R (1978) Morphological evaluation of canine autogenous vein grafts in the arterial circulation. Surgery 84:253–264
9. Angelini GD, Bryan AJ, Williams HMJ et al. (1992) Timecourse of medial and intimal thickening in pig arteriovenous bypass grafts: relationship to endothelial injury and cholesterol accumulation. J Thorac Cardiovasc Surg 103:1093–1103
10. Zwolak RM, Adams MC, Clowes AW (1987) Kinetics of vein graft hyperplasia: association with tangential stress. J Vasc Surg 5:126–136
11. Pederson DC, Bowyer DE (1985) Endothelial injury and healing in vitro: studies using an organ culture system. Am J Pathol 119:264–272
12. Soyombo AA, Angelini GD, Bryan AJ, Jasani B, Newby AC (1990) Intimal proliferation in an organ culture of human saphenous vein. Am Pathol 237:1401–1410
13. Angelini GD, Breckenridge IM, Butchart EG et al. (1985) Metabolic damage to human saphenous vein during preparation for coronary artery bypass grafting. Cardiovasc Res 19:326–334
14. Angelini GD, Passani SL, Breckenridge IM, Newby AC (1987) Nature and pressure dependence of damage induced by distension of human saphenous vein coronary artey bypass grafts. Cardiovasc Res 21:902–907
15. Angelini GD, Breckenridge IM, Psaila JV, Williams HM, Henderson AH, Newby AC (1987) Preparation of human saphenous vein for coronary artery bypass grafting impairs its capacity to produce porstacyclin. Cardiovasc Res 21:28–33
16. Angelini GD, Breckenridge IM (1985) Is there a rationale for treatment with aspirin before coronary surgery? Lancet ii:843
17. Cooper JP, Newby AC (1991) Monocyte adhesion to human saphenous vein in vitro. Atherosclerosis 91:85–95
18. Francis SE, Hunter S, Holt CM, Gadsdon PA, Angelini GD (1992) Growth factor activity detected in serum-free culture of pig arteriovenous bypass grafts. J Cell Biochem S16A:28
19. Holt CM, Francis SE, Rogers S et al. (1992) Intimal proliferation in an organ culture of human internal mammary artery. Cardiovasc Res 26:1189–1194
20. Ross R (1986) The pathogenesis of atherosclerosis- an update. N Engl J Med 314:488–500
21. Ip JH, Fuster V, Badimon L, Badimon J, Taubman MB, Chesebro JH (1990) Syndromes of accelerated atherosclerosis: role of vascular injury and smooth muscle cell proliferation. J Am Coll Cardiol 15:1667–1687
22. Lindner V, Reidy MA (1991) Proliferation of smooth muscle cells after vascular injury is inhibited by an antibody against basic fibroblast growth factor. Proc Natl Acad Sci USA 88:3739–3743
23. Angelini GD, Breckenridge IM, Williams HM, Newby AC (1987) A surgical preparative technique for human saphenous vein coronary bypass grafts which preserves medial and endothelial functional integrity. J Thorac Cardiovasc Surg 94:393–398
24. Angelini GD, Soyombo AA, Newby AC (1991) Smooth muscle cell proliferation in response to injury in an organ culture of human saphenous vein. Eur J Vasc Surg 5:5–12
25. Cooper JP, Soyombo A, Williams A, Newby AC (1992) Monocytes inhibit intimal smooth muscle proliferation: in vitro studies with human saphenous vein. Br Heart J 68:93
26. Holt CM, Francis SE, Clelland C, Violaris AG, Angelini GD (1992) Neointimal proliferation and endogenous growth factor release in an organ culture of human coronary artery. J Cell Biochem S16A:11
27. Francis SE, Holt CM, Taylor T, Gadsdon PA, Angelini GD (1992) Another cautionary note on the use of PCNA. J Pathol 166:418

28. Buck RC (1977) Organ cultures of rat aorta: a scanning and transmission electron microscopic study. Exp Mol Pathol 26:260–276
29. Gotlieb AI, Boden P (1984) Porcine aortic organ culture: a model to study the cellular response to vascular injury. In Vitro 20:535–542
30. Fingerle J, Kraft T (1987) The induction of smooth muscle cell proliferation in vitro using an organ culture system. Int Angiol 6:65–72
31. Koo EWY, Gotlieb AI (1989) Endothelial stimulation of intimal cell proliferation in a porcine aortic organ culture. Am J Pathol 134:497–503
32. Soyombo A, Newby AC (1991) Inhibition of smooth muscle proliferation by cyclic nucleotides in an organ culture of human saphenous vein. J Mol Cell Cardiol 23 [Suppl V]:S114
33. Francis SE, Holt CM, Taylor T, Gadsdon P, Angelini GD (1992) Heparin and intimal thickening in an organ culture of human saphenous vein. Atherosclerosis 93:155–156
34. Thyberg J, Hedin U, Sjölund M, Palmberg L, Bottger BA (1990) Regulation of differentiated properties and proliferation of arterial smooth muscle cells. Arteriosclerosis 10: 966–990
35. Southgate KM, Davies M, Booth RFG, Newby AC (1992) Involvement of extracellular matrix degrading metalloproteinases in rabbit aortic smooth muscle cell proliferation. Biochem J 288:93–99
36. Unemori EN, Bouhanna KS, Werb Z (1990) Vectorial secretion of extracellular matrix proteins, matrix-degrading proteinases, and tissue inhibitor of metalloproteinases by endothelial cells. J Biol Chem 265:445–451
37. Reidy MA, Silver M (1985) Endothelial regeneration – lack of intimal proliferation after defined injury to rat aortas. Am J Pathol 118:173–177
38. Clowes AW, Clowes MM, Fingerle J, Reidy MA (1989) Kinetics of cellular proliferation after arterial injury – role of acute distension in the induction of smooth muscle proliferation. Lab Invest 60:360–364
39. Henney AM, Wakely PR, Davies MJ et al. (1991) Localization of stromelysin gene expression in atherosclerotic plaques by in situ hybridization. Proc Natl Acad Sci USA 88:8154–8158
40. Bonchek LI (1980) Prevention of endothelial damage during preparation of saphenous veins for bypass grafting. J Thorac Cardiovasc Surg 79:911–915
41. Angelini GD, Bryan AJ, Hunter S, Newby AC (1992) A simple preparative technique which preserves human saphenous vein functional integrity during coronary artery bypass grafting. Ann Thoracic Surg 53:871–874
42. Boerboom LE, Olinger GN, Bonchek LI et al. (1985) The relative influence of arterial pressure versus intraoperative distention on lipid accumulation in primate vein bypass grafts. J Thorac Cardiovasc Surg 90:756–764
43. Blankenhorn DH, Nessim SA, Johnson RL, Sanmarco ME, Azen SP, Cashin-Hemphill L (1987) Beneficial effect of combined colestipolniacin therapy on coronary atherosclerosis and coronary venous bypass grafts. J Am Med Assoc 257:3233–3240
44. Anderson JL, Baim DS, Fein SA, Goldstein RA, LeJemtel TH, Likoff MJ (1987) Efficacy and safety of sustained (48 hour) intravenous infusions of milrinone in patients with severe congestive heart failure: a multicentre study. J Amer Coll Cardiol 9:711–722

Chronic Changes in Venous Grafts After Implantation

D.A. Lewis and V.M. Miller

Introduction

Autogenous blood vessels are the material of choice for replacement of diseased arteries. However, the long-term patency of vascular grafts, in particular vein grafts, is limited due to progressive narrowing of the lumen by myointimal hyperplasia [63]. This review focuses on the function of endothelial cells in vein grafts, in particular, how this function is affected by stimuli in the local environment, and how these stimuli might contribute to the development of myointimal hyperplasia.

A central theme for intimal hyperplasia and alternatively occlusion of vein grafts is injury to endothelial cells; this injury need not necessarily be a denuding injury [12]. Mechanical damage to the endothelial cells results from the operative procedure. In addition, changes in the chemical and physical environment (for example, pressure, flow, and oxygen tension) to which the veins are exposed chronically in the arterial system alter functional properties of the venous endothelium and smooth muscle [18].

Vascular endothelial cells produce factors which regulate tone and growth of underlying smooth muscle, aggregation of platelets, and adherence and migration of leukocytes [3–5, 30, 57, 61, 62, 84]. Substances produced by endothelial cells function antagonistically. For example, nitric oxide, a factor proposed to be the endothelium-derived relaxing factor, originally described by Furchgott [29, 79], causes relaxation of vascular smooth muscle and inhibits its proliferation [35]. In contrast, the endothelins, an endothelium-derived family of isopeptides, cause contraction and promote mitogenesis of the smooth muscle [34, 59, 87, 88]. Alterations in the balance between this functional antagonism could result in vasospasm and/or vascular occlusive disease [53].

Comparison of Endothelium-Derived Vasoactive Factors in Arteries and Veins

Before considering stimuli which might affect the function of the venous endothelium, it is first necessary to understand some differences in func-

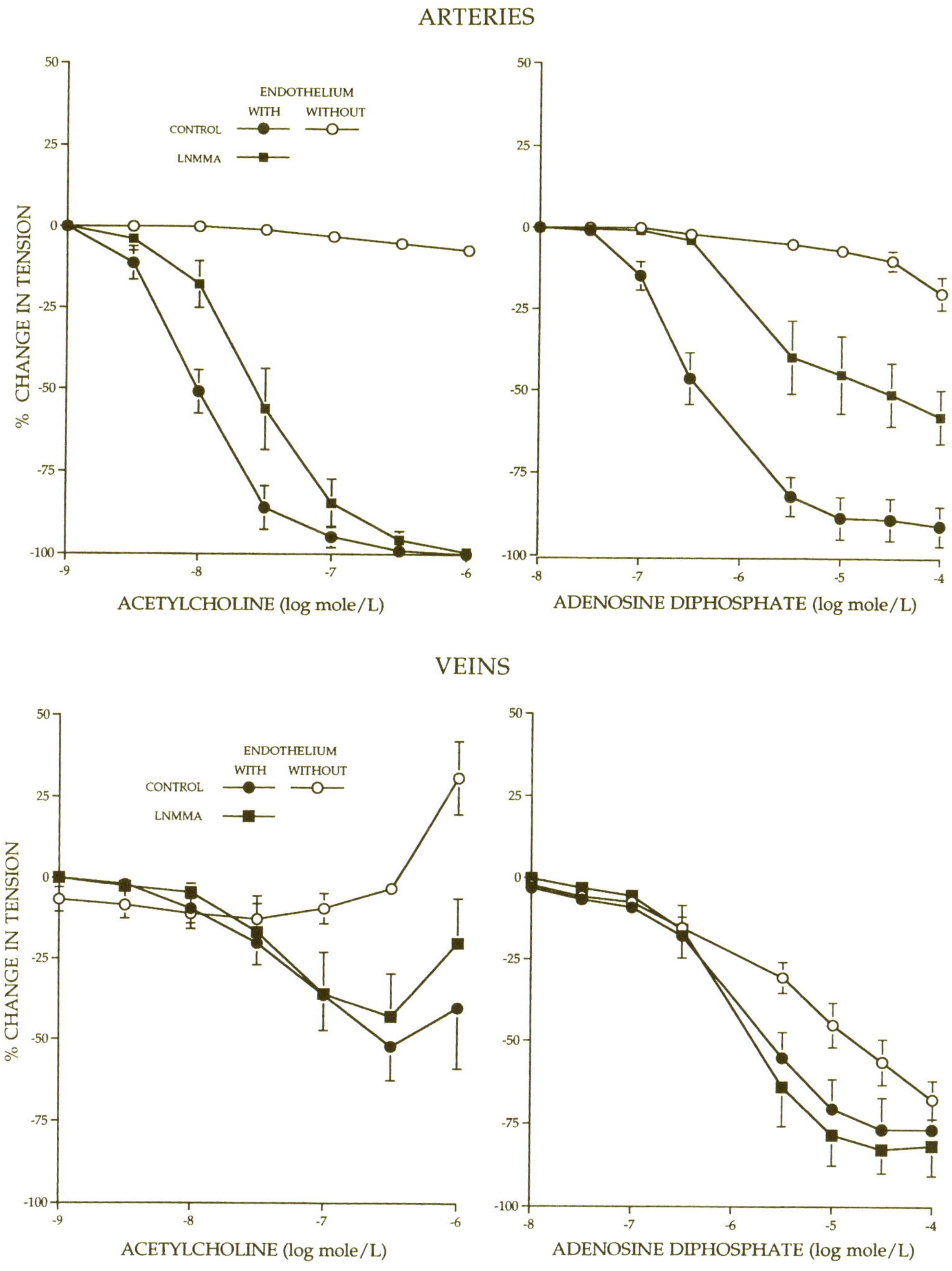

Fig. 1. Responses to acetylcholine (*left panels*) and adenosine-5-diphosphate (*right panels*) in canine femoral arteries (*top panels*) and veins (*bottom panels*), with and without endothelium, in the absence (*control*) and presence of a synthetic analog of L-arginine, (N^G-monomethyl-L-arginine, *LNMMA*; 1×10^{-4} *M*). Rings of blood vessels were suspended for the measurement of isometric force in organ chambers. Data are expressed as percentage change in tension from a contraction to prostaglandin $F_{2\alpha}$ (2×10^{-6} *M*). Values are shown as mean ± SEM, $n = 6$ in each group. Endothelium-dependent relaxations to acetylcholine are greater in arteries than in veins. Inhibition of production of nitric oxide by LNMMA did not decrease relaxations to either acetylcholine or adenosine diphosphate in veins

tional characteristics between arterial and venous endothelium. In general, endothelium-dependent relaxations to acetylcholine are more difficult to demonstrate in veins compared to arteries (Fig. 1) [20, 31, 32, 58, 85]. This represents a difference, in part, in the production of endothelium-derived nitric oxide. Nitric oxide is synthesized enzymatically from L-arginine. In endothelial cells constitutive nitric oxide synthase requires the cofactors calcium-calmodulin and nicotinamide adenine dinucleotide phosphate [7, 10, 20, 39, 41, 76, 77]. While synthetic analogs of L-arginine and inhibitors of the cofactors inhibit most endothelium-dependent relaxations in arteries, they are much less effective in veins (Fig. 1) [64, 72]. However, contractions of venous smooth muscle are inhibited by exogenously administered nitric oxide as well as by other nitrovasodilators [73]. The identity of endothelium-derived relaxing factor(s) insensitive to inhibition by analogs of L-arginine is not known. This substance(s) is probably not a metabolite of arachidonic acid by either cyclo-oxygenase, lipoxygenase, or cytochrome P450 as inhibitors of these enzymes also do not inhibit endothelium-dependent relaxations in veins [27, 55, 90] (Figs. 2, 3).

Both arterial and venous endothelial cells produce contractile factors. Although venous and arterial endothelial cells metabolize arachidonic acid

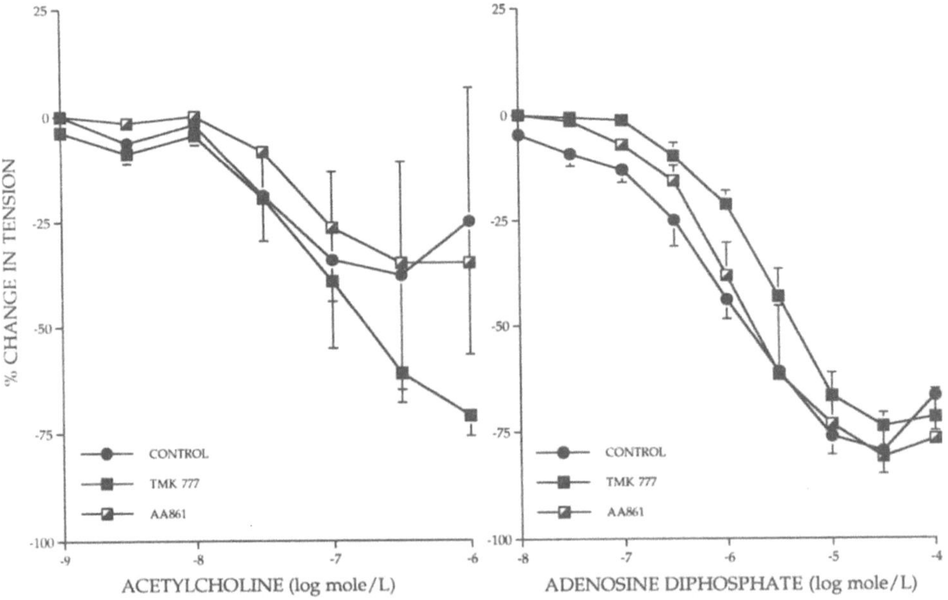

Fig. 2. Responses to acetylcholine and adenosine-5-diphosphate in canine femoral veins, with endothelium, in the absence (*control*) and presence of two inhibitors of lipo-oxygenase (AA861, $1 \times 10^{-5} M$; TMK 777, $1 \times 10^{-6} M$). Rings of blood vessels were suspended for the measurement of isometric force in organ chambers. Data are expressed as percentage change in tension from a contraction to prostaglandin $F_{2\alpha}$ ($2 \times 10^{-6} M$). Values are shown as mean ± SEM, n = 6 in each group

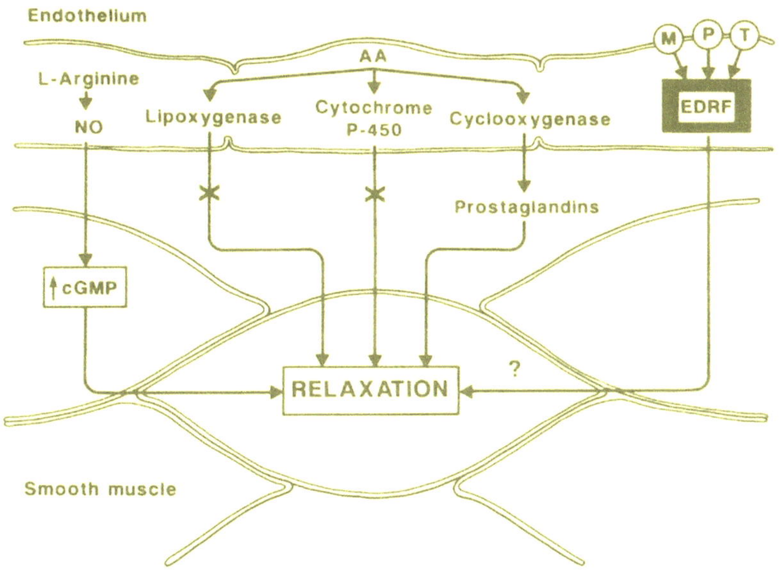

Fig. 3. Schematic of endothelium derived relaxing factors in veins. Muscarinic (*M*), purinergic (*P*), and thrombin (*T*) receptors are located on the endothelial cell surface. These receptors release endothelium-derived relaxing factors (*EDRF*) in veins which cannot be totally explained by nitric oxide or by products of arachidonic acid (*AA*) metabolism by cyclo-oxygenase, lipooxygenase, or cytochrome P-450. EDRF, in turn, produces relaxation in smooth muscle cells by as yet undefined mechanisms

by cyclo-oxygenase, the ratio of vasoconstrictor to vasodilator prostanoids is greater in veins than in arteries [20, 71, 89]. The production of endothelins has not been compared between arterial and venous endothelium. However, venous smooth muscle is more sensitive than arterial smooth muscle to the contractile effects of endothelin-1 [69]. This probably represents differences in both receptors and receptor-activated signal transduction pathways which activate contractile proteins. Two endothelin receptors (types A and B) have been identified by molecular cloning techniques [40, 56, 81, 82]. A selective antagonist of endothelin type A receptors (BQ 123) does not inhibit contractions to endothelin-1 in veins (Fig. 4) as it does in arteries [42]. This observation supports a heterogeneous distribution of endothelin receptors throughout the vasculature. Further, the subtypes of endothelin receptors may be coupled preferentially to specific intracellular mechanisms [14]. This would in part explain observations that membrane depolarization to endothelin-1 is greater in venous compared to arterial smooth muscle [69], and that contractions to endothelin-1 in veins are not sensitive to antagonists of voltage-dependent calcium channels [74].

Collectively, these results indicate that functions of both endothelial and smooth muscle cells of veins and arteries are not the same. This is not sur-

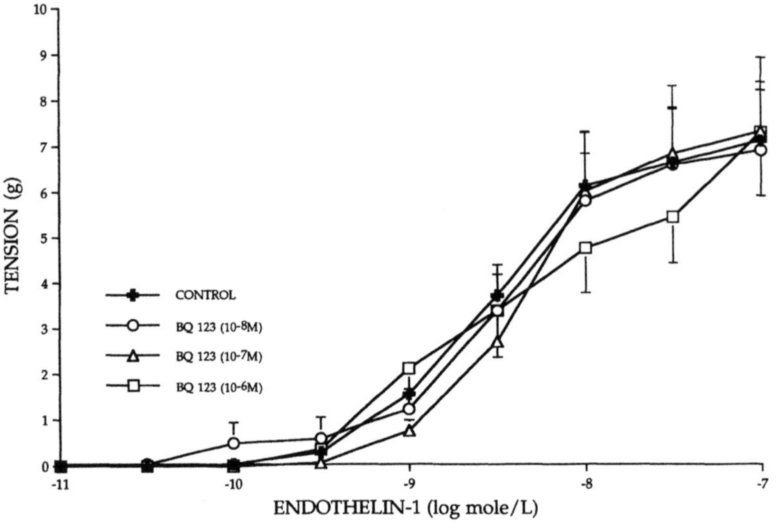

Fig. 4. Contractions to endothelin-1 in canine femoral veins, without endothelium, in the absence (*control*) and presence of a selective antagonist of endothelin type A receptors, BQ 123. Data are expressed as grams increase in tension. Values are shown as mean ± SEM, $n = 6$ in each group. BQ 123 did not inhibit contractions to endothelin-1 in these veins

prising as the blood vessels not only perform different functions in the circulation but are also exposed chronically to different environmental (mechanical and chemical) stimuli. When a vein is placed in the arterial circulation as a graft, pressure, flow, oxygen tension, and circulating hormones affect the metabolism of venous endothelial cells and potentially alter the balance between inhibitory/contractile and anti-mitogenic/mitogenic factors.

Modulation of Venous Endothelium

Mechanical Damage

The manner in which a blood vessel is harvested for use as a graft is important in maintaining a viable and intact endothelial lining. When blood vessels are excised so as to maintain in situ diameter and length, there is minimal endothelial cell loss [54]. The "no touch" method is used routinely to harvest saphenous veins for coronary and femoral popliteal bypass grafts. However, this method can result in up to 70% loss of endothelial cells, which represents about a 60% loss in endothelial-derived relaxing factors, including prostacyclin [2].

Distention of veins may lessen vasospasm prior to implantation. However, this procedure may lower patency rates because of mechanical injury to both endothelial and smooth muscle cells [1]. When saphenous veins are distended to arterial pressures, loss of endothelial cells ranges from 2% to 70%. This is compared to a 4% loss of endothelial cells in arteries distended to the same pressure [63]. Venous endothelial cells also exhibit fewer and more shallow cytoplasmic processes following distension [63]. After implantation of these distended vessels, large thrombogenic defects with exposed collagenous fibrils were found in the veins, while the internal mammary arteries showed little damage [52]. These studies suggest that veins are more susceptible to mechanical damage than arteries following harvesting for grafting.

In addition to harvesting technique, the medium in which the vein is stored prior to implantation may contribute to preserving endothelial integrity. Loss of endothelial cells from human saphenous veins was less than 10% when nitroglycerin was added to a balanced pH electrolyte storage solution [21]. Based upon histological examination of the tissue, veins stored in arterial, heparinized blood (20°–37°C) for up to 90 min showed little structural damage [91]. However, veins stored in heparinized blood had a time-dependent loss in endothelium-dependent relaxations compared to veins stored in physiological salt solution [2]. Therefore, both structural and functional characteristics of the tissue must be determined when evaluating the effectiveness of techniques for harvesting blood vessels for grafting.

Blood Flow and Oxygen Tension

Increases in blood flow stimulate production of endothelium-derived relaxing factors, including nitric oxide, in arterial endothelial cells [9, 19, 28, 68] and inhibit production of endothelins [68, 86]. In veins proximal to an arteriovenous fistula, where blood flow is increased three- to fivefold and the partial pressure of oxygen is increased to arterial levels, endothelium-dependent relaxations mediated by nitric oxide are increased [65] (Fig. 5). Production of endothelin in venous endothelial cells exposed to increases in blood flow and oxygen tension has not been measured directly. However, preliminary experiments from our laboratory suggest that the tissue content of endothelin-1 is reduced in fistula- compared to sham-operated veins by about 33% (unpublished observation). These results suggest that flow and oxygen tension regulate the production of nitric oxide and endothelins in veins as in arteries, and that nitric oxide may provide negative feedback for the production of endothelin in veins. Contractions to endothelin-1 are reduced in fistula-operated venous smooth muscle (unpublished observation). Whether this results from a change in density or sensitivity of endothelin receptors or intracellular mechanisms is not known. However, if endothelin receptors are associated with both contractile and proliferative processes, these results suggest that blood flow and oxygen tension have the potential to alter the proliferative process also. Therefore, it might be

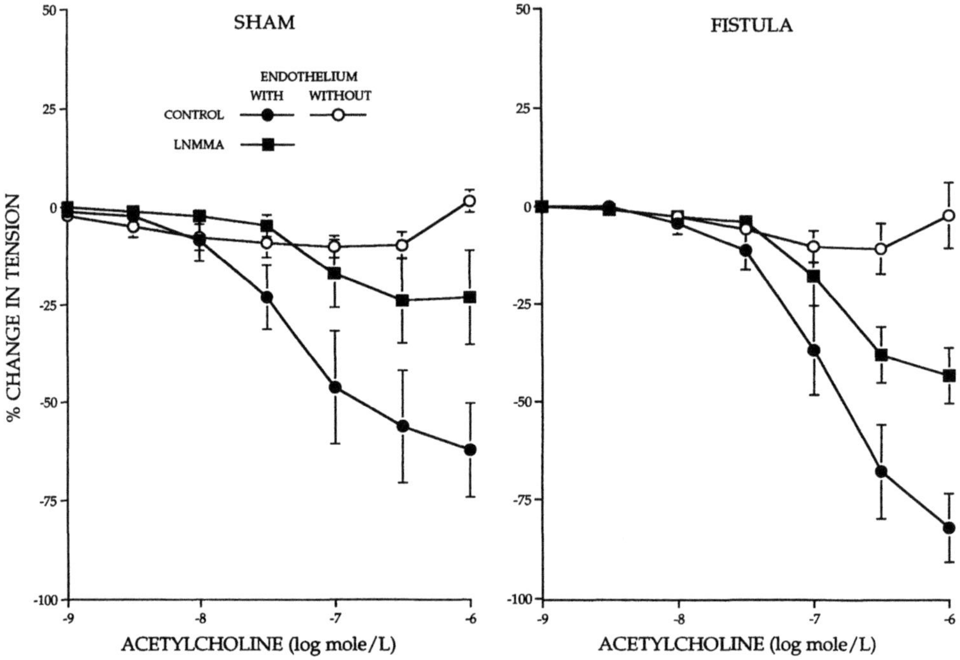

Fig. 5. Responses to acetylcholine in sham- and fistula-operated canine femoral veins, with and without endothelium, in the absence (*control*) and presence of the synthetic analogue of L-arginine (*LNMMA*; 1×10^{-4} *M*). Rings of blood vessels were suspended for the measurement of isometric force in organ chambers. Data are expressed as percentage change in tension from a contraction to prostaglandin $F_{2\alpha}$ (2×10^{-6} *M*). Values are shown as mean ± SEM, $n = 6$ in each group. Relaxations were greater in fistula-operated veins. Inhibition of the relaxations by LNMMA suggests that nitric oxide is one mediator of the relaxation under conditions of chronic increases in blood flow and oxygen tension in veins

expected that the rate of blood flow through the vein graft could affect both anatomical and functional characteristics of that graft (see below).

Endothelium of Vein Grafts

Anatomical and functional changes in veins placed in the arterial circulation have been described as occurring in three phases [1]. First, from day 0 to day 7 there is an initial rapid proliferation of smooth muscle cells with an increase in cell numbers. This may result from an increase in wall stress or cyclical stretching as well as from growth factors released by platelets at sites of endothelial cell denudation or injury. Endothelial cells form a confluent lining in 1 week [1]. The second phase, from week 1 to week 4, includes rapid medial and intimal thickening. This represents no further increase in cell number and a reduction in cell density [1], suggesting cell migration, hypertrophy, and production of extracellular matrix. Finally in the third phase, from week 4 to week 39, there is a slower increase in medial and intimal size with a parallel increase in cell numbers but not cell density [1]. In addition, small, nonmyelinated, but not myelinated nerve endings penetrate the graft [60].

A common feature of reversed and in situ (nonreversed) vein grafts from animals studied after 4 weeks is the selective loss of endothelium-dependent relaxations to acetylcholine [17, 22, 48, 67, 70]. Endothelium-dependent relaxations to adenosine diphosphate, thrombin, and calcium ionophore are preserved in grafts [8, 26]. Whether this is due to a selective loss of muscarinic receptors or coupling of the receptors to synthesis of endothelium-derived factors is not known. In addition, changes in the smooth muscle occur as cyclic guanosine monophosphate (cGMP), which mediates relaxations to nitric oxide, is reduced in the smooth muscle of vein grafts [17, 48]. In spite of some clinical evidence to suggest that long term patency for nonreversed (in situ) grafts is better than reversed grafts [8, 26], no differences were observed in endothelium-dependent responses between the two types of grafts [67]. Indomethacin, an inhibitor of cyclo-oxygenase, increased endothelium-dependent relaxations to the calcium ionophore in non-reversed grafts [67]. These results suggest that contractile substances are produced by endothelial cells of vein grafts, as has been observed in unoperated veins [71]. Methylene blue, an inhibitor of cGMP, also increased relaxations in vein grafts. This ovservation supports the existence of a mechanism other than nitric oxide/cGMP-mediated relaxations in vein grafts (see Fig. 3) [67].

In contrast to grafts taken from experimental animals, explanted, long-term (7 months–12 years) saphenous vein coronary artery bypass grafts from humans demonstrated endothelium-dependent relaxations to acetylcholine, as well as to A23187, thrombin, and histamine [49]. There was an inverse correlation between the magnitude of relaxations to thrombin and the degree of intimal hyperplasia. No such correlation was observed in response to acetylcholine or A23187 [49]. The reasons for differences in response between grafts from humans and animals are not clear. However, the age of the grafts and the anatomical location of the graft (peripheral compared to coronary) may affect endothelium-dependent responses. In addition, human grafts were obtained from explanted hearts of coronary transplant recipients in congestive heart failure. These patients received the "usual medications" for this condition [49], which could include converting enzyme inhibitors, digoxin, and diuretics. Therefore, the chronic effects of circulating hormones and medication in patients with cardiac myopathies necessitating transplant can not be excluded as stimuli affecting the function of endothelial cells in these grafts.

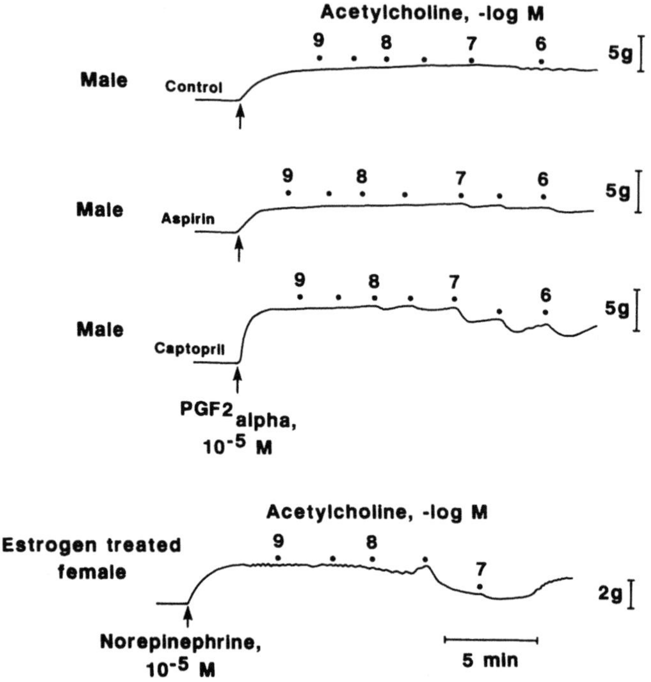

Fig. 6. Representative traces of responses to acetylcholine in rabbit autogenous vein grafts with endothelium. Jugular veins were placed in the carotid arteries as reversed interpositional grafts. After 4 weeks the grafts were removed, and rings were suspended for the measurement of isometric force in organ chambers. *Traces 1–3*, responses to acetylcholine of vein grafts contracted with prostaglandin $F_{2\alpha}$ from untreated, aspirin-treated, and captopril-treated, male rabbits. Note the marked relaxation to acetylcholine in grafts from captopril-treated rabbits. *Bottom trace*, response of a vein graft from an estrogen-treated female rabbit. Again, note the marked relaxation to acetylcholine which is not present in grafts from control male (*top trace*) or ovariectomized-female rabbits (not shown)

Modulation of Graft Patency and Function

Medications

Aspirin is used routinely for antiplatelet therapy after graft surgery [13, 33, 36, 51]. Aspirin may also affect prostanoid production in the endothelium. However, chronic treatment with aspirin did not increase endothelium-dependent relaxations of jugular veins placed as reversed interpositional grafts in carotid arteries of rabbits (unpublished data; see Fig. 6).

The renin-angiotensin pathway is endogenous to the vascular wall [46], and angiotensin II has been implicated as a factor which promotes vascular growth [15, 16, 37]. In addition to reducing mean arterial pressure, converting enzyme inhibitors reduce intimal hyperplasia following vascular injury [16, 37]. Converting enzyme inhibitors which prevent the conversion of angiotensin I to angiotensin II increase formation of eicosanoids from the endothelium via local kinin accumulation and prevent polymorphonuclear accumulation in injured tissue [83].

Chronic treatment with captopril (a converting enzyme inhibitor) restored or protected endothelium-dependent relaxations to acetylcholine in reversed autogenous jugular veins placed into the carotid arteries of male rabbits (Fig. 6). These results may explain why relaxations to acetylcholine were observed in the human coronary grafts, as captopril may be used in the treatment of congestive heart failure.

Hormones

Gender, which is often used in assessing risk for cardiovascular disease may also affect the function of vein grafts [45, 80, 92]. A comparison of reversed vein grafts in ovariectomized female rabbits with and without estrogen supplements showed that only grafts from rabbits treated with estrogen relaxed to acetylcholine (Fig. 6).

Blood Flow and Oxygen Tension

As discussed above, increases in blood flow can initiate release of endothelium-derived factors. Several studies have described structural changes in vein grafts when blood flow through the graft is altered. In general, when blood flow is increased, hyperplasia is decreased [25, 75, 78]. In response to low shear, smooth muscle cells of grafts differentiate into secretory cells. Thus, the intima would be lined with modified smooth muscle cells which could enhance platelet aggregation. In contrast, grafts exposed to high shear had an intima lined with endothelial cells and less intimal hyperplasia [75, 78]. In coronary arterial grafts acute increases in blood flow either by tachycardia or isosorbide dinitrate produced an increase in vasodilation in the mammary arterial grafts, but none in saphenous vein grafts [38]. In reversed femoral vein grafts endothelium-dependent relaxations were determined after blood flow was increased via a fistula distal to the caudal anastomoses. In these grafts, small relaxations to acetylcholine were observed while none were seen in grafts with normal flow (Fig. 7). However, relaxations to adenosine diphosphate and thrombin were increased compared to grafts with normal flows [11]. Relaxations to adenosine diphosphate and thrombin may be mediated by an endothelium-derived factor other than nitric oxide (see Fig. 3). This factor or the receptor-coupled mechanisms associated with its release appears to be more stable than those of acetylcholine/nitric oxide systems. These data suggest that

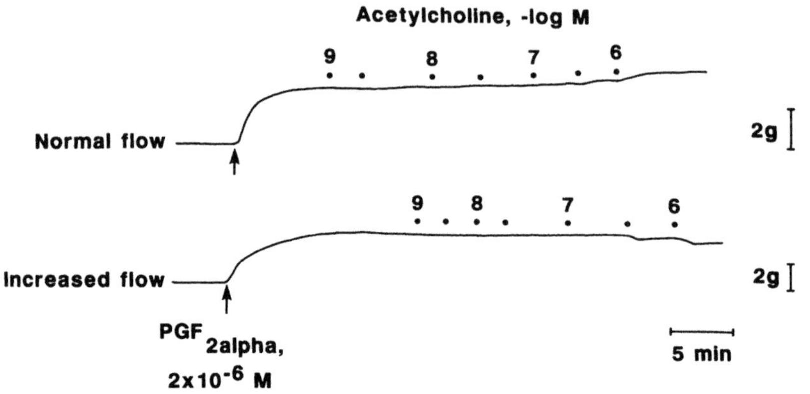

Fig. 7. Representative traces of responses to acetylcholine in canine autogenous vein grafts with endothelium. Femoral veins were placed in femoral arteries as reversed interpositional grafts. After 6 weeks the grafts were removed and rings suspended in organ chamber for the measurement of isometric force. *Top trace*, response of a ring cut from a canine vein graft with normal flow (120 ml/min). *Bottom trace*, response of a canine vein graft in which a fistula was placed distal to the caudal anastomosis (increased flow, 560 ml/min). Note the small relaxation to acetylcholine in the graft with increased flow

expression of receptor-operated, endothelium-dependent relaxations in vein grafts may be related to blood flow. Therefore, since endothelium-derived factors may also affect thrombosis and mitogenesis, blood flow may influence early and long-term patency of vein graft.

Endothelial Function In Alternative Graft Materials

Polymeric Grafts

Often patients with peripheral occlusive disease lack vessels which are suitable for grafting. Synthetic materials provide an alternative form of graft material. The two most common types of materials are dacron and expanded polytetra-fluoroethylene (ePTFE). In order to improve the patency of small diameter synthetic grafts, endothelial cells have been seeded or sodded onto the inner lumen of the synthetic wall. The seeded endothelium produces platelet-derived growth factor (PDGF) at midgraft but not at either anastomosis [44]. Some consider the sodded endothelium functional by the number of adhered thrombi and by the anatomical features of the endothelium [93]. Preliminary data from our laboratory show that autogenous endothelial cells derived from the falciform fat pad and sodded onto ePTFE grafts produce endothelium-derived relaxing factors in response to acetylcholine, ADP, and thrombin when implanted into canine carotid arteries for 4 weeks. Cells lining unsodded grafts did not produce bioassayable relaxing factors in response to these agents.

These results indicate that endothelial cells sodded onto synthetic graft material retain viable, receptor-coupled mechanisms for release of endothelium-derived factors.

Shear stress may also affect patency of synthetic grafts as it does in natural grafts. Dogs with unsodded ePTFE grafts in femoral and carotid arteries had greater pseudointimal thickening and greater neointimal thickening at the anastomosis under low shear stress, while high shear stress in smaller diameter grafts (3 mm) had poorer patency [6]. Unsodded ePTFE grafts in baboons developed less intimal hyperplasia when blood flow through the grafts was increased via a fistula distal to the grafts. When the fistulae were ligated, reducing blood flow, an increase in intimal hyperplasia developed after 1 month [47].

The inherent thrombotic potential (platelet aggregability and prostaglandin synthesis) of the graft recipient may also play a role in the patency of synthetic grafts. Dogs with either high thrombogenic potential or low thrombogenic potential received bilateral dacron grafts in the carotid arteries. Patency rates for the high thrombogenic group that was treated with aspirin and dazmegral, and the low thrombogenic group were 100% while the untreated high thrombogenic group was only 10% [43].

Cryopreserved Natural Veins

Another alternative graft material is frozen, natural blood vessel. Canine coronary arteries were slowly frozen in fetal calf serum and stored for 7 days. Subsequent studies showed that the cryopreserved arteries were able to relax and contract to certain vasoactive agents [50]. The endothelium of cryopreserved canine saphenous veins produces an endothelium-derived relaxing factor and prostanoids, but the ability of the cell to synthesize nitric oxide is probably reduced [24]. Comparison of cryopreserved and freshly harvested saphenous veins used as arterial autografts showed that cryopreservation did not affect early patency, blood flow, or platelet deposition in the grafts at 4 weeks post-operatively [23]. Functional nerve terminals were not present in either fresh or cryopreserved grafts, and endothelium-dependent relaxations to acetylcholine were absent in both types of grafts. However, endothelium-dependent relaxations to ADP and the calcium ionophore A23187 were present in both types of grafts [23]. Results from this study suggest that some endothelial function is retained in cryopreserved veins when used as autografts. However, most often cryopreserved grafts would be used as allografts. These grafts would be subject to factors associated with rejection in addition to other stimuli associated with vein-artery transplant. Canine cryopreserved veins used as arterial allografts remained patent after 4 weeks when the dogs were treated with a combination of antiplatelet and immunosuppressive drugs. However, the grafts lost function al smooth muscle, which precluded assessment of endothelium using organ chambers techniques [66].

Summary

The vascular endothelium produces substances which regulate tone and growth of the underlying smooth muscle. Venous and arterial endothelium differ in production of endothelium-derived factors and in the receptor-coupled mechanisms activating production of these factors. Endothelium of veins used as replacements for diseased arteries may be damaged by mechanical manipulation of the tissue. In addition, pressure, flow, and oxygen tension of the arterial circulation may potentially alter the ratio in production of inhibitory (antithrombogenic antimitogenic, vasodilatory): stimulatory (prothrombogenic, promitogenic, vasoconstrictor) endothelium-derived factors. Careful manipulation of the tissue as well as new therapies directed toward increasing production of antimitogenic endothelium-derived factors may extend the long-term patency of vein grafts.

References

1. Angelini GD, Bryan AJ, Williams HMJ, Soyombo A, Tovey J, Newby AC (1992) Time-course of medial and intimal thickening in pig venous arterial grafts: relationship to endothelial injury and cholesterol accumulation. J Thorac Cardiovasc Surg 103:1093–1103
2. Angelini GD, Christie MI, Bryan AJ, Lewis MJ (1989) Surgical preparation impairs release of endothelium-derived relaxing factor from human saphenous vein. Ann Thorac Surg 48:417–420
3. Azuma H, Ishikawa M, Sekizaki S (1986) Endothelium-dependent inhibition of platelet aggregation. Br J Pharmacol 88:411–415
4. Azuma H, Ishikawa M, Sekizaki S (1986) Endothelium-dependent inhibition of platelet aggregation. Br J Pharmacol 88:441–445
5. Bath PMW, Hassall DG, Gladwin A-M, Palmer RMJ, Martin JF (1991) Nitric oxide and prostacyclin. Divergence of inhibitory effects on monocyte chemotaxis and adhesion to endothelium in vitro. Arterioscler Thromb 11:254–260
6. Binns RL, Ku DN, Stewart MT, Ansley JP, Coyle KA (1989) Optimal graft diameter: effect of wall shear stress on vascular healing. J Vasc Surg 10:326–337
7. Bredt DS, Snyder SH (1990) Isolation of nitric oxide synthetase, a calmodulin-requiring enzyme. Proc Natl Acad Sci USA 87:682–685
8. Buchbinder D, Rollins DL, Semrow CM, Schuler JJ, Meyer JP, Flanigan DP (1988) In situ tibial reconstruction. State-of-the-art or passing fancy. Ann Surg 207:184–188
9. Buga GM, Gold ME, Fukuto JM, Ignarro LJ (1991) Shear strss-induced release of nitric oxide from endothelial cells grown on beads. Hypertension 17:187–193
10. Busse R, Mulsch A (1990) Calcium-dependent nitric oxide synthesis in endothelial cytosol is mediated by calmodulin. FEBS Lett 265:133–136

11. Cambria RA, Lowell RC, Gloviczki P, Miller VM (1994) Chronic changes in blood flow alter endothelium-dependent responses in vein grafts in dogs. J Vasc Surg (in press)
12. Chervu A (1990) Myo-intimal hyperplasia. Semin Vasc Surg 3:21–28
13. Chesebro JH, Fuster V (1986) Platelet-inhibitor drugs before and after coronary artery bypass surgery and coronary angioplasty: the basis of their use, data from animal studies, clinical trial data, and current recommendations. Cardiology 73(4–5):292–305
14. Cioffi CL, Neale RF, Jackson RH, Sills MA (1992) Characterization of rat lung endothelin receptor subtypes which are coupled to phosphoinositide hydrolysis. J Pharmacol Exp Ther 262:611–618
15. Clozel J-P, Hess P, Michael C, Schietinger K, Baumgartner HR (1991) Inhibition of converting enzyme and neointima formation after vascular injury in rabbits and guinea pigs. Hypertension 18:II–55–II–59
16. Clozel M, Kuhn H, Hefti F (1990) Effects of angiotensin-converting enzyme inhibitors and of hydralazine on endothelial function in hypertensive rats. Hypertension 16:532–540
17. Cross KS, El-Sanadiki MN, Murray JJ, Mikat EM, McCann RL, Hagen P-O (1988) Functional abnormalities of experimental autogenous vein graft neoendothelium. Ann Surg 208:631–638
18. Davies PF, Tripathi SC (1993) Mechanical stress mechanisms and the cell. An endothelial paradigm. Circ Res 72:239–245
19. DeForrest JM, Hollis TM (1978) Shear stress and aortic histamine synthesis. Am J Physiol 234:H701–H705
20. DeMey JG, Vanhoutte PM (1982) Heterogeneous behavior of the canine arterial and venous wall. Circ Res 51:439–447
21. Dries D, Mohammad SF, Woodward SC, Nelson RM (1992) The influence of harvesting technique on endothelial preservation in saphenous veins. J Surg Res 52:219–225
22. El-Khatib H, Lupinetti FM, Sanofsky SJ, Behrendt DM (1991) Production of endothelium-dependent relaxation responses by saphenous vein grafts in the canine circulation. Surgery 110:523–528
23. Elmore JR, Gloviczki P, Brockbank KGM, Miller VM (1991) Cryopreservation affects endothelial and smooth muscle function of canine autogenous saphenous vein grafts. J Vasc Surg 13:584–592
24. Elmore JR, Gloviczki P, Brockbank KGM, Miller VM (1992) Functional changes in canine saphenous veins after cryopreservation. Int Angiol 11:26–35
25. Faulkner SC, Fisher RD, Conkle DM, Page DL, Bender HW Jr (1975) Effect of blood flow rate on subendothelial proliferation in venous autografts used as arterial substitutes. Circulation [Suppl I]:163–172
26. Fogle MA, Whittemore AD, Couch NP, Mannick JA (1987) A comparison of in situ and reversed saphenous vein grafts for infrainguinal reconstruction. J Vasc Surg 5:46–52
27. Forstermann U, Alheid U, Frolich JC, Mulsch A (1988) Mechanisms of action of lipoxygenase and cytochrome P-450-mono-oxygenase inhibitors in blocking endothelium-dependent vasodilatation. Br J Pharmacol 93:569–578
28. Frangos JA, Eskin SG, McIntire LV, Ives CL (1985) Flow effects on prostacyclin production by cultured human endothelial cells. Science 227:1477–1479
29. Furchgott RF, Zawadski J (1980) The obligatory role of epithelial cells in the relaxation of arterial smooth muscle by acetylcholine. Nature 288:373–376
30. Furlong B, Henderson AH, Lewis MJ, Smith JA (1987) Endotherlium-derived relaxing factor inhibits in vitro platelet aggregation. Br J Pharmacol 90:687–692
31. Furuta T, Hayakawa A, Iida N, Inagaki A, Shigei T (1987) Distribution of cholinesterase in canine venous system. Jpn J Pharmacol 43:237–241
32. Furuta T, Shigei T (1987) A regional difference in endothelium-dependent relaxation responses to acetylcholine in the canine venous system. Jpn J Pharmacol 44:207–210
33. Fuster V, Dyken ML, Vokonas PS, Hennekens C (1993) Aspirin as a therapeutic agent in cardiovascular disease. Circulation 87:659–675

34. Gal CS, Herbert JM, Garcia C, Boutin M, Maffrand JP (1990) Importance of the phenotypic state of vascular smooth muscle cells on the binding and the mitogenic activity of endothelin. Peptides 12:575–579
35. Garg UC, Hassid A (1989) Nitric oxide-generating vasodilators and 8-bromo-cyclic guanosine monophosphate inhibit mitogenesis and proliferation of cultured rat vascular smooth muscle cells. J Clin Invest 83:1774–1777
36. Gavaghan TP, Gebski V, Baron DW (1991) Immediate postoperative aspirin improves vein graft patency early and late after coronary artery bypass graft surgery. A placebo-controlled, randomized study. Circulation 83(5):1526–1533
37. Griffin SA, Brown WCB, MacPherson F, McGrath JC, Wilson VG, Korsgaard N, Mulvany MJ, Lever AF (1991) Angiotensin II causes vascular hypertrophy in part by a non-pressor mechanism. Hypertension 17:626–635
38. Hanet C, Schroeder E, Michel X, Cosyns J, Rion R, Verhelst R, Wijns W (1991) Flow-induced vasomotor response to tachycardia of the human internal mammary artery and saphenous vein grafts late following bypass surgery. Circulation 84:III-286–III-274
39. Hecker M, Mitchell JA, Harris HJ, Katsura M, Thiemermann C, Vane JR (1990) Endothelial cells metabolize N^G-monomethyl-L-arginine to L-citrulline and subsequently to L-arginine. Biochem Biophys Res Commun 167:1037–1043
40. Hosoda K, Nakao K, Arai H, Suga S, Ogawa Y, Mukoyama M, Shirakami G, Saito Y, Nakanishi S, Imura H (1991) Cloning and expression of human endothelin-1 receptor cDNA. FEBS Lett 287:23–26
41. Ignarro LJ (1990) Biosynthesis and metabolism of endothelium-derived nitric oxide. Annu Rev Pharmacol Toxicol 30:535–560
42. Ihara M, Noguchi K, Saeki T, Fukuroda T, Tsuchilda S, Kimura S, Fukami T, Ishikawa K, Nishikibe M, Yano M (1992) Biological profiles of highly potent novel endothelin antagonisits selective for the ET_A receptor. Life Sci 50:247–255
43. Kaplan S, Marcoe KF, Sauvage LR, Zammit M, Wu H-D, Mathisen SR, Walker MW (1986) The effect of predetermined thrombotic potential of the recipient on small-caliber graft performance. J Vasc Surg 3:311–321
44. Kaufman BR, Fox PL, Graham LM (1992) Platelet-derived growth factor production by canine aortic grafts seeded with endothelial cells. J Vasc Surg 15:699–707
45. Khan SS, Nessim S, Gray R, Czer LS, Chaux A, Matloff J (1990) Increased mortality of women in coronary artery bypass surgery: evidence for referral bias. Ann Intern Med 112:561–567
46. Kifor I, Dzau VJ (1987) Endothelial renin-angiotensin pathway: evidence for intracellular synthesis and secretion of angiotensins. Circ Res 60:422–428
47. Kohler TR, Kirkman, TR, Kraiss LW, Zierler BK, Clowes AW (1991) Increased blood flow inhibits neointimal hyperplasia in endothelialized vascular grafts. Circ Res 69:1557–1565
48. Komori K, Schini VB, Gloviczki P, Bourchier RG, Vanhoutte PM (1991) The impairment of endothelium-dependent relaxations in reversed vein grafts is associated with a reduced production of cyclic guanosine monophosphate. J Vasc Surg 14:67–75
49. Ku DD, Caulfield JB, Kirklin JK (1991) Endothelium-dependent responses in long-term human coronary artery bypass grafts. Circulation 83:402–411
50. Ku DD, Willis WL, Caulfield JB (1990) Retention of endothelium-dependent vasodilatory responses in canine coronary arteries following cryopreservation. Cryobiology 27:511–520
51. Landymore RW, MacAulay MA, Manku MS (1990) The effects of low, medium and high dose aspirin on intimal proliferation in autologous vein grafts used for arterial reconstruction. Eur J Cardiothorac Surg 4(8):441–444
52. Lehmann KH, von Segesser L, Muller-Glauser W, Siebenmann R, Schneider K, Luscher TF, Turina M (1989) Internal mammary coronary artery grafts: is their superiority also due to a basically intact endothelium? Thorac Cardiovasc Surg 37:187–189
53. Lerman A, Burnett JC Jr (1992) Intact and altered endothelium in regulation of vasomotion. Circulation III:12–19

54. Lewis DA, Loomis JL, Segal SS (1991) Preservation of endothelial cells in excised rat carotid arteries. Effects of transmural pressure and segment length. Circ Res 69:997–1002
55. Lewis DA, Miller VM (1992) Role of lipoxygenase and cytochrome-P450 in the production of endothelium-derived relaxing factors in canine femoral veins. J Cardiovasc Pharmacol 20:401–407
56. Lin HY, Kaji EH, Winkel GK, Ives HE, Lodish HF (1991) Cloning and functional expression of a vascular smooth muscle endothelin 1 receptor. Proc Natl Acad Sci 88:3185–3189
57. Lipowsky H, Chien S (1989) Role of leukocyte-endothelium adhesion in affecting recovery from ischemic episodes. Ann NY Acad Sci 565:308–315
58. Luscher TF, Diederich D, Siebenmann R, Lehmann K, Stulz P, von Segesser L, Yang Z, Turina M, Gradel E, Weber E, Buhler FR (1988) Difference between endothelium-dependent relaxation in arterial and in venous coronary bypass grafts. N Engl J Med 319:462–467
59. Masaki T, Kimura S, Yanagisawa M, Goto K (1991) Molecular and cellular mechanism of endothelin regulation. Implications for vascular function. Circulation 84:1457–1477
60. McGeachie JK, Meagher S, Prendergast FJ (1989) Vein-to-artery grafts: the long-term development of neo-intimal hyperplasia and its relationship to vasa vasorum and sympathetic innervation. Aust N Z J Surg 59:59–65
61. Mehta JL, Lawson DL, Nichols WW, Mehta P (1989) Modulation of vascular tone by neutrophils: dependence on endothelial integrity. Am J Physiol 257:H1315
62. Mehta JL, Lawson DL, Nicolini FA, Ross MH, Player DW (1991) Effects of activated polymorphonuclear leukocytes on vascular smooth muscle tone. Am J Physiol 261:H327–H334
63. Merrilees MJ, Shepphard AJ, Robinson MC (1988) Structural features of saphenous vein and internal thoracic artery endothelium: correlates with susceptibility and resistance to graft atherosclerosis. J Cardiovasc Surg 29:639–646
64. Miller VM (1991) Selective production of endothelium-derived nitric oxide in canine femoral veins. Am J Physiol 261:H677–H682
65. Miller VM, Aarhus LL, Vanhoutte PM (1986) Modulation of endothelium-dependent responses by chronic alterations of blood flow. Am J Physiol 251:H520–H527
66. Miller VM, Bergman RT, Gloviczki P, Brockbank KGM (1992) Cryopreserved venous allografts: effects of immunosuppression and antiplatelet therapy on patency and function. J Vasc Surg (in press)
67. Miller VM, Bower TC, McCullough JL, Gloviczki P, Vanhoutte PM (1990) Endothelium-dependent responses in nonreversed (in situ) vein grafts. J Vasc Biol Med 2:155–162
68. Miller VM, Burnett JC Jr (1992) Modulation of nitric oxide and endothelin by chronic increases in blood flow in canine femoral arteries. Am J Physiol 263:H103–H108
69. Miller VM, Komori K, Burnett JC Jr, Vanhoutte PM (1989) Differential sensitivity to endothelin in canine arteries and veins. Am J Physiol 257:H1127–H1131
70. Miller VM, Reigel MM, Hollier LH, Vanhoutte PM (1987) Endothelium-dependent responses in autogenous femoral veins grafted into the arterial circulation of the dog. J Clin Invest 80:1350–1357
71. Miller VM, Vanhoutte PM (1985) Endothelium-dependent contractions to arachidonic acid are mediated by products of cyclo-oxgenase. Am J Physiol 248:H432–H437
72. Miller VM, Vanhoutte PM (1989) Is nitric oxide the only endothelium-derived relaxing factor in canine femoral veins? Am J Physiol 257:H1910–H1916
73. Miller VM, Vanhoutte PM (1990) Relaxations to SIN-1, nitric oxide, and sodium nitroprusside in canine arteries and veins. J Cardiovasc Pharmacol 14:S67–S71
74. Miller VM, Vanhoutte PM (1990) Contractions to endothelin in canine veins: effects of calcium antagonists and inhibitors of endothelium-derived relaxing factor(s). In: Rubanyi GM, Vanhoutte PM (eds) Endothelium-derived contracting factors. Karger, Basel, pp 80–87

75. Morinaga K, Eguchi H, Miyazaki T, Okadome K, Sugimachı K (1987) Development and regression of intimal thickening of arterially transplanted autologous vein grafts in dogs. J Vasc Surg 5:719–730
76. Mulsch A, Bassenge E, Busse R (1989) Nitric oxide synthesis in endothelial cytosol: evidence for a calcium-dependent and a calcium-independent mechanism. Naunyn Schmiedebergs Arch Pharmacol 340:767–770
77. Nishida K, Harrison DG, Navas JP, Fisher AA, Dockery SP (1992) Molecular cloning and characterization of the constitutive bovine aortic endothelial cell nitric oxide synthase. J Clin Invest 90:2092–2096
78. Okadome KT, Yukizane T, Mii S, Sugimachi K (1990) Ultrastructural evidence of the effects of shear stress variation on intimal thickening in dogs with arterial transplanted autologus vein grafts. J Cardiovasc Surg 31:719–726
79. Palmer RMJ, Ferrige AG, Moncada S (1987) Nitric oxide release accounts for the biological activity of the endothelium-derived relaxing factor. Nature 327:524–526
80. Roberts WC, Kragel AH, Potkin BN (1990) Ages at death and sex distribution in age decade in fatal coronary artery disease. Am J Cardiol 66:1379–1381
81. Sakamoto A, Yanagisawa M, Sakuraj T, Takuwa Y, Yanagasawa H, Masaki T (1991) Cloning and functional expression of human cDNA for the ET_B endothelin receptor. Biochem Biophys Res Commun 178:656–663
82. Sakurai T, Yanagisawa M, Takuwa Y, Miyazaki H, Kimura S, Goto K, Masaki T (1990) Cloning of cDNA encoding a non-isopeptide-selective subtype of the endothelin receptor. Nature 348:732–735
83. Schror K (1992) Role of prostaglandins in the cardiovascular effects of bradykinin and angiotensin-converting enzyme inhibitors. J Cardiovasc Pharmacol 20:S68–S73
84. Scott-Burden T, Schini VB, Elizondo E, Junquero DC, Vanhoutte PM (1992) Platelet-derived growth factor suppresses and fibroblast growth factor enhances cytokine-induced production of nitric oxide by cultured smooth muscle cells. Circ Res 71:1088–1100
85. Seidel CL, LaRochelle J (1987) Venous and arterial endothelia: different dilator abilities in dog vessels. Circ Res 60:626–630
86. Sharefkin JB, Diamond SL, Eskin SG, McIntire LV, Dieffenbach CW (1991) Fluid flow decreases preproendothelin mRNA levels and suppresses endothelin-1 peptide release in cultured human endothelial cells. J Vasc Surg 14:1–9
87. Shichiri M, Hirata Y, Nakajima T, Ando K, Imai T, Yanagisawa M, Masaki T, Marumo F (1991) Endothelin-1 is an autocrine/paracrine growth factor for human cancer cell lines. J Clin Invest 87:1867–1871
88. Simonson MS, Jones JM, Dunn MJ (1992) Differential regulation of fos and jun gene expression and AP-1 cis-element activity by endothelin isopeptides. J Biol Chem 267:8643–8649
89. Skidgel RA, Printz MP (1978) PGI_2 production by rat blood vessels: diminished prostacyclin formation in veins compared to arteries. Prostaglandins 16:1–16
90. Vanhoutte PM, Miller VM (1985) Heterogeneity of endothelium-dependent responses in mammalian blood vessels. J Cardiovasc Pharmacol 7:S12–S23
91. Wagner R (1990) Intimal protection of bypass-veins during intraoperative storage in blood or Euro-Collins-solution: the role of medium, temperature, and time. Thorac Cardiovasc Surg 38:151–156
92. Wenger NK (1990) Gender, Coronary artery disease, and coronary bypass surgery (editorial). Ann Intern Med 112:557–558
93. Williams SK, Schneider T, Kapelan B, Jarrell BE (1991) Formation of a functional endothelium on vascular grafts. J Elect Micro Tech 19:239–451

Pharmacological Intervention

Lipids and Lipid-Lowering Drugs and Graft Function

H. Drexel and F.W. Amann

Nature and Time Course of Graft Changes

There is a relationship between the type of graft changes and the time since operation. (a) Thrombotic events are almost exclusively responsible for early graft closures and account for an attrition rate of 10% by 1 month after operation [16]. (b) By the end of the first postoperative year a further 10% loss of patent bypasses has occurred because of intimal fibromuscular hypertrophy. (c) Atherosclerotic plaque, in contrast, is not detectable prior to the end of the first year after operation and is rarely observed before the end of the second or third year [1, 2, 23, 30–32]. Plaques are observed histologically in 21% of grafts at a mean of 5 years after operation; about one-third of grafts at this time have more than 75% atherosclerotic obstructions, and a further one-third have total occlusions secondary to atherosclerosis. In one study, atherosclerosis – defined as intimal foam cell accumulation or frank plaques – was found only 39 or more months after operation and was present in 79% of such cases [29]. Consistent with the temporal sequence of graft changes, all atherosclerotic grafts show some degree of intimal fibromuscular proliferation.

The atherosclerotic lesions observed in vein grafts differ morphologically from lesions in arteries in two respects: (a) foam cells are the principal or even the only cell in the lesion, and (b) the foam cells appear to erode the thickened intima. Thus, these lesions resemble more the experimentally induced atherosclerotic lesions in animals than "native" fatty streak or plaque lesions in human arteries; consequently they appear more closely related to lipids and lipid-laden cells than "native" human atherosclerotic lesions. Otherwise, the atherosclerotic lesions are indistinguishable from those occurring in native arteries, and occlusions result from the typical complications, thrombi, or intimal dissections with intramural hematomas. The thin fibrous cap of the lipid-rich lesions makes them fragile, and this explains the occurrence of rupture and thrombosis.

In good agreement with the above-mentioned histological findings, angiographically detectable atherosclerotic graft changes usually do not develop earlier than 3 years, and the majority of angiographically visible graft stenoses appear between 5 and 12 years after grafting [12, 13]. In keeping with this notion, a bypass patency rate of about 80% is almost unchanged from 1 to 5 years postoperatively [10]. However, between years 6 and 11, a drop occurs from 80% to 63% of grafts. During this period, the average luminal diameter reduction increases from 40% to 60%, and the proportion of grafts with significant (≥50%) stenosis increases from 33% to 70%. In an autopsy study about 50% of patients had evidence of atherosclerosis in at least one of their grafts after 10–12 years [10]. Angiographic evidence of atherosclerosis had a major impact on prognosis: patients with lesions had at least twice the risk of graft occlusion between 10 and 12 years after bypass surgery than those without. In summary, the typical lag time of atherosclerosis manifestation in grafts is about 5 years. This time pattern of lesion development permits to take preventive steps aimed against graft atherosclerosis. Under the ideal (but unrealistic) assumption that graft atherosclerosis is totally preventable (e.g., by lipid intervention), one could expect to be able to abolish specifically the atherosclerosis-related attrition occurring between years 1 and 10, but not the attrition attributable to thrombosis and fibrointimal proliferation during year 1. Consequently, an increase in patency rate from 67% to only 80% but not 100% would be achieved. This should be kept in mind when considering interventions.

The above observations apply only for saphenous vein grafts (SVGs) and not for internal mammary artery (IMA) grafts. Interestingly, IMA grafts rarely develop atherosclerosis, even late postoperatively. In comparison, the patency rate 10 years after operation is about 90% with IMA grafts versus 50% with SVGs [19]. Specifically, atherosclerotic occlusions were reported by the same authors in only 5% of patients with IMA grafts as opposed to 53% with SVGs. In line with these findings, the incidence of late cardiac events is also lower with IMA grafts as compared to SVGs, and long-term (10-year) survival of patients is significantly ($p < 0.0001$) better than with SVGs [14, 24].

It is also interesting to compare progression of atherosclerosis in grafts with that occurring in coronary branches unrelated to grafts in the same patients. At 11 years 10% of the unrelated branches show disease progression, thus considerably less than the 37% in grafts [9]. This finding is strongly supported by experimental evidence in hypercholesterolemic animals showing a greater tendency to develop atheroma in vein grafts than in native coronary arteries [17, 22, 26–28], or grafted internal thoracic arteries [8, 20, 26]. In contrast to native arteries IMA grafts SVGs venous grafts thus appear especially prone to atheroma, while progression of atherosclerosis is in the same order of magnitude in native arteries and in IMA grafts. In other words, SVGs require more aggressive preventive steps against atherosclerosis.

Graft Atherosclerosis: A Lipid-Related Disease?

Before discussing these data one should emphasize that patients undergoing coronary artery bypass grafting have one selection criterion in common: they are prone to atherosclerotic vascular lesions. Thus, the selection of these patients is systematically biased towards atherogenic risk factors [25].

Strong evidence for dyslipidemia as a risk factor for human venous graft atherosclerosis also comes from follow-up studies. Angiographic evidence of atherosclerosis in bypass grafts is not related to age, gender, or commonly identified risk factors such as cigarette smoking after operation, hypertension, and diabetes mellitus [11, 13].

In contrast, total serum cholesterol and serum triglycerides are higher in patients with atherosclerotic grafts than in patients with unchanged grafts 10–12 years after bypass surgery [13]. Also, high-density lipoprotein (HDL) cholesterol is lower and low-density lipoprotein (LDL) cholesterol higher in patients with grafts developing atherosclerotic lesions than in patients without lesions [13]. Interestingly, in the same patients none of the risk factors (including lipids) was predictive of simultaneous disease progression in native arteries. This again underlines that the SVGs are more prone to atherosclerosis; the reason for this is that they are more vulnerable to dyslipidemia than native vessels. The lack of correlations between nonlipid risk factors – such as diabetes mellitus or cigarette smoking – and subsequent events may be due to the small patient numbers studied [11] and should not be mistaken as arguing against intervention of multiple risk factors. However, it appears justified to distinguish between stronger (i.e., lipid) and weaker (i.e., non-lipid) risk factors.

In a retrospective autopsy study Atkinson et al. [1] examined the relationship between lesion morphology and risk factors. This series contained 90% men. Cholesterol and blood pressure measurements were performed five and four times per patient, respectively. Atherosclerotic grafts had been in place longer than those with fibrointimal proliferation. High-degree stenoses and occlusions were mostly atherosclerotic. A strong association of hypercholesterolemia (defined as >240 mg/dl) was found with graft atherosclerosis, whereas fibrointimal proliferation was increased in patients with hypertension. It is noteworthy that the differences in lipids between the two cohorts were large. Patients with atherosclerotic grafts had mean cholesterol levels of around 315 mg/dl (8.1 mmol/l) compared to 170 mg/dl (4.4 mmol/l) in patients with fibrointimal proliferation only. Patients with and without fibrointimal proliferation differed significantly in their mean systolic blood pressure levels: 160 versus 135 mmHg. Again, no relationships were found between diabetes mellitus or smoking and histologic graft changes. The authors concluded that the presence of risk factors may determine the type of change that occurs in saphenous vein bypass grafts. Since morphologic lesions varied from graft to graft even in the same patient, the authors also concluded that other risk factors, such as technical, hemodynamic factors, as well as preexisting changes might have been contributory in their patients.

One study found no clear association of plasma lipids with graft atherosclerosis [18]. Even in this study, although not significantly different to patients without progression of graft atherosclerosis, those with occlusion at 6 years had high triglyceride (295 ± 222 mg/dl) and cholesterol levels (267 ± 57 mg/dl). No lipoprotein levels were reported from this study.

Lipid Metabolism: A Brief Overview of the Clues to Atherosclerosis

The principal question now is whether the relationship of elevated plasma cholesterol and triglyceride levels to graft atherosclerosis is causal. To answer this question, a look at lipoprotein metabolism is helpful [21].

Apolar lipids (triglycerides and cholesteryl esters) are insoluble in aqueous fluids such as blood. Hence, lipid transport can be achieved only via "solubilization" of lipids by lipoproteins. These macromolecules carry the apolar lipids in their core, which is wrapped by a surface film consisting of a monolayer of phospholipids and proteins. The surface film has thus the structure of half a cell membrane. The specific requirements for lipid transport are met by the protein component, the so-called apolipoproteins (apo). These molecules accomplish three important metabolic steps: secretion of lipoprotein, activation of lipolytic enzymes, and binding to specific lipoprotein receptors.

In the fasted (postabsorptive) state, the liver is the only site of lipoprotein secretion (Fig. 1). Hepatic triglycerides and cholesteryl esters are packed into very low density lipoproteins (VLDL); each VLDL particle carries one molecule apo B 100, which is one of the largest mammalian proteins (>500 kDa).

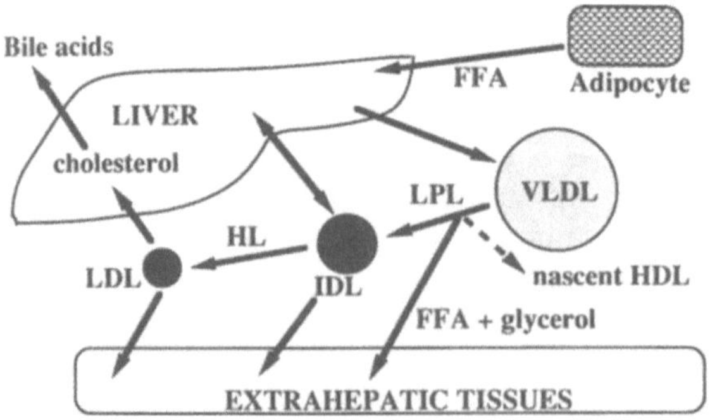

Fig. 1. Schematic model of lipid metabolism. *LDL*, Low-density lipoprotein; *IDL*, intermediate-density lipoprotein; *VLDL*, very-low-density lipoprotein; *HDL*, high-density lipoprotein; *HL*, hepatic lipase; *LPL*, lipoprotein lipase; *FFA*, free fatty acids

Table 1. Enzymes and transfer proteins involved in lipid metabolism

Enzyme	Main site of action	Mode of action	Molecular weight (kDa)
Lipoprotein lipase	Muscle endothelium	Triglyceride hydrolysis	50
Hepatic lipase	Liver endothelium	Triglyceride hydrolysis	53
Lecithin: cholesteryl acyltransferase	Circulating blood	Cholesteryl esterification	47
Cholesteryl ester transfer protein	Circulating blood	Lipid exchange	74

Circulating VLDL offer triglycerides to nonhepatic tissues. A major proportion of the VLDL triglycerides is hydrolyzed by lipoprotein lipase (Table 1). This enzyme (50 kDa) is found abundantly in the capillary bed of skeletal muscle, myocardium, and adipose tissue. Via fatty acids, triglyceride hydrolysis provides these tissues with energy. Concomitantly, lipolysis gives rise to smaller and relatively cholesterol-enriched intermediate-density lipoproteins (IDL). VLDL and IDL adsorb apo E in the circulation, by which IDL can bind to the membranes of hepatic and nonhepatic cells via the so-called apo B/E receptor.

A further step in triglyceride hydrolysis is mediated by hepatic lipase (53 kDa) which is located at sinusoidal capillaries (Table 1). IDL are the main substrate of hepatic lipase. Triglyceride removal increases their relative cholesterol content and density, the particles being transformed to LDL. LDL are taken up by hepatic and extrahepatic cells via the apo B/E receptor.

HDL are closely linked to triglyceride metabolism. Firstly, by the hydrolysis of triglycerides lipoprotein lipase diminishes the core mass of VLDL. In consequence, a respective part of the surface film dissociates from the particle. By interaction between hydrophobic surfaces discoidal bilayers of protein and phospholipids are formed. These discs represent nascent HDL and encompass all necessary components of mature lipoproteins except core lipids. In addition to these VLDL-derived nascent HDL, similar or identical particles are also secreted by liver and intestine. Nascent HDL are transformed to mature HDL particles by uptake of lipids, mainly cholesterol. The term "reverse cholesterol transport" refers to a putative pathway that includes transfer of free cholesterol from peripheral tissues onto HDL, cholesterol esterification at the surface of the HDL particle by lecithin: cholesterol acyltransferase (47 kDa), transport of HDL cholesteryl esters to the liver, and hepatic uptake of the cholesteryl esters (Fig. 2). It can be seen in Fig. 2 that triglycerides also intervene with HDL metabolism by the action of cholesteryl ester transfer protein (74 kDa) which catalyzes an exchange of VLDL triglyceride and HDL cholesterol, thus causing a net transfer of triglyceride from VLDL to HDL and one of cholesterol in the opposite direction from HDL to VLDL. This explains,

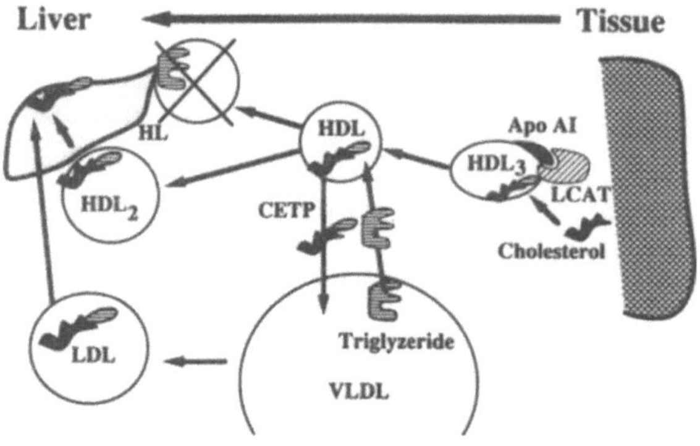

Fig. 2. Reverse cholesterol transport. *HL*, hepatic lipase; *Apo*, apolipoprotein; *CETP*, cholesteryl ester transfer protein; *LCAT*, lecithin:cholesteryl acyltransferase; *HDL*, high-density lipoprotein; *LDL*, low-density lipoprotein; *VLDL*, very-low-density lipoprotein

together with the connection between lipolysis and nascent HDL, why increased VLDL and decreased HDL often coexist in individuals, or, conversely, why subjects with effective triglyceride removal (and low plasma triglyceride levels) such as endurance athletes typically have high HDL levels.

IDL and LDL are considered directly atherogenic. VLDL probably are not atherogenic per se. However, by intervening with the reverse cholesterol transport, VLDL can be seen as being indirectly atherogenic. HDL are associated with protection against atherosclerosis, and one way to explain this is reverse cholesterol transport with removal of excess cholesteryl esters from nonhepatic tissues such as the arterial wall.

In summary, the accumulation of cholesterol in the peripheral tissue is positively related to IDL and LDL levels and negatively related to HDL levels. This view of the fasting lipid transport should be widened by considering postprandial lipid transport. Alimentary triglycerides and cholesterol are secreted by chylomicrons whose triglycerides serve as substrate for lipoprotein lipase in a manner identical to VLDL triglycerides. After lipolysis, a particle class arises which, similarly to IDL, is cholesterol enriched and referred to as chylomicron remnants. The latter complete the picture of cholesterol movements in the blood: LDL and IDL in the fasting state and chylomicron remnants in the postprandial state cover the cholesterol demand of peripheral tissues. However, if increased, these lipoproteins overload tissues with cholesterol. HDL eventually counterbalance this overload by taking up the excess cholesterol. Various disturbances of this lipid homeostasis increase the risk for atherosclerotic vascular disease.

A further independent and direct atherosclerotic risk lies in lipoprotein (a). This LDL-like particle is characterized by covalent linkage of apo B to the so-called apolipoprotein (a) which is a glycoprotein biochemically resembling plasminogen. Its plasma concentration is mainly determined genetically, and levels higher than 300 mg/l are considered atherogenic. Because, at the time of this writing, there is no effective means of lowering apolipoprotein (a) levels, this independent lipid risk factor will not be further considered here. In view of the fact that the hallmark of human atherosclerosis is cholesteryl ester accumulation in the arterial intima it is not surprising that all defects in the transport of cholesteryl esters ultimately are involved in atherogenicity.

Regarding patients with graft atherosclerosis, both hypercholesterolemia (>300 mg/dl) and hypertriglyceridemia (>200 mg/dl) are risk factors. Hypercholesterolemia in this range is caused by LDL or IDL, and triglycerides in this range are most often associated with low HDL levels. Thus, in any of these cases there is an atherogenic lipoprotein pattern, and our current understanding of lipoprotein metabolism provides the link to explain graft atherosclerosis.

If the arterial wall is exposed to such dyslipidemias, lipid deposition (atheroma) and fibrous tissue growth (sclerosis) [3] occur. There are numerous indications that autologous venous grafts succumb to this atherosclerotic action of dyslipidemias. Indeed, as mentioned above, it appears that grafts are more vulnerable than natural arteries.

Selected Aspects of Clinical Pharmacology of Lipid-Lowering Drugs

Grossly, two types of drugs affecting lipid metabolism can be distinguished: those mainly lowering triglyceride levels (and increasing HDL levels) and those triggering LDL cholesterol removal from the plasma and thus mainly lowering cholesterol levels. Among the former nicotinic acid and its derivatives (e.g., acipimox) decrease VLDL synthesis and increase VLDL catabolism. VLDL and its products (IDL and LDL) are decreased and HDL is increased. Fibric acid derivatives (clofibrate, bezafibrate, gemfibrozil) have a similar mode of action and mainly increase lipoprotein lipase acitivity thereby decreasing VLDL and increasing HDL; lowering of LDL is less pronounced.

Bile acid sequestrant resins such as colestyramine or colestipol increase cholesterol removal. By adsorption of bile acids in the bowel lumen and interruption of their enterohepatic circle, the resins increase bile acid synthesis from cholesterol and decrease hepatic intracellular cholesterol levels. Secondary to the decrease in the intracellular cholesterol pool, the cell increases LDL receptor number at its surface, and more LDL are bound. Thus, resins ultimately lower LDL cholesterol and consequently total cholesterol. Inhibitors of hydroxy-methyl-glutaryl coenzyme A reductase (lovastatin, pravastatin, simvastatin) directly inhibit de novo synthesis of cholesterol at an early rate-limiting step in the synthetic pathway. This lowers intra-

Table 2. Effectiveness of lipid-lowering drugs

Compound	Cholesterol (%)	Triglycerides (%)	HDL cholesterol (%)	LDL cholesterol (%)
Resins[a]	−15	+10	+5	−20
Statins[b]	−30	−10	+10	−40
Niacin	−20	−30	+20	−15
Fibrates[c]	−10	−40	+15	−5
Probucol	−10	−10	−25	−10

[a] e.g., colestyramine, colestipol.
[b] e.g., lovastatin, pravastatin, simvastatin.
[c] e.g., clofibrate, bezafibrate, fenofibrate, gemfibrozil.

cellular cholesterol, increases LDL receptor number, and stimulates LDL uptake.

Probucol is a unique drug in that it lowers both LDL and HDL cholesterol. Because of the HDL-lowering effect and storage of the drug in adipose tissue for many years there are some concerns about the use of this compound. On the other hand, it offers the possibility of additional benefit by inhibiting oxidation of lipoproteins. Oxidative modification of lipoproteins (especially LDL) is thought to play a major role in foam cell formation.

Table 2 summarizes the effectiveness of these five classes of lipid-lowering drugs.

Lipid-Lowering Drugs for Prevention and Regression of Graft Atherosclerosis

Because in humans SVG atherosclerosis is frequently associated with high serum cholesterol and elevated serum triglyceride levels or both [1, 2, 23, 30], it is promising to treat hyperlipidemia in an attempt to prevent graft atheroclerosis. Evidence that this treatment is effective comes mainly from two reports [4, 15] of the Cholesterol Lowering Atherosclerosis Study (CLAS) that was conducted in Los Angeles. In this trial 188 patients were randomized to receive combined colestipol (30 g/day) and niacin (4 g/day) therapy plus diet or placebo plus diet. Only patients who had undergone coronary bypass surgery at least 3 months before entering the trial were included; entry into the CLAS occurred an average of 3.3 years after coronary bypass surgery. CLAS-I [4] had a 2-year follow-up and CLAS-II a 4-year follow-up [15]; thus on average CLAS-I covered the time 3.3–5.3 years after surgery and CLAS II that 3.3–7.3 years after surgery. After an interval of 2 years (CLAS-I) 162 of the 188 patients had a second follow-up angiogram.

Drug therapy resulted in a 25% reduction in total cholesterol, 43% reduction in LDL cholesterol, 37% increase in HDL cholesterol levels, and 57% decrease in the LDL/HDL cholesterol ratio. The active treatment also resulted in a greater weight loss than placebo (from 117% to 113% ideal body weight, compared to a decrease from 119% to 118%). A global change score ranging from −3 to +3 was used to assess progression/regression of atherosclerotic lesions per patient. This score was later shown to correlate well with computer-derived quantitative coronary angiography [7].

The study showed a dramatic (40%) reduction in the percentage of patients with new lesions and with progression of disease in SVGs. The reduction in numbers of new lesions in native coronary arteries was of comparable magnitude as in SVGs. However, no difference was observed in the incidence of new SVG closures in the treated versus the placebo group. Treatment benefit was observed in both low- and high-cholesterol subgroups although it was more pronounced in the latter.

The treatment group developed more skin-related and gastointestinal adverse effects. However, more than 90% of treated patients adhered to the drug regimen: five drug-treated and two placebo-treated patients dropped out because of non-compliance. Nevertheless, the authors cautioned that their aggressive regimen requires close supervision because of recognized side effects. The authors concluded from these data that, "The clinical implication of CLAS coronary results are that therapy after coronary bypass surgery should routinely include measures to lower blood cholesterol levels. At this time, we advocate measures to lower blood cholesterol levels in all post-coronary bypass patients." This was the first and hitherto only study to show a significant benefit of lipid-lowering on the course of SVG atherosclerosis. The success of the study is explained by three features: (a) the study minimized effects of other, nonlipid risk factors by including only currently normotensive nonsmokers; (b) greater changes in blood lipid levels were achieved for longer times than in any previous trial, especially regarding the over 50% decrease in LDL/HDL cholesterol ratio; and (c) more subjects completed two angiograms than in any previous trial.

It is interesting that the same intervention also proved beneficial in significantly preventing progression of femoral atherosclerosis in the same patients. However, the effect on femoral arteries was less marked than the strong and consistent benefit on native coronary arteries and bypass grafts [6].

In a further report after 4 years (CLAS-II) 103 patients not requiring further bypass surgery (56 on colestipol/niacin and 47 on placebo) were reevaluated by a third angiogram [15] (70% of drug- and 79% of placebo-treated patients also were on aspirin). Changes in blood lipid, lipoprotein, and apo levels were maintained, and at 4 years significantly more drug-treated subjects demonstrated nonprogression (52% drug- versus 15% placebo-treated) and regression (18% versus 6%) in native arteries. More importantly, only 16% of drug-treated versus 38% of placebo-treated patients developed new lesions in their bypass grafts, the difference being highly significant both at 2 years ($p = 0.01$) and at 4 years ($p = 0.006$), with a more pronounced benefit after 4 than after 2. The placebo-treated group evidenced significant atherosclerotic progression from 2 to 4 years while the drug-treated group did not. However, again, there was no significant difference between drug-treated and placebo-treated patients in progression of existing graft lesions and graft closures. These data suggest that new graft lesion may be lipid driven, but that progression and occlusion of existing vein graft lesion may be thrombosis driven and not preventable by lipid-lowering interventions. Again, the beneficial effect of drugs was apparent in both high- and low-cholesterol subgroups. A causal relationship between lipid-lowering and beneficial effects on atherosclerosis was further emphasized by the finding of a significant ($p < 0.007$) interaction between treatment and time. In CLAS-II fewer side effects from lipid-lowering drugs were observed than in CLAS-I. This is not astonishing because a decreased frequency of side effects is a frequent clinical observation with long-term niacin therapy, and because aspirin, which reduces some of the niacin-related side effects, was coadministered. The authors concluded that beneficial effects of lipid-lowering intervention continue for 4 years, and that the need for early initiation of vigorous long-term lipid-lowering therapy in coronary bypass subjects was reaffirmed.

It must be noted that the CLAS studies included only men. Thus, there is no direct information about the effects of lipid-lowering on bypass atherosclerosis in women.

A number of other studies have also provided evidence that lipid-lowering drugs can prevent or reverse angiographically detectable atherosclerotic lesions in native coronary arteries. However, because none of these reports include specific data on the course of graft atherosclerosis they are not considered here. A study addressing the efficacy of 3-hydroxy-3-methylglutaryl coenzyme A reductase inhibitor for preventing graft atherosclerosis (the National Institutes of Health Post-Coronary Artery Bypass Graft Study) is now underway.

Together the above data indicate that SVG atherosclerosis is a potentially preventable lipid-related disease which should be prevented and treated by aggressive lipid-lowering therapy. The fact that IMA grafts are relatively resistant favors the use of IMA grafts whenever possible. Finally, we would emphasize that platelet inhibitors and calcium channel blockers may also intervene with cholesteryl ester accumulation and thus with the formation of bypass atheroma. The place of these drugs in prevention of bypass changes is discussed, respectively, by J.H. Chesebro et al. and S.O. Gottlieb (this volume).

Acknowledgements. We are indebted to Gabriela M. Kuster for careful reading of the manuscript.

References

1. Atkinson JB, Forman MB, Perry JM (1985) Correlation of saphenous vein bypass graft angiograms with histologic changes at necropsy. Am J Cardiol 55:952–955
2. Atkinson JB, Forman MB, Vaughn WK (1985) Morphologic changes in long-term saphenous vein bypass grafts. Chest 88:341–348
3. Blankenhorn DH, Kramsch DM (1989) Reversal of atherosis and sclerosis. The two components of atherosclerosis. Circulation 79:1–7
4. Blankenhorn DH, Nessim SA, Johnson RL, Sanmarco ME, Azen SP, Cashin-Hemphill L (1987) Beneficial effects of combined colestipol-niacin therapy on coronary atherosclerosis and coronary venous bypass grafts. J Am Med Assoc 257:3233–3240
5. Blankenhorn DH, Alaupovic P, Wickham E, Chin HP, Azen SP (1990) Prediction of angiographic change in native human coronary arteries and aortocoronary bypass grafts. Lipid and nonlipid factors. Circulation 81:470–476
6. Blankenhorn DH, Azen SP, Crawford DW, Nessim SA, Selzer RH, Shircore AM, Wickham EC (1991) Effects of colestipol-niacin therapy on human femoral atherosclerosis. Circulation 83:438–447
7. Blankenhorn DH, Selzer RH, Mack WJ, Crawford DW, Pagoda J, Lee PJ, Shircore AM, Azen SP (1992) Evaluation of colestipol/niacin therapy with computer-derived coronary end-point measures. A comparison of different measures of treatment effect. Circulation 86:1701–1709
8. Bonchek LI, Boerboom LE, Olinger GN (1982) Prevention of lipid accumulation in experimental vein bypass grafts by anti-platelet therapy. Circulation 66:338–341
9. Bourassa MG, Enjalbert M, Campeau L (1984) Progression of atherosclerosis in coronary arteries and bypass grafts. Ten years later. Am J Cardiol 53:102C–107C
10. Bourassa MG, Fisher LD, Campeau L (1985) Long-term fate of bypass grafts. The Coronary Artery Surgery Study and Montreal Heart Institute experiences. Circulation 72:V-71–V-78
11. Bourassa MG, Campeau L, Lesperance J (1991) Changes in grafts and in coronary arteries after coronary bypass surgery. In: Waters DD, Bourassa MG (eds) Care of the patient with previous coronary bypass surgery. Cardiovascular clinics 21/2. Davis, Philadelphia, pp 83–100
12. Campeau L, Enjalbert M, Lesperance J (1983) Atherosclerosis and late closure of aortocoronary saphenous vein grafts. Sequential angiographic studies at 2 weeks, 1 year, 5 to 7 years, and 10 to 12 years after surgery. Circulation 68:II-1–II-7
13. Campeau L, Enjalbert M, Lesperance J (1984) The relation of risk factors to the development of atherosclerosis in saphenous vein bypass grafts and the progression of disease in the native circulation. A study 10 years after aortocoronary bypass surgery. N Engl J Med 311:1329–1332
14. Cameron A, Kemp HG Jr, Green GE (1986) Bypass surgery with the internal mammary artery graft 15 year follow-up. Circulation 74:III-30–III-36
15. Cashin-Hemphill L, Mack WJ, Pogoda JM, Sanmarco ME, Azen SP, Blankenhorn DH (1990) Beneficial effects of colestipol-niacin on coronary atherosclerosis. J Am Med Assoc 264:3013–3017
16. European Coronary Surgery Study Group (1982) Long-term results of prospective randomized study of coronary artery bypass surgery in stable angina pectoris. Lancet 2:1173–1180
17. Friedman M (1963) Spontaneous atherosclerosis and experimental thromboatherosclerosis. Arch Pathol 76:571–577
18. Grondin CM, Campeau L, Lesperance J (1979) Atherosclerotic changes in coronary vein grafts six years after operation. Angiographic aspect in 110 patients. J Thorac Cardiovasc Surg 77:24–31

19. Grondin CM, Campeau L, Lesperance J (1984) Comparison of late changes in internal mammary artery and saphenous vein grafts in two consecutive series of patients 10 years after operation. Circulation 70:208–212
20. Harper LA, Ross R, Slichter SJ (1976) Homocystine-induced atherosclerosis. J Clin Invest 58:731–741
21. Havel RJ, Kane JP (1989) Structure and metabolism of plasma lipoproteins. In: Scriver CR, Beaudet AL, Sly WS, Valle D (eds) Metabolic basis of inherited disease. McGraw-Hill, New York, pp 1129–1138
22. King P, Royle JP (1972) Autogenous vein grafting in atheromatous rabbits. Cardiovasc Res 6:627–633
23. Lie JT, Lawrie GM, Morris GC Jr (1977) Aortocoronary bypass saphenous vein graft artherosclerosis. Anatomic study of 99 vein grafts from normal and hyperlipoproteinemic patients up to 75 months postoperatively. Am J Cardiol 40:906–914
24. Loop FD, Lytle BW, Cosgrove DM (1986) Influence of the internal mammary-artery graft on 10 year survival and other cardiac events. N Engl J Med 314:1–6
25. Roberts WC (1989) Lipid-lowering therapy after an atherosclerotic event (editorial). Am J Cardiol 64:693–695
26. Rossiter SJ, Brody WR, Kosek JC, Liptom MJ, Angell WW (1974) Internal mammary artery versus autogenous vein for coronary artery bypass graft. Circulation 50:1236–1243
27. Sako Y (1961) Susceptibility of autologous vein grafts to atheromatous degeneration. Surg Forum 12:247–249
28. Scott HW Jr, Morgan CV, Bolasny BL, Lainer VC, Younger RK, Butts W (1970) Experimental atherosclerosis in autogenous venous grafts. Arch Surg 101:677–682
29. Smith SH, Geer JC (1983) Morphology of saphenous vein coronary artery bypass grafts. Arch Pathol Lab Med 107:13–18
30. Solymoss BC, Nadeau P, Millette D (1988) Late thrombosis of saphenous vein coronary bypass grafts related to risk factors. Circulation 78:I-140–I-143
31. Spray TL, Roberts WC (1977) Status of the grafts and the native coronary arteries proximal and distal to coronary anastomotic sites of aortacoronary bypass grafts. Circulation 55:741–749
32. Vlodaver Z, Edwards JE (1973) Pathologic analysis in fatal cases following saphenous vein coronary arterial bypass. Chest 64:555–563

Treatment of Severe Hypercholesterolemia in Patients with Coronary Heart Disease by Means of Lipoprotein Apheresis

D. Seidel

Introduction

Diseases resulting from premature atherosclerosis are the most common cause not only of death but also of early retirement [1–2]. Today, the major therapeutic interventions for atherosclerotic coronary disease are percutaneous transluminal coronary angioplasty and coronary bypass graft surgery (see chapter by F. Loop, this volume). At the time of these therapeutic interventions, however, the disease has already become clinically very relevant and, within its own natural history, is at a very late stage. Hence early risk factor intervention is of particular importance to prevent the disease. Nevertheless, even in patients who have undergone coronary bypass surgery, risk factor intervention, in particular treatment of hypercholesterolemia is crucial to maintain functionally vital grafts (see also chapter by H. Drexel and F. Amman, this volume).

Results of many studies have shown that there are a large number of factors involved in atherogenesis. While disturbances in lipid metabolism [hyperbetalipoproteinemia, hypoalphalipoproteinemia, accumulation of chylomicron and/or very low density lipoprotein (VLDL) remnants], structural abnormalities of lipoproteins, and family history of myocardial infarction are the most important risk factors. Hypertension, smoking, elevated blood glucose, and overweight also have an impact on early cardiovascular events. More recently lipoprotein(a) [Lp(a)], fibrinogen, and the biological modification of lipoproteins have been added to the list of risk factors for atherosclerosis [3–7].

In many patients suffering from coronary heart disease (CHD) low-density lipoprotein (LDL), Lp(a), and fibrinogen are elevated at the same time and may potentiate the cardiovascular risk derived from each factor alone. It is obvious that these risk factors remain important and unaffected by revascularization procedures, and by coronary bypass surgery in particular. Most forms of hypercholesterolemia result from a defect in the removal of LDL from plasma by the liver, and the LDL receptor is now recognized as the crucial element in the control of LDL cholesterol homeostasis [8, 9]. If the physiological clearing mechanisms for LDL are insufficient, diet and drug therapy alone are often ineffective. This also holds true for Lp(a) and fibrinogen, either of which at present can hardly be lowered by diet or drugs.

In humans plasma LDL cholesterol levels below 110 mg/dl seem to be necessary to inhibit the development of atherosclerosis or to induce regression of the vessel wall lesions [10]. This has been impressively demonstrated in six different secondary intervention studies ([11–16] and D.H. Blankenhorn et al., personal communication). Although the therapeutic approach and strategy were different in these studies, the outcomes were similar and promising: lowering of LDL cholesterol by 35%–50% was followed by a two fold increase in the progression/regression ratio compared to controls. These beneficial effects of lipid-lowering interventions also apply for the progression of coronary artery bypass graft disease (see also chapter by H. Drexel and F. Amman).

The cornerstone of strategies to reduce the risk of coronary heart disease and coronary graft disease after surgery in the population is undoubtedly diet. With the advent of the 3-hydroxy-3-methylglutaryl coenzyme A (HMG-CoA) reductase inhibitors, a new class of powerful lipid-lowering drugs was introduced with great potential in the treatment of hypercholesterolemia. The use of these drugs is now increasing, and confirmation of their long-term safety will be of profound importance for their general use in the treatment of atherosclerotic disease. More radical measures such as partial ileal bypass [17], portocaval shunt [18], liver transplantation [19] plasma exchange [20, 21], and LDL apheresis [22] have also been introduced for the treatment of severe hypercholesterolemia.

Plasma exchange has proven particularly successful in the management of severe hypercholesterolemia such as homozygous familial hypercholesterolemia (FH) [20, 21]. Since this therapy requires substitution of plasma fractions, with its inherent danger, several LDL apheresis procedures with varying degrees of selectivity and efficiency have subsequently been developed, some of which are at present being evaluated in clinical trials.

While the use of such therapies for the primary prevention of CHD is restricted largely to the most severe forms of hypercholesterolemia, in secondary prevention, in particular also in patients who have undergone bypass surgery, the combination of diet and drugs together with plasmapheresis seems an attractive therapeutic possibility if diet and drug therapy alone are not sufficient to achieve the therapeutic goal of LDL cholesterol levels below 110 mg/dl. The combination of plasma LDL apheresis with diet and drugs now allows a maximal lowering of LDL cholesterol of up to 80%. This is also the case in patients who only a few years ago were classified as resistant to treatment of hypercholesterolemia. Besides LDL, some apheresis procedures also eliminate other risk factors of clinical importance for CHD, such as Lp(a) and or fibrinogen, and can greatly improve the hemorrheological status of the patients.

LDL Apheresis Procedures

In the past decade several systems have been developed for the extracorporeal elimination of LDL cholesterol from plasma. These procedures are collectively referred to as LDL apheresis. Today, LDL apheresis has largely replaced plasma exchange therapy as introduced by DeGennes [20] and Thompson [21]. Now, with the experience gathered over several years of clinical use, the efficiency, specificity, and safety of the various LDL apheresis methods can be compared. Three methods of LDL apheresis have been clinically established and are now used for the treatment of severe hypercholesterolemia: (a) various LDL immuno adsorption techniques, using immobilized mono- or polyclonal antibodies to apolipoprotein (apo) B100 [23, 24], (b) LDL binding by dextrane sulfate attached to cellulose [25], and (c) heparin induced extracorporeal LDL precipitation [26, 27]. Plasma membrane filtration has also been proposed, but this retains in addition to LDL other macromolecules such as high-density lipoprotein (HDL), immunoglobulins, and albumin and therefore cannot be considered specific. This technique closely resembles plasma exchange, with its disadvantages for long-term therapy.

In addition to the marked reduction in LDL cholesterol concentrations achieved by all procedures, it has become apparent that at least one – that of heparin-induced extracorporeal LDL plasmapheresis (H.E.L.P.) – results in an equally significant change in hemorrheology. This system has been widely used. Its efficiency and safety, alone and in combination with HMG-CoA reductase inhibitors, has been investigated in great detail. Therefore this review focuses on the H.E.L.P. system as a new therapeutic tool to lower LDL, Lp(a), and fibrinogen at the same time, to improve hemorrheology and to achieve regression of coronary sclerosis in patients who are otherwise refractory to the treatment of severe hypercholesterolemia.

The H.E.L.P. Apheresis System

H.E.L.P. operates by increasing the positive charges on LDL and Lp(a) particles at low pH, allowing them to specifically form a network with heparin and fibrinogen in the absence of divalent cations [26, 28, 29]. Only a limited number of other heparin-binding plasma proteins are coprecipitated by heparin at low pH. Other proteins, such as apo A_1, apo A_2, albumin, and immunoglobulins, do not significantly bind to heparin at low pH and are not precipitated in the system [27, 28]. Complement activation takes place in all extracorporeal therapy systems. However, as a specific feature of H.E.L.P. activated complement C3 and C4 as well as the terminal complement complex are largely adsorbed to the precipitation filter, resulting in plasma concentrations which are actually below those measured before apheresis [30]. Leukocytopenia, a hallmark of complement activation, has not been observed under H.E.L.P. therapy.

The H.E.L.P. system (Braun, Melsungen, Germany) has unique features:

- It removes LDL, Lp(a), and fibrinogen with high efficiency.
- It does not remove HDL.
- It does not alter or modify plasma lipoproteins.
- It does not change plasma concentrations of cell mediators.
- It avoids the use of compounds with immunogenic or immunostimulatory activity.
- It uses only disposable material and avoids regeneration of any of the used elements.
- It is a technically safe and well-standardized procedure.
- In short- and long-term treatment, tolerance and benefit are excellent.

The major steps of the H.E.L.P. system in removing the atherogenic compounds are illustrated in Fig. 1. In the first step, plasma is obtained by filtration of whole blood through a plasma separator. This is then mixed continuously with a 0.3 *M* acetate buffer of pH 4.85 containing 100 IU heparin/ml. The sudden precipitation occurs at a pH of 5.12, and the suspension is circulated through a 0.4 μm polycarbonate filter to remove the precipitated LDL, Lp(a), and fibrinogen. Excess heparin is adsorbed by passage through an anion-exchange column which binds only heparin at the given pH. The plasma buffer mixture is finally subjected to a bicarbonate

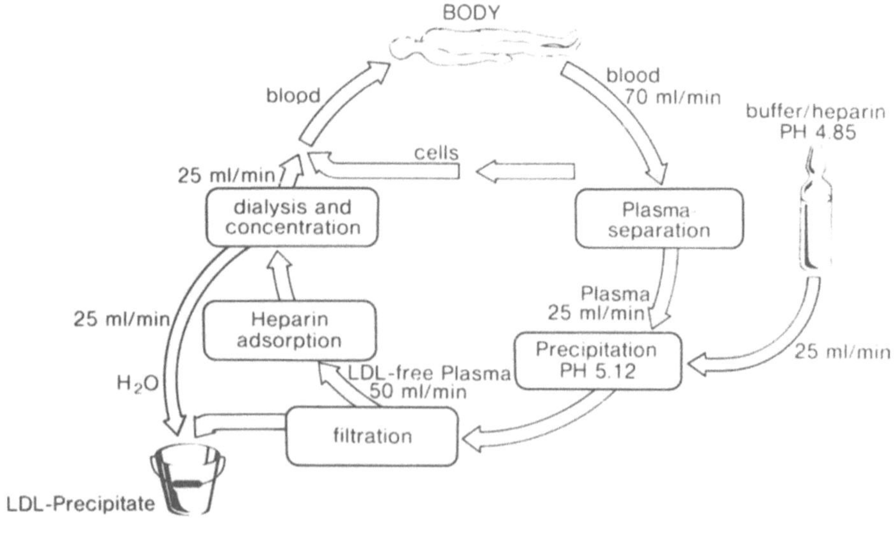

Fig. 1. Flow sheet of the H.E.L.P. procedure

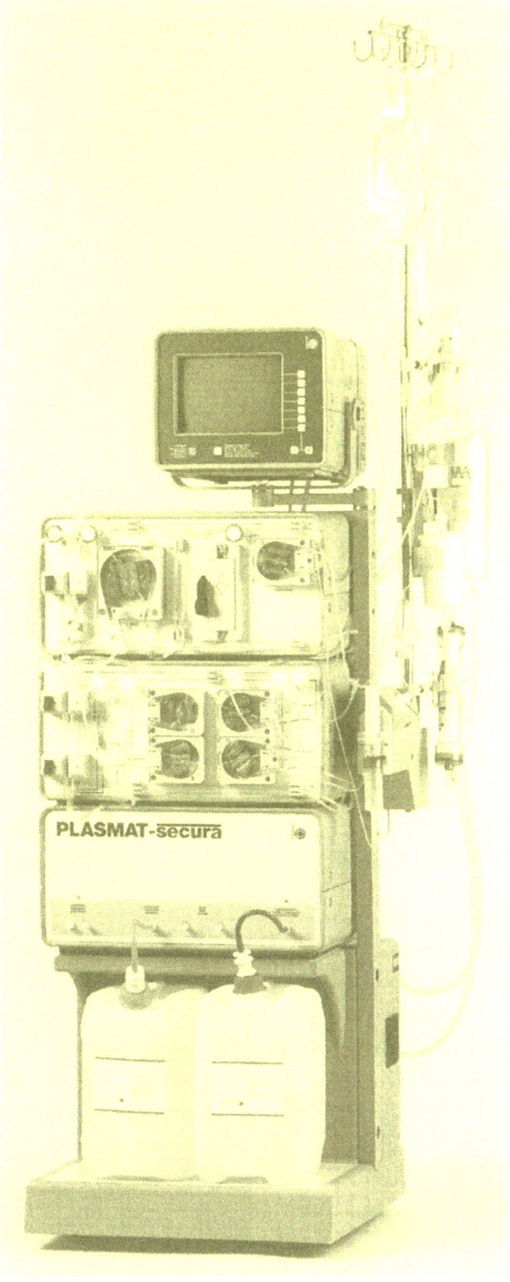

Fig. 2. HD Secura H.E.L.P. system (Braun Melsungen, Germany)

dialysis and ultrafiltration to remove excess fluid and to restore the physiological pH, before the plasma is mixed with the blood cells and returned to the patient. All filters and tubings required for the treatment are sterile and disposable and are intended for single use only. This makes it easy and reliable to work with the system and guarantees a steady quality for each treatment, independent of the clinic performing the procedure. Safety is assured by a visual display and two microprocessors operating in parallel (Fig. 2). Due to the excellent tolerance of the procedure the patients leave the hospital shortly after the end of the treatment session.

Clinical Experience with the H.E.L.P. System

The clinical experience with the H.E.L.P. system goes back to 1985. By 1992 approximately 300 patients had been treated in over 30000 single treatments. Some patients have been treated for more than 5 years. Currently, the system operates in approximately 100 centers in Germany, Italy, the United States, Austria, and Ireland.

The efficiency of the system is 100% for the elimination of LDL, Lp(a), and fibrinogen. Per single treatment (lasting 1.5–2h), 2.8–31 plasma is treated, causing a reduction of approximately 50% of these three compounds in plasma of the treated patients.

The rates of return to preapheresis concentrations for LDL differ between normocholesterolemics and heterozygous as well as homozygous FH patients, while they are almost identical for Lp(a) [31, 32]. Normocholesterolemics return rather quickly towards the steady-state pretreatment levels. Heterozygous FH patients display a rate of return between those of normocholesterolemic and a homozygous FH patient, the latter being slowest in her rate of return to pretreatment LDL concentrations. In biweekly treatment intervals the pretreatment values usually reach a new steady state after four to eight treatments.

Long-term effects of the H.E.L.P. treatment based on interval values between two treatments (cholesterol after H.E.L.P. + cholesterol before H.E.L.P. divided by 2) and expressed as percentage of concentrations at the start are shown in Table 1.

H.E.L.P. treatment also significantly improves plasma viscosity (−15%), erythrocyte aggregation (−50%), and erythrocyte filtration (+15%), which is followed by an acute (20%–30%) increase in the oxygen tension in

Table 1. Long-term effects of H.E.L.P. therapy: mean ± SD interval values of approximately 6000 treatments

LDL cholesterol	−51% ± 14
Lipoprotein (a)	−45% ± 5
Fibrinogen	−46% ± 15
Apolipoprotein B100	−45% ± 15
HDL cholesterol	+12% ± 2
Apolipoprotein A_1	+9% ± 2

muscle tissue [33, 34]. The changes in plasma viscosity are due to the reduction in both LDL and fibrinogen. The change in erythrocyte aggregation is due primarily to fibrinogen reduction. Changes in erythrocyte filtrability correlate with an improvement in the cholesterol/phospholipid ratio of cell membranes [33]. It is conceivable to associate the rheological findings with the impressive relief from angina, together with the improvement in exercise ECG and in physical capacity that we observe in most (over 90%) of the patients shortly (2–3 months) after start of the therapy [29, 33, 34].

The first coronary angiographies 2 years after H.E.L.P. treatment in over 50 patients (to be reported elsewhere by the H.E.L.P. multicenter study group [15]) lend support to the hope that regression of coronary heart disease is possible in humans [16]. First evaluation of the 2-year follow-up by blinded angiograms revealed a regression of the coronary artery disease twofold more than progression.

HMG-CoA reductase inhibitors were not available when the H.E.L.P. multicenter study was started. In the meantime, since these compounds are now on the market, we and others have investigated the effect of a combined therapy using lovastatin, simvastatin, or pravastatin together with the H.E.L.P. apheresis system.

Experience with Combined H.E.L.P. and HMG-CoA Reductase Inhibitor Therapy

With plasma cholesterol levels exceeding 300 mg/dl, the use of specific diets and drugs may not be sufficient when LDL concentrations are below 110 mg/dl, and/or regression of CHD is aimed at as a means of secondary intervention. We have investigated the efficacy of a combined therapy, using HMG-CoA reductase inhibitors (lovastatin, simvastatin, pravastatin) [35] together with H.E.L.P. and treated approximately 20 patients with severe FH on a long-term basis. These compounds significantly decrease the rate of

Table 2. Long-term effects of H.E.L.P. and HMG-CoA reductase inhibitor treatment: mean ± SD interval values of approximately 1400 treatments

	HMG-CoA reductase inhibitor	H.E.L.P. + HMG-CoA reductase inhibitor
LDL cholesterol	−38% ± 12%	−69% ± 12%
HDL cholesterol	+10% ± 9%	+14% ± 6%
Apolipoprotein B100	−30% ± 9%	−53% ± 8%
Apolipoprotein A_1	+13% ± 4%	+12% ± 9%
Lipoprotein (a)	No change	−43% ± 7%
Fibrinogen	No change	−44% ± 10%

return after H.E.L.P. in both heterozygous and homozygous FH patients by 20%–30% [29, 31, 32]. When the two treatments are combined, a reduction of the interval LDL cholesterol level of 70% may be achieved while Lp(a) and fibrinogen are not further affected (over the effect by the H.E.L.P. treatment alone; see Table 2). In the combined form therapy intervals between two H.E.L.P. treatments may in many cases be extended from 7 to 14 days, depending on the synthetic rates for LDL or the severity of CHD.

Treatment Tolerance and Safety of H.E.L.P.

Overall treatment tolerance has been very good, and no major complications have been observed after 30000 treatments in approximately 300 patients. The treatment effects have been maintained on long-term treatment for over 6 years. At the end of the H.E.L.P. therapy, plasma concentrations of proteins that are not selectively precipitated by heparin at low pH are generally in the range of 80%–90% of the initial values and return to their original level no later than 24 h after the end of treatment [27, 29, 36]. No substitution of any kind has been necessary in 6 years of clinical experience. In contrast to some other LDL apheresis systems the H.E.L.P. procedure does not alter the physicochemical characteristics of LDL, nor does it alter the ligand quality of LDL for lipoprotein receptors [37].

Special attention has been focussed on the effect of H.E.L.P. on hemostasis. All posttreatment controls have been typical for extracorporeal procedures, and no critical bleeding complications have been observed. Complement activation is found in all extracorporeal procedures. However, as a specific feature of the H.E.L.P. system activated complement C3 and C4 and the terminal complement complex are largely adsorbed to the filter system of H.E.L.P., resulting in plasma concentrations which are actually below those measured before LDL apheresis. C5a is not retained in the filter system, but plasma levels at the end of the treatment are within the normal range and leukocytopenia, a hallmark of complement activation, has never been observed under H.E.L.P. treatment [30]. Plasma electrolyte, hormone, vitamin, enzyme, and immunoglobulin concentrations as well as hematological parameters remain virtually unchanged at the end of each treatment and on long-term application [29, 35, 36] (Table 3).

Typical Case Reports

Case 1. A typical follow-up kinetic for LDL and Lp(a) under H.E.L.P. treatment of a patient with severe progressive coronary heart disease is shown in Fig. 3. At the start of our therapy the 33-year-old patient with

Table 3. H.E.L.P. therapy in combination with HMG-CoA reductase inhibitor (24 months; mean ± SD)

Parameters	Baseline		Simvastatin + H.E.L.P.		Parameters	Baseline		Simvastatin + H.E.L.P.	
	Mean	SD	Mean	SD		Mean	SD	Mean	SD
Substrates					Hematological indices				
Sodium	140.0	0.7	141.0	0.3	Hemoglobin	14.0	0.44	14.3	0.07
Potassium	3.9	0.12	4.0	0.05	Hematocrit	41.8	1.1	42.0	0.73
Calcium	9.2	0.11	8.9	0.1	Erythrocytes	4.4	0.14	4.6	0.1
Phosphate	3.7	0.16	3.3	0.03	Thrombocytes	226.0	10.2	220.0	9.5
Iron	88.2	9.3	95.5	3.9	Leukocytes	5.18	0.39	5.22	0.48
Creatinine	0.85	0.04	0.9	0.02	Lymphocytes	37.4	2.76	33.3	2.1
BUN	15.2	1.7	14.5	0.4	Monocytes	7.2	1.02	6.2	2.45
Uric acid	5.3	0.4	5.3	0.4	Neutrophils	51.3	3.16	57.4	3.12
Glucose	94.0	0.9	100.0	6.4	Eosinophils	2.6	0.43	1.8	0.61
Total bilirubin	0.43	0.03	0.56	0.4	Basophils	0.7	0.18	0.7	0.1
Total protein	7.0	0.1	6.9	0.1	Hemostasis				
Albumin (%)	61.6	1.73	61.4	0.42	Quick test (PT) (%)	98.0	0.25	99.0	0.91
α_1-Protein (%)	3.6	0.3	3.6	0.1	TT (s)	14.0	0.12	14.0	0.21

Table 3. H.E.L.P. therapy in combination with HMG-CoA reductase inhibitor (24 months; mean ± SD)

Parameters	Baseline		Simvastatin + H.E.L.P.		Parameters	Baseline		Simvastatin + H.E.L.P.	
	Mean	SD	Mean	SD		Mean	SD	Mean	SD
α-Protein (%)	8.0	0.42	8.3	0.14	Endocrinological indices				
β_2-Protein (%)	13.0	0.56	12.0	0.03	Cortisol	12.6	1.05	13.3	1.15
γ-Protein (%)	13.7	0.99	14.8	0.14	Testosterone	6.7	1.07	6.4	0.26
Enzymes					ACTH	40.3	3.78	40.4	6.18
ALAT (GOT)	10.0	0.4	13.5	0.4	LH[a]	15.9	8.36	11.1	5.91
ASAT (GPT)	11.0	2.0	19.0	1.0	FSH[a]	16.0	0.22	28.0	10.3
γ-GT	21.0	5.8	25.0	2.1	T3	133.5	7.35	123.5	12.4
CK	45.0	7.0	45.0	2.0	T4	7.0	0.61	7.3	0.1
LDH	143.0	10.8	151.0	4.6	FT4	7.5	0.62	7.5	0.6
Amylase	16.0	2.7	16.0	0.3	FT3	142.5	7.64	137.5	6.01
CHS	5151.0	525.0	5455.0	530.0					
ALP	101.0	6.6	110.0	2.8					

ALAT (GOT), Alanine aminotransferase (glutamic oxaloacetic transaminase); ASAT (GPT), asparate aminotransferase (glutamic pyruvic transaminase); BUN, blood urea nitrogen; γ-GT, γ-glutamyltransferase; CK, creatine kinase; LDH, lactate dehydrogenase; CHS, cholinesterase; ALP, alkaline phosphate; PT, prothrombin time; TT, thromboplastin time; ACTH, adrenocorticotropic hormone; LH, luteinizing hormone; FSH, follicle-stimulating hormone; T3, triiodothyronine; T4, thyroxine; FT4, free thyroxine; FT3, free triiodothyronine.

[a] Only in men and premenopausal women.

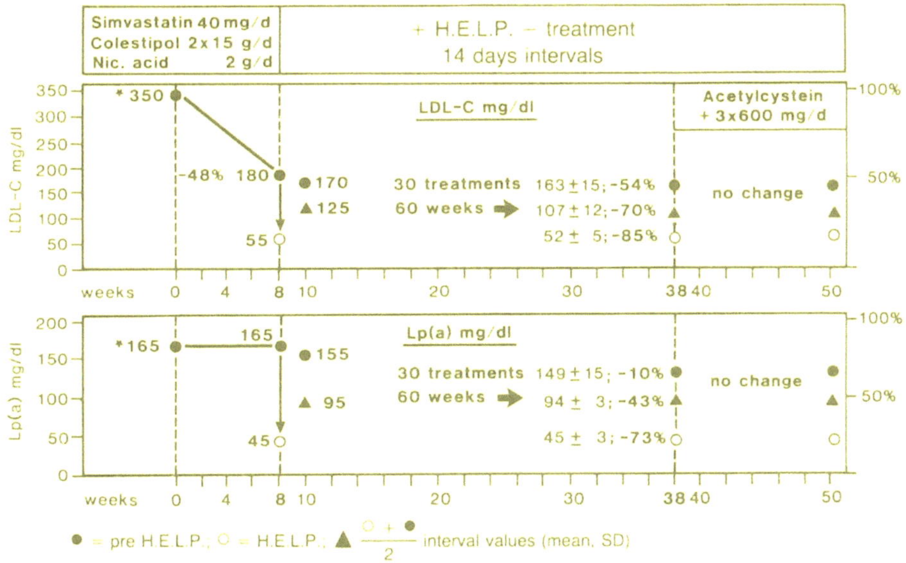

Fig. 3. Maximal treatment of FH and elevated plasma Lp(a) concentrations in a 33-year-old man. Baseline LDL cholesterol (*LDL-C*) 350 mg/dl, Lp(a) 165 mg/dl. Well-maintained PTCA results after 1 year of treatment and no further progression of CHD

myocardial infarction had a history of a coronary bypass and PTCA. He showed LDL cholesterol levels of 350 mg/dl and a marked Lp(a) elevation of 165 mg/dl. LDL cholesterol was lowered with an HMG-CoA reductase inhibitor (simvastatin) by about 48% to 170 mg/dl, but no effect on Lp(a) levels was observed. In the combination with regular H.E.L.P. treatment we were able to maintain LDL concentration at an interval value of 110 mg/dl. In addition, H.E.L.P. treatment resulted in a marked decrease (−70%) of postapheresis Lp(a) concentrations. The interval Lp(a) levels remained around 90 mg/dl. Fibrinogen was lowered from a baseline value of 317 mg/dl to a H.E.L.P. interval value of 177 mg/dl, which is a 44% reduction. Control angiography after 2 years revealed that the combined treatment had stopped the very progressive CHD which was developing in the patient previous to the opherisis. The clinical situation had also considerably improved.

Case 2. Experience with the H.E.L.P. treatment in a homozygous form of FH is presented in Fig. 4. Early death from cardiac consequences of premature coronary sclerosis and aortic stenoses is the usual outcome of homozygous FH [38]. Inherited as an autosomal dominant defect of the LDL receptor gene, this disease is characterized by very high plasma LDL cholesterol concentrations (between 200 and 1000 mg/dl) and the development of severe cutaneous and tendon xanthomata in childhood. All conventional lipid-lowering treatments with diet and medication are completely insufficient. Since 1985 we have been following and treating an FH patient, born

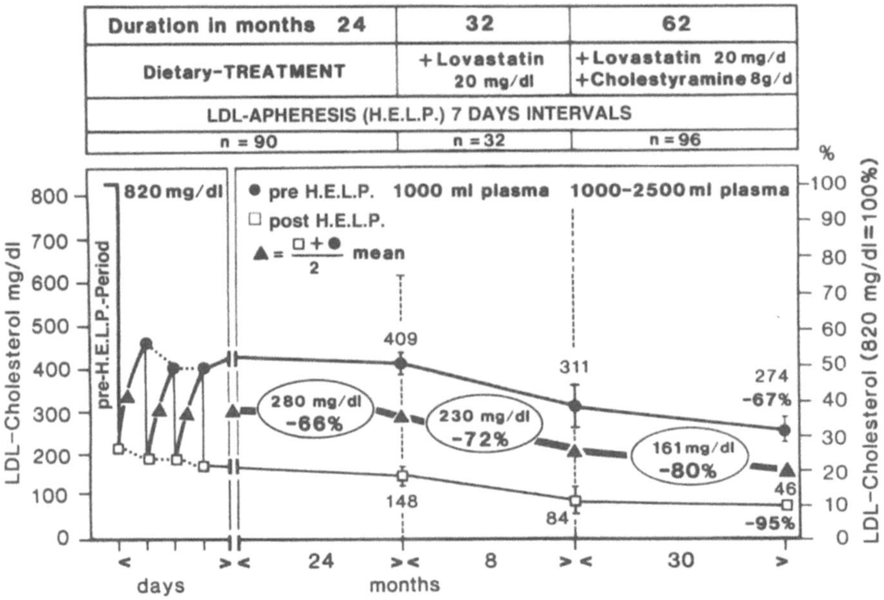

Fig. 4. Maximal treatment of homozygous FH in a 7-year-old girl. Follow-up of LDL cholesterol (*LDL-C*). Baseline LDL-C 820 mg/dl

in 1979, with the H.E.L.P. apheresis procedure [32]. LDL cholesterol concentrations before the start of treatment exceeded 800 mg/dl. The follow-up of LDL concentrations under H.E.L.P. treatment alone and in combination with lovastatin and regular cholestyramine is shown in Fig. 4. The girl was treated for 2 years by weekly H.E.L.P. apheresis. Under this procedure the LDL cholesterol interval levels were maintained below 280 mg/dl. At this time a rapid regression of multiple xanthomata was observed. Additional medication of lovastatin and cholestyramine achieved a further LDL decrease to 180 mg/dl. The treated plasma volume was recently enhanced from 1.5 to 2.5 l. This has now resulted in a mean LDL cholesterol level of 160 mg/dl, which is equivalent to a decrease of 80% as compared to pretreatment values. The therapy was excellently tolerated. The girl is well and shows normal growth and development. No signs of cardiovascular symptoms have been noted.

H.E.L.P. Treatment in Heart-Transplant Patients with Severe Hypercholesterolemia: Report of a Proceeding Study

The goal of this proceeding trial is to decrease recurrent CHD of heart grafts. In this study the patients are followed for 4 years. LDL cholesterol concentrations in all patients are maintained at a level below 120 mg/dl.

Treatment was started from a baseline LDL cholesterol concentration above 280 mg/dl with simvastatin, which resulted in a reduction in LDL cholesterol by 40% but exceeded 170 mg/dl LDL. In the combination of simvastatin and H.E.L.P. treatment LDL cholesterol level below 120 mg/dl was achieved. As in other H.E.L.P. patients overall treatment tolerance in this group ($n = 5$) has been very good, and no major complications have been observed in the first 6 months of therapy. Special attention has been given to the tolerance and pharmacokinetics of both simvastatin and cyclosporine A. No signs of myopathy have been observed. No change of cell mediators such as interleukin-2 receptor, interleukin-6 receptor, interferon-γ, or tumor necrosis factor before and after H.E.L.P. treatment have been observed.

From our first clinical experience in heart-transplanted patients with severe hypercholesterolemia the additional therapy with H.E.L.P. may be not only useful but necessary to achieve long-lasting benefit from the transplantation. Annual examination by angiograms of the patients should provide an explanation for the drastic LDL-lowering therapy in the prevention of graft atherosclerosis in heart-transplant patients.

Comparison of Techniques to Lower LDL by Apheresis

Three methods for the selective removal of LDL from plasma have been established and are now used for treatment of severely hypercholesterolemic patients: (a) LDL immunoadsorption using immobilized anti-apo B antibodies for LDL binding [23, 24], (b) LDL binding to dextran sulfate cellulose (DSC) [25], and (c) heparin induced extracorporeal LDL precipitation (H.E.L.P.) [26, 27]. Two recent reviews [39, 40] have compared the various procedures with regard to their efficiency in lowering LDL concentrations and safety. All three procedures achieved an approximately 60% decrease in LDL plasma concentrations in the course of a single LDL apheresis session. The reduction in HDL lipoprotein levels and immunoglobulins was usually less than 20%, with no significant difference between the three LDL apheresis methods. These apparent losses may to some extent be due to nonspecific plasma dilution by the saline priming solution from the extracorporeal plasma circuit.

Double plasma filtration, although also effective in reducing LDL, was not selective. Total plasma protein loss (HDL, immunoglobulins, and albumin) was significant, and concomitant albumin substitution was regularly required. Therefore, double plasma filtration occupies a position close to plasma exchange. This technique should not be recommended for FH treatment.

Immunoabsorption and DSC apheresis are highly specific for apo B containing lipoproteins which include VLDL, intermediate density lipoproteins, and Lp(a). It has recently been demonstrated that increased Lp(a) concentrations are significantly correlated with increased risk for CHD.

Immunoadsorption, DSC LDL apheresis, and H.E.L.P. apheresis all eliminate Lp(a) to about the same extent as LDL. In contrast to immunoadsorption and DSC apheresis, H.E.L.P. also eliminates fibrinogen. Parallel measurements of plasma viscosity and erythrocyte aggregation before and after H.E.L.P. LDL apheresis revealed a significant reduction of 15% and 50%, respectively [33]. The muscle oxygen tension was found to be significantly higher directly after treatment compared with pretreatment values, probably as a result of improved microcirculation under H.E.L.P. therapy [33, 34].

Results from multicenter studies using the H.E.L.P. and the DSC LDL apheresis as a means of drastic lipid-lowering therapy are now available [16, 36, 41, 42]. In the H.E.L.P. multicenter study 51 participants were examined by coronary angiography at the start and after 2 years of the treatment. First evaluations of the angiograms with quantitative determination of stenosis revealed a twofold higher regression than progression rate of the coronary arteries in the patients under H.E.L.P. therapy. Close to 40% of all patients showed a clear tendency of stenosis regression [15, 36]. Another small study of seven patients with heterozygous FH produced evidence that H.E.L.P. LDL apheresis administered once a week for 7–24 months induced regression of carotid atherosclerotic plaques [16]. Plaques were evaluated by a three-dimensional reconstruction of ultrasound images. Of 21 observed plaques only 1 progressed, 12 did not change, and 8 regressed within 6–12 months.

Data of one multicenter study using DSC LDL apheresis [41] are at present available only in preliminary form. Here 64 patients with FH (54 heterozygous and 10 homozygous) were treated at 7- to 14-day intervals for 18 weeks. Baseline LDL cholesterol concentrations were 243 mg/dl and 447 mg/dl, respectively. Time-averaged LDL cholesterol levels on treatment were 139 mg/dl in heterozygotes and 210 mg/dl in homozygotes. HDL cholesterol increased slightly, but the changes were not significant. Lp(a) levels were reduced markedly, but long-term concentrations were not given.

The second DSC LDL Apheresis Multicenter Study [42] used LDL apheresis combined with cholesterol-lowering drugs to treat homozygous or heterozygous FH. By visual judgement or computer analysis the coronary angiograms revealed a regression in 38%, no change in 49%, and progression in 14%, indicating an encouraging result of aggressive cholesterol-lowering therapy in coronary atherosclerosis of FH patients.

LDL immunoadsorption, DSC LDL apheresis, and H.E.L.P. apheresis are all safe and equally potent methods of extracorporeal LDL elimination. Lp(a) can also be removed specifically from plasma by these procedures. In addition, H.E.L.P. apheresis selectively reduces plasma fibrinogen, to a beneficial effect on the microcirculation. Long-term observations show that besides the marked reduction in LDL cholesterol some increase of HDL cholesterol occurs which may add to the antiatherogenic effect of LDL apheresis treatment.

Conclusion

Hypercholesterolemia is an important risk factor for coronary artery disease and also graft dysfunction and closure after bypass surgery (see also chapter by H. Drexel and F. Amman, this volume). Hence, effective control of hypercholesterolemia remains an important therapeutic goal, even after revascularization procedures such as percutaneous transluminal angioplasty or bypass surgery.

LDL apheresis is the most potent technique to eliminate LDL and Lp(a) when physiological clearing mechanisms are insufficient. The H.E.L.P. system can also very efficiently remove fibrinogen and thus improve plasma viscosity and microcirculation. Long-term observations show that, in addition to the marked reduction in LDL cholesterol, a remarkable increase of HDL occurs which may add to the antiatherogenic effect of the extracorporeal procedures. For the future, the availability of safe and efficient apheresis techniques in the treatment of severe hypercholesterolemia in patients with coronary heart disease, including those who have already undergone bypass surgery, may provide new dimensions.

References

1. Castelli WP, Wilson PWF, Levy D, Anderson K (1990) Serum lipids and risk of coronary artery disease. In: Leaf A, Weber PC (eds) Atherosclerosis reviews, vol 21. Raven, New York, pp 7–19
2. Cremer P, Muche R (1990) Göttinger Risiko-, Inzidenz- und Prävalenzstudie (GRIPS) Empfehlungen zur Pravention der koronaren Herzkrankheit. Ther Umsch 6:482–491
3. Seidel D, Neumeier D, Cremer P, Nagel D (1992) Lipoprotein(a) in internal medicine. 9th international symposium on atherosclerosis, Rosemont-Chicago, 6–11 Oct 1991
4. Koenig W, Ernst E (1992) The possible role of hemorrheology in atherothrombogenesis. Atherosclerosis 94(2,3):93–107
5. Smith EB (1990) Transport, interactions and retention of plasma proteins in the intima: the barrier function of the internal elastic lamina. Eur Heart J 11 [Suppl E]:72–81
6. Smith EB (1986) Fibrinogen, fibrin and fibrin degradation products in relation to atherosclerosis. In: Fidge NH, Nestel PJ (eds) Atherosclerosis VI. Elsevier, Amsterdam, pp 459–462
7. Kienast J, Berning B, van de Loo J (1990) Fibrinogen als Risikoindikator bei arteriosklerotischen Veränderungen und Koronararterien-Erkrankungen. Diagn Lab 40:162
8. Brown MS, Goldstein JL (1986) A receptor mediated pathway for cholesterol homeostasis. Science 232:34–37
9. Seidel D, Cremer P, Thiery J (1985) Plasmalipoproteine und Atherosklerose. Intern Welt 5:114–124, 6:159–165
10. Cremer P, Nagel D, Labrot B, Muche R, Elster H, Mann H, Seidel D (1991) Göttinger Risiko-, Inzidenz- und Prävalenzstudie (GRIPS). Springer, Berlin Heidelberg New York
11. Ornish D, Brown SE, Scherwitz LW, Billings JH, Armstrong WT, Ports TA, McLanahan SM, Kirkeeide RT, Brand RJ, Gould KL (1990) Can lifestyle changes revers coronary heart disease? Lancet 336:129–133

12. Buchwald H, Varco RL, Matts JP, Long JM, Fitch LL, Campbell GS, Pearce MB, Yellin AE, Edmiston WA, Smink RD Jr, Sawin HS Jr, Campos CT, Hansen BJ, Tuna N, Karnegis JN, Sanmarco ME, Amplatz K, Castaneda-Zuniga WR, Hunter DW, Bissett JK, Weber FJ, Stevenson JW, Leon AS, Chalmers TC, and the POSCH Group (1990) Effect of partial ileal bypass surgery on mortality and morbidity from coronary heart disease in patients with hypercholesterolemia. N Engl J Med 323:946–955
13. Brown BG, Albers JJ, Fisher LD, Schaeffer SM, Lin JT, Kaplan C, Zhao XQ, Bisson BD, Fitzpatrick VF, Dodge HT (1990) Regression of coronary artery disease as a result of intensive lipid lowering therapy in men with high levels of apolipoprotein B. N Engl J Med 323:1289–1298
14. Blankenhorn D, Nessim S, Johnson R, Sanmarco ME, Azen SP et al. (1987) Beneficial effects of combined colestipol-niacin therapy on coronary atherosclerosis and coronary venous bypass grafts. JAMA 257:3233–3240
15. Gohlke H, Bestehorn H-P, Braunagel K, Bauer M, Betz P, Schuff-Werner P, Seidel D for the H.E.L.P. – Study Group (1992) H.E.L.P. – Therapie Lührt zu Regression der KHK bei patienten mit therapierefraktärer lamiliärer Hypercholesterinämie. Z Kardiol 81:66
16. Hennerici M, Kleophas W, Gries FA (1991) Regression of carotid plaques during low density lipoprotein cholesterol elimination. Stroke 22:989–992
17. Buchwald H (1964) Lowering of cholesterol adsorption and blood levels by ileal exclusion. Circulation 29:713–720
18. Starzl TE, Chase HP, Ahrens EH, McNamara DJ, Bilheimer DW, Schaefer EF, Rey J, Porter KA, Stein E, Francavilia A, Benson LN (1983) Portocaval shunt in patients with familial hypercholesterolemia. Ann Surg 198:273–283
19. Starzl LE, Bilheimer DW, Bahnson HT, Shaw BW, Hardesty RL, Griffith BP, Iwatsuki S, Zitelli BJ, Gartner JC, Malatack JJ, Urbach AH (1984) Heart-liver transplantation in a patient with familial hypercholesterolemia. Lancet 1:1382–1383
20. De Gennes J, Touraine R, Maunard B et al. (1976) Formes homozygotes cutaneotendineuses de xanthomatose hypercholesterolemique dans une observation familiale exemplaire. Essai de plasmapherese à titre de traitement heroique. Bull Mem Soc Hop Paris 118:1377–1402
21. Thompson GR, Lowenthal R, Myant NB (1975) Plasma exchange in the management of homozygous familial hypercholesterolemia. Lancet 1:1208–1211
22. Lupien PJ, Moojani S, Award J (1976) A new approach to the management of familial hyperchlesterolemia: removal of plasma cholesterol based on the principle of affinity chromatography. Lancet 1:1261–1265
23. Stoffel W, Demant T (1981) Selective removal of apolipoprotein B-containing serum lipoproteins from blood plasma. Proc Natl Acad Sci USA 78:611–615
24. Riesen WT, Imhof C, Sturzenegger E, Descoeudres C, Mordasini R, Oetliker OH (1986) Behandlung der Hypercholesterinämie durch extrakorporale Immunabsorption. Schweiz Med Wochenschr 116:8
25. Yokoyama S, Hayashi R, Satani M, Yamamoto A (1985) Selective removal of low density lipoprotein by plasmapheresis in familial hypercholesterolemia. Atherosclerosis 5:613
26. Seidel D, Wieland H (1982) Ein neues Verfahren zur selektiven Messung und extrakorporalen Elimination von Low-Density-Lipoproteinen. J Clin Chem Clin Biochem 20:684–685
27. Eisenhauer T, Armstrong VW, Wieland H, Fuchs C, Scheler F, Seidel D (1987) Selective removal of low density lipoproteins (LDL) by precipitation at low pH: first clinical application of the H.E.L.P. system. Klin Wochenschr 65:161–168
28. Armstrong VW (1987) Die säureinduzierte Präzipitation von Low-Density-Lipoproteinen mit Heparin. Grundlagen zum H.E.L.P.-Verfahren. Habilitationsschrift, Göttingen
29. Seidel D (1990) The H.E.L.P. system: an efficient and safe method of plasmatherapy in the treatment of severe hypercholesterolemia. Ther Umsch 47:514–519
30. Würzner R, Schuff-Werner P, Franzke A, Nitze R, Oppermann M, Armstrong VW, Eisenhauer T, Seidel D, Götze O (1991) Complement activation and depletion during

LDL-apheresis by heparin-induced extracorporeal LDL-precipitation (H.E.L.P.). Eur J Clin Invest 21:288–294

31. Armstrong VW, Schleef J, Thiery J, Muche R, Schuff-Werner P, Eisenhauer T, Seidel D (1989) Effect of H.E.L.P.-LDL apheresis on serum concentrations of human lipoprotein(a): kinetic analysis of the post-treatment return to baseline levels. Eur J Clin Invest 19:235–240
32. Thiery J, Walli AK, Janning G, Seidel D (1990) Low density lipoprotein plasmapheresis with and without lovastatin in the treatment of the homozygous form of familial hypercholesterolemia. Eur J Pediatr 149:716–721
33. Schuff-Werner P, Schütz E, Seyde WC, Eisenhauer T, Janning G, Armstrong VW, Seidel D (1989) Improved haemorheology associated with a reduction in plasma fibrinogen and LDL in patients being treated by heparin-induced extracorporeal LDL precipitation (H.E.L.P.). Eur J Clin Invest 19:30–37
34. Kleophas W, Leschke M, Tschöpe D, Martin J, Schauseil S, Schottenfeld Y, Strauer BE, Gries FA (1990) Akute Wirkungen der extrakorporalen LDL-Cholesterin- und Fibrinogen-Elimination auf Blutrheologie und Mikrozirkulation. Dtsch Med Wochenschr 115:7–11
35. Thiery J, Armstrong V, Bosch T, Eisenhauer T, Schuff-Werner P, Seidel D (1990) Maximaltherapy der Hypercholesterinämie bei koronarer Herzerkrankung. Ther Umsch 47(6):520–529
36. Seidel D, Armstrong VW, Schuff-Werner P for the H.E.L.P. Study Group (1991) The H.E.L.P.-LDL-Apheresis Multicenter Study, an angiographically assessed trial on the role of LDL-apheresis in the secondary prevention of coronary heart disease. I. Evaluation of safety and cholesterol-lowering effects during the first 12 months. Eur J Clin Invest 21:375–383
37. Schultis H-W, v Bayer H, Neitzel H, Riedel E (1990) Functional characteristics of LDL particles derived from various LDL-apheresis techniques regarding LDL-drug-complex preparation. J Lipid Res 31:2277–2284
38. Goldstein JL, Brown MS (1983) Familial hypercholesterolemia. In: Starnbury JB, Wyngaarden JB, Fredrickson DS, Goldstein JL, Brown MS (eds) The metabolic basis of inherited disease. 5th Edition, McGraw-Hill, New York, pp 672–712
39. Keller C (1991) LDL-apheresis: results of long-term treatment and vascular outcome. Atherosclerosis 86:1–8
40. Demant T, Seidel D (1992) Recent developments in low-density lipoprotein apheresis. Curr Opin Lipidol 3:43–48
41. Gordon BR, Bilheimer DW, Brown DC, Dau PC, Gotto AM, Illingworth DR, Jones PH, Kelsey SF, Leitman SF, Stein EA, Stern TN, Zavoral JH, Zwiener J, for Liposorber Study Group (1991) Multicenter study of the treatment of familial hypercholesterolemia (FH) by LDL-apheresis using the liposorber LA-15 system (abstract). Arterioscler Thromb 11:1409
42. Tatami R, Inoue N, Itoh H, Kishino B, Koga N, Nakashima Y, Nishide T, Okamura K, Saito Y, Teramoto T, Yasugi T, Yamamoto A and Goto Y for the LARS Investigators (1992) Regression of coronary atherosclerosis by combined LDL-apheresis and lipid-lowering drug therapy in patients with familial hypercholesterolemia: a multicenter study. Atherosclerosis 95:1–13
43. Greten H, Bleifeld W, Beil FU, Daerr W, Strauer BE, Kleophas W, Gries FA, Schuff-Werner P, Thiery J, Seidel D (1992) LDL-Apheresis. Ein therapeutisches Verfahren bei schwerer Hypercholesterinämie. Dtsch Arztebl Arztl Mitt 89(1/2):48–49

Antiplatelet Drugs

J.H. Chesebro, B.J. Meyer, A. Fernandez-Ortiz, I.K. Jang, and V. Fuster

Thrombus and platelet deposition in vein grafts begins intraoperatively as soon as blood begins to flow through the graft [1]. This knowledge led to antithrombotic therapy being started perioperatively and to the first convincing platelet inhibitor trial in coronary bypass graft operations [2, 3]. Prior studies had started the same therapy several days after operation when thrombus had already formed, and thus they were unsuccessful [4]. In the first several months after operation, occlusion is related to thrombosis that is, in part, due to vein graft injury, technical problems, and associated coronary artery disease with small coronary arteries and low vein-graft blood flow [1–3, 5–7]. Asymptomatic mural thrombosis within vein grafts appears considerable, is probably underestimated at angiography, and is only recognized in its most extensive form (Fig. 1).

Structure and Pharmacodynamics of Antiplatelet Therapies

Aspirin

Aspirin is acetylsalicylic acid, which is an ester of acetic acid. It has a molecular weight of 180 and is a weak acid with a pK_a 3.5. Aspirin is an acetyl donor to the platelet membrane and irreversibly acetylates the platelet enzyme cyclooxygenase which inhibits formation of thromboxane A_2. Non-acetylated salicylates have no significant effect on platelet aggregation. Other nonsteroidal anti-inflammatory agents inhibit cyclooxygenase in a reversible fashion.

Aspirin inhibits the platelet aggregation caused by thromboxane A_2 and arachidonic acid, but only partially inhibits the aggregation induced by adenosine diphosphate, collagen, or a low concentration of thrombin. Aspirin does not inhibit the adherence of a primary layer of platelets to the sub-endothelium, but usually reduces the number of platelet layers above the initial layer by blocking thromboxane A_2 synthesis. Aspirin may reduce but does not largely prevent the release of contents of platelet granules, and thus growth factors which are chemoattractants and mitogens, such as platelet-derived growth factor (PDGF) or transforming growth factor-beta,

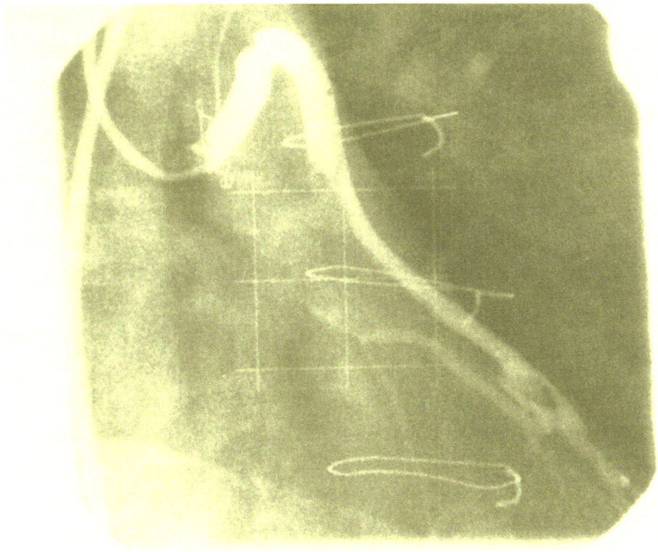

Fig. 1. Vein graft angiogram of the left anterior descending coronary artery in asymptomatic patient 8 days after operation. Note the diffuse narrowing of the mid and distal graft (with hazy irregular borders) and filling defect adjacent to the distal anastomosis which are hallmarks of mural thrombosis. (Reprinted with permission from [8])

may still be secreted from platelets. By reducing the extent of thrombosis, aspirin may reduce neointima formation and the extent of smooth muscle cell proliferation [1, 6, 9].

Although aspirin permanently acetylates cyclooxygenase for the lifetime of the platelet, its effect on the cyclooxygenase of vascular endothelium is not permanent because endothelial cells synthesize additional cyclooxygenase. Daily administration of 1 mg/kg aspirin inhibits formation of platelet cyclooxygenase and thromboxane A_2 and the production of vascular prostacyclin [10–12]. A loading dose of 160 mg aspirin is sufficient to inhibit platelet thromboxane A_2, and 80 mg/day aspirin is sufficient to maintain this inhibition [12].

Initially, higher doses of aspirin were used until it was realized that lower doses also achieve an antithrombotic affect but avoid the toxic side effects of higher doses. Aspirin at 1 mg/kg per day reduces but does not eliminate mural thrombosis after deep arterial injury [13]. Clinically, aspirin at a dosage of 80–325 mg/day achieves an antithrombotic affect [14–17]. Side effects are dose-related and mainly involve the gastrointestinal tract [18]. Thus today aspirin doses of 80–325 mg/day are used as antithrombotic therapy.

Combined use of low-dose aspirin (80–160 mg/day) and an anticoagulant such as heparin and warfarin in sequence, appear to provide superior antithrombotic protection [17, 19–24]. Thus combined use appears rational in patients at a high risk of thrombosis, such as those with mechanical prosthetic heart valves combined with aortocoronary bypass grafts, unstable angina (especially patients who present on daily aspirin), and patients with acute myocardial infarction undergoing thrombolysis, or those who have previously shown a high thrombotic tendency. Aspirin (160 mg) plus heparin (activated partial thromboplastin time, aPTT, 60–85 s) reduce the incidence of reocclusion after thrombolysis with recombinant tissue plasminogen activator or streptokinase (administered for acute myocardial infarction) to 4.9%–6.4% as documented by the angiographic substudy of the GUSTO trial [24a].

The absorption of aspirin after oral administration is rapid and complete, but there may be slight variations according to dosage form, tablet dissolution rate, and gastric pH. Food decreases the rate but not the extent of absorption, and the absorption of enteric-coated preparations is usually delayed. After rectal administration, the absorption of aspirin is delayed and incomplete compared with the absorption achieved with oral administration of equal doses.

The physical half-life of the aspirin molecule is only 15–20 min since it is rapidly hydrolyzed to salicylate by deacylation in the liver, and free salicylic acid and conjugated metabolites are excreted by the kidney [25]. The initial antithrombotic protection afforded by oral dosing of 160 mg is obtained within 15–30 min.

Dipyridamole

Dipyridamole is a vasodilator with pharmacologic actions similar to papaverine. It is lipophilic and has a molecular weight of 505 and a pK_a 6.1. It only slightly changes systemic blood pressure or peripheral blood flow in usual doses. The action of dipyridamole is linked to its effect on the metabolism and transport of adenosine.

Dipyridamole increases platelet cyclic adenosine monophosphate by three mechanisms: first, by inhibiting phosphodiestrase and thus the breakdown of cyclic adenosine monophosphate; second, by inhibiting the uptake of adenosine by vascular endothelium and erythrocytes; and third, by activating adenylate cyclase and effecting a prostacyclin mechanism on the platelet membrane [26–28].

Dipyridamole has better antithrombotic effects against prosthetic surfaces such as artificial heart valves and arteriovenous shunts than it does against biologic surfaces. Experimentally, aspirin has been found to potentiate dipyridamole by preventing thromboembolism from originating on prosthetic surfaces [29]. Aspirin has been found to be as effective as combined aspirin and dipyridamole against biologic surfaces in experimental and clinical studies [13, 30–32]. Because cardiopulmonary bypass involves prosthetic surfaces, a dipyridamole infusion may be advantageous perioperatively, especially when high-risk aortocoronary vein grafts, are involved such as those with low flow and those which anastamose to distal arteries less than 1.5 mm in diameter [33, 34]. Unfortunately, early postoperative vein graft occlusion rates were not examined in either of the two studies [33, 34], although these would have given the greatest chance of showing a difference if one exists.

Oral absorption of dipyridamole is slow and subject to individual variability. The bioavailability varies from 27% to 66%, and protein binding is very high at 91%–99%. It is transformed in the liver to the glucuronic acid conjugate. The initial distribution half-life after oral administration is 40–90 min, and the elimination half-life is 10–12 h. The time to peak plasma concentration after oral administration is 1–3 h (usually about 75 min). Elimination is primarily biliary, and up to 20% enterohepatic recirculation may occur. At the usual preoperative doses of 100 mg four times daily, dipyridamole very seldom induces angina (one of 202, 0.5% [2], and seven of 1149, 0.6% [35]).

Sulfinpyrazone

Sulfinpyrazone is a uricosuric agent which is structurally related to phenylbutazone but does not have significant anti-inflammatory effects. It competitively inhibits platelet cyclooxygenase but its mechanism of action is uncertain [36]. It reduces thrombus formation on subendothelium, inhibits platelet adhesion to collagen, and may protect endothelium against chemical injury [37]. Like dipyridamole, sulfinpyrazone is more beneficial against prosthetic than against biologic surfaces, and similarly it has been found reduce experimental thromboembolism in artificial cannulae in a dose-dependent fashion as well as to reduce thrombus in arteriovenous cannulae, and to improve platelet survival to normal in patients with prosthetic heart valves [37, 38]. As was also found for dipyridamole, sulfinpyrazone did not reduce quantitative ^{111}In-platelet deposition onto deeply injured arteries in the pig [13]. No placebo-controlled prospective trials have been done to document reduced thromboembolism in patients with prosthetic heart valves; the only data in these patients have been obtained by retrospective or cohort observations [38]. Clinical benefits in patients with coronary artery disease have been variable, with questionable benefit after myocardial infarction, no benefit in patients with unstable angina, and probably some small benefit in preventing aortocoronary vein graft occlusion [34–43].

Ticlopidine

Ticlopidine appears to block the interaction of von Willibrand factor and fibrinogen with platelets and thus may alter the reactivity of the platelet membrane. Ticlopidine inhibits platelet aggregation induced by even high concentrations of adenosine diphosphate and that induced by low concentrations of thrombin, collagen, thromboxane A_2 and platelet-activating factor, but not by high concentrations of these agonists. It also prolongs the bleeding time and shortens prolonged platelet survival [44, 45].

It may take several days for maximal antithrombotic effects to occur, and inhibition may persist for more than 3 days after stopping therapy, with a return to baseline values after 4–10 days [44, 46]. There is a direct, dose-dependent relationship between the ex vivo inhibition of adenosine diphosphate-induced platelet aggregation and the dose of ticlopidine. (NB: Inhibition of platelet aggregation is not useful for predicting in vivo antithrombotic effectiveness.) Maximal effect is reached at a dose of 500 mg daily [46]. Ticlopidine does not inhibit synthesis of prostacyclin, but, at a dosage of 250 mg twice daily in patients with unstable angina, it reduces the incidence of myocardial infarction, vascular mortality, and total coronary events by 50% [47]. At a dosage of 500–750 mg/day, ticlopidine also markedly reduced the incidence of abrupt thrombotic occlusion after percutaneous transluminal coronary angiography (PTCA), but did not reduce the rate of restenosis [48, 49]. It has also been effective in reducing aorto-coronary vein graft occlusion both early and late after operation [50].

Eighty percent of a ticlopidine dose is absorbed rapidly. Absorption is increased by about 20% after a meal and is decreased by about the same after antacids containing aluminum and magnesium. Protein binding is high (98%), primarily to lipoproteins and albumin. Hepatic metabolism is extensive, resulting in approximately 20 metabolites. The elimination half-life of a single 250 mg dose is 7.9 h in subjects aged 20–43 years and 12.6 hours in subjects aged 65–76 years. After repeated dosing twice daily, the elimination half-life is about 4 days in those aged 20–43 years and about 5 days in those aged 65–76 years. The onset of action determined by inhibition of platelet aggregation begins within 2 days, but apparent clinically significant inhibition (more than 50%) occurs within 4 days. Time to peak concentration is 2 h after a 250 mg dose. Ticlopidine elimination is 60% renal and 23% biliary/fecal. Repeated administration of 250 mg twice daily results in a steady state concentration after 14–21 days. Maximal inhibition of platelet aggregation (60%–70%) occurs within 8–11 days. After stopping treatment, bleeding time and platelet function tests return to pretreatment levels within 1–2 weeks [25].

Most side effects which include neutropenia, agranulocytosis, thrombocytopenia, gastrointestinal disturbances, and skin rash occur within the first 3 months of treatment. Some occur or recur months later. Rarely, neutropenia, thrombocytopenia, or thrombocytopenic purpura occur after years of treatment. Fatalities have been associated with severe neutropenia or thrombocytopenic purpura [25]. Gastrointestinal disturbances have occurred in up to 40% of patients, are usually mild, and usually disappear within 1–2 weeks after stopping therapy. About 13% of patients have withdrawn from clinical studies because of side effects [25]. Skin rash occurs in about 5% of patients on ticlopidine. This may disappear within several days after stopping treatment and may not recur after restarting therapy. The incidence of intracerebral bleeding was 0.5%, epistaxis 0.5%–1%, itching 1.3%, neutropenia 2.4% overall and 0.8% severe (including agranulocytosis, fever, chills, pharyngitis, other signs of infection, ulcers, sores, or white spots in the mouth). Purpura, ranging from pinpoint to large bruises (red or purple) may occur in 2% of patients. Diarrhea may occur in 13%, indigestion in 7%, nausea in 7%, and abdominal pain in 4%. Cholestatic jaundice or hepatitis is rare. Hives have occurred in 0.5%–1%. Asymptomatic thrombocytopenia may occur in 0.4% [25].

Direct Thrombin Inhibitors

Hirudin is a polypeptide of 65 amino acids which was isolated from the salivary glands of the European leech (*Hirudo medicinalis*). The selectivity and affinity for α-thrombin with which it binds in a 1:1 noncovalent complex is exceptional ($K_d = 2 \times 10^{-14} M$); for recombinant hirudin C6P39393, $K_d = 2 \times 10^{-13} M$). The marked specificity and affinity for thrombin appears to be due to multiple molecular contacts rather than a small number of strong interactions. The molecular weight is 7000 [51–57].

Hirudin blocks thrombin-mediated platelet activation and deposition at higher doses and the conversion of fibrinogen to fibrin at lower doses [58–61]. Because platelets are extremely sensitive to minute amounts of thrombin [61], there is a very sharp demarcation of dose–activity response of hirudin for totally preventing mural thrombosis onto deeply injured arteries in vivo; thrombosis occurs at an aPTT of 1.7 × control but is totally blocked at ≥2.0 × control [59]. Because more thrombin appears to be generated after deep or plaque injury than after mild injury [60], more hirudin is necessary to prevent thrombosis after deep or plaque injury. Hirudin limits platelet deposition to a single layer or less after deep arterial injury [59]. Since hirudin is a direct thrombin inhibitor, it inhibits clot-bound thrombin at the same dose which inhibits thrombin in plasma [62].

Thrombosis and thrombolysis are dynamic and simultaneous processes, thus blocking thrombosis will accelerate thrombolysis. It appears that the most potent antithrombotic therapy, hirudin, maximally accelerates thrombolysis (compared with aspirin or heparin) [63]. This has also been evident in humans where a 5-day infusion of hirudin in patients with unstable angina and aortocoronary vein graft occlusion resulted in recanalization of a totally occluded graft, and in two out of the three patients thus treated, aPTT was 2.5–3.0 × control (J.H. Chesebro, unpublished data) in the absence of any thrombolytic therapy. The opposite relationship between thrombosis and thrombolysis is also applicable; blocking thrombolysis, for example with aprotinin, promotes thrombosis of vein grafts and myocardial infarction and is dangerous to humans [64].

Thus these very preliminary data suggest that the direct thrombin inhibitor hirudin may be helpful in treating acutely occluded aortocoronary bypass grafts and may have a role in future perioperative therapy in aortocoronary bypass graft operations. A phase 1 study of the intravenous infusion of hirudin in humans showed that the best laboratory test for monitoring hirudin dosage and blood levels was the aPTT ($r = 0.88$) [65]. Hirudin does not significantly prolong bleeding time in humans [65], which is no longer during hirudin therapy it is than with heparin or any other antithrombotic therapy. Experimentally, hirudin has been found to block thrombosis within the vascular lumen but not within fissures or tears of the arterial wall (J.H. Chesebro, unpublished data); the latter protects against bleeding.

Rationale for Antithrombotic Therapy

Perioperative antithrombotic therapy is critical for preventing thrombosis in vein grafts because platelet deposition begins as soon as blood starts to flow through the vein graft [1, 2]. Second, prevention of acute thrombosis in the vein graft markedly reduces subsequent neointimal proliferation 2–3 months after operation in the canine model (see I.K. Jang and V. Fuster, this volume) [66]. Thus antithrombotic therapy to reduce acute mural and occlusive thrombus appears capable of reducing occlusion both in the acute phase and between the acute phase and 1 year later [2, 3, 73]. Tabulation of several clinical trials where antithrombotic therapy was started at variable times before and after operation showed the importance of early therapy (at least within 48 h of operation) in reducing the vein graft occlusive process both early and a year after operation (Fig. 2). Vein graft occlusion cannot be successfully prevented if therapy is started more than 48 h after operation.

Dipyridamole alone does not significantly reduce platelet deposition or mural thrombus formation on deeply injured arteries, but it does appear to reduce platelet deposition on artificial materials in vivo [13, 74]. In experiments, dipyridamole was found to decrease platelet activation and maintain the platelet count during cardiopulmonary bypass when given as an infusion during the operation [75, 76]. In humans, dipyridamole maintained platelet counts above $150 \times 10^9/l$ in 71% of patients compared with only 28% in control patients when dipyridamole was administered preoperatively at 100 mg four times a day and during operation as an infusion at 0.24 mg/kg per hour. In addition, the total blood loss from the chest tubes was reduced from 1550 ml in the control group to 850 ml in the dipyridamole group, and packed red blood cell transfusions were reduced from 3.31 to 1.91 per patient in the treated group [77]. Thus oral plus intraoperatively administered intravenous dipyridamole may be a possible approach for reducing bleed-

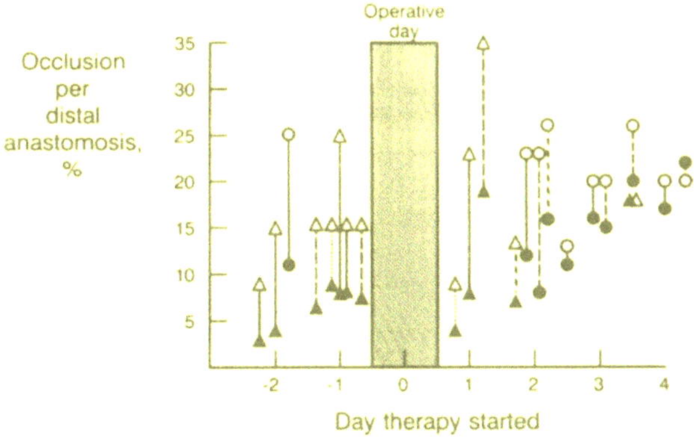

Fig. 2. Relationship of vein graft occlusion to the day of starting antiplatelet therapy before (day minus 2 or 1) or after (day 1, 2, 3, or 4) operation. Studies in which therapy was started before or at least within 48 hours after operation were the most successful in preventing subsequent vein graft occlusion. The time of angiography is shown by the shape of the symbol (*triangle*, at or before 6 months; *circle*, at 12 months or later). The drugs administered are shown by the type of lines between symbols (*continous line*, acetylsalicylic acid plus dipyridamole; *dashed line*, acetylsalicylic acid; *dotted line*, sulfinpyrazone; *diagonally dashed line*, ticlopidine). *Open symbols* depict placebo; *closed symbols* depict treatment. (Data from studies reported in [2–4, 31, 32, 41, 42, 49, 67–72]. Modified from [98] with permission)

ing and platelet consumption in vein grafts and cardiopulmonary bypass oxygenator apparatus. More clinical trials with intravenous perioperative dipyridamole are needed in humans to better evaluate the effectiveness on bleeding and reduction of blood transfusions and platelet activation.

The intraoperative and early postoperative use of compounds which block fibrinolysis to decrease intraoperative blood loss promotes thrombosis. This is not only an acute danger to the patient (increased Q-wave myocardial infarction from 9% in placebo to 14% and 18% in aprotinin groups in repeat coronary artery bypass graft patients) because of vein graft occlusion (50% of vein grafts occluded at autopsy in aprotinin groups and none in placebo group) [64], but also may enhance mural thrombosis in vein grafts, which may increase vein graft occlusion days, months, or years after the operation. Increasing coagulation factors such as with desmopressin (desamino-8-arginine vasopressin, DDAVP) may alao enhance mural thrombosis and create a risk. The danger of increasing thrombosis and occlusion is very real, since thrombosis enhances neointimal proliferation [1, 6, 66] (see I.K. Jang and V. Fuster, this volume). If these approaches to reducing bleeding are to be used in patients, they should first be tested in animals to more precisely examine mechanisms and risks. Unfortunately desmopressin does not have any effect in animals and cannot be tested in this fashion.

Platelet Inhibitor Dosages and Incidence of Vein Graft Occlusion

Therapeutic dosages of platelet inhibitor therapy were originally based on a given therapy prolonging a shortened platelet survival in patients with thromboembolic disease [78–81]. The dosages for the first two major platelet inhibitor trials were chosen on this basis [2, 3, 32, 43]. These trials were also based on pathophysiologic principles from animal studies (see I.K. Jang and V. Fuster, this volume) [1, 6, 66]. Therapy was administered for 2 days and at 2 h before operation and continued immediately after operation (dipyridamole via the nasogastric tube, as outlined in Tables 1 and 2. The therapy currently recommended is only slightly modified from these studies. Angiographic evaluation was performed approximately 1 week and 1 year after operation.

Early Occlusion

In three very large trials, vein graft angiography was performed within a mean of 8–10 days after operation. The results from the Mayo Clinic study

Table 1. Antiplatelet therapy in the Mayo Clinic Study

Two days before operation
Dipyridamole (Persantin, 100 mg, orally four times daily
On day of operation
2 h before operation: dipyridamole, 100 mg, orally
1 h after operation: dipyridamole, 100 mg, via nasogastric tube (clamp, 1.5 h)
7 h after operation: dipyridamole, 75 mg, and aspirin, 325 mg via nasogastric tube (clamp, 1.5 h)
On day after operation and daily thereafter
Dipyridamole, 75 mg, and aspirin, 325 mg orally three times daily

No other aspirin or prostaglandin-inhibiting drugs, especially nonsteroidal anti-inflammatory agents – sulindac (Clinoril) would least interfere – inhibitors of gastric acid secretions (for example, cimetidine or ranitidine) or simultaneous antacid should be given. For patients with only internal mammary artery bypass grafts and no vein grafts, empiric therapy is advised for 3 months to allow healing at anastomotic sites.

Table 2. Antiplatelet therapy in the Veterans Administration Cooperative Study

All drugs started before operation
Aspirin 325 mg daily
Aspirin 325 mg three times daily
Aspirin 325 mg and dipyridamole 75 mg, both three times daily
Sulfinpyrazone 267 mg three times daily

All therapy was started 48 h before operation except aspirin which was administered as a single dose 12 h before operation. The first dose of therapy was administered 6 h after operation by a nasogastric tube which was then clamped for 1.5 h. Therapy was continued every 8 h down the nasogastric tube until regular oral dosing could be substituted.

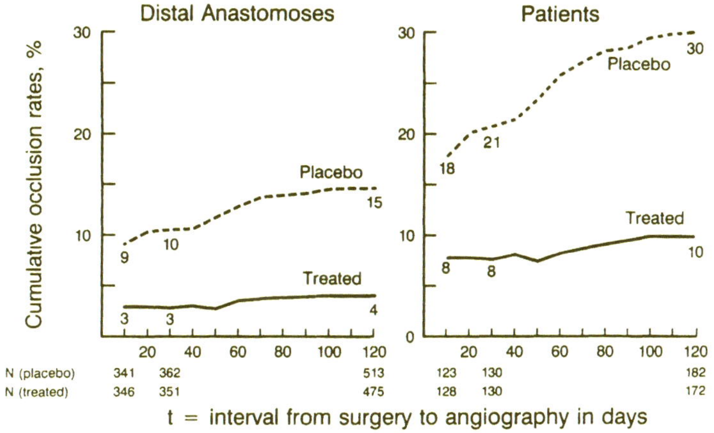

Fig. 3. Occlusion rate of vein graft-coronary artery distal anastomoses totally occluded on angiography at t days after operation (*left*) and of patients with one or more distal anastomoses occluded on angiography at t days after operation (*right*). For group difference, p value and 95% confidence limits were as follows: at $t = 10$, $p = 0.003$, 5%–22%; at $t = 30$, $p = 0.0004$, 7%–23%; at $t = 120$, $p < 10^{-6}$, 14%–30%). The range of t was 7–180 days. The occlusion rates did not change from 120 to 180 days after operation, when only six more patients underwent angiography. N = total number of distal anastomoses or patients in treated and placebo groups at 10, 30 and 120 days after operation. (Reprinted with permission from [2])

are summarized in Fig. 3. Angiography was performed in 88% of patients at a median of 8 days after operation. There was a reduction in the frequency of vein graft occlusion from 10% in the placebo group to 3% in the treated group (rising to 15% in the placebo group within 30 days, and to 4% in the treated group within 6 months). These reductions in occlusion were present in more than 50 subgroups, including patients at higher and lower risk for occlusion as determined by distal coronary artery lumen diameter, vein graft blood flow, or presence or absence of coronary endarterectomy [2]. The results from the Veteran's Administration Cooperative Study (angiography in 72% of patients at a mean of 9 days and all within 60 days after operation) are summarized in Fig. 4. In the combination group, the preoperative dose of dipyridamole was 225 mg/day rather than the 400 mg/day needed to normalize a shortened platelet survival in patients without aspirin [78] as in the Mayo study. Occlusion rates were not different in any of the groups with aspirin (7.4% versus 15% of grafts in the placebo group). Occlusion rates in the treated groups were all higher (approximately two-fold) than in the Mayo Clinic study. Sulfinpyrazone resulted in only borderline benefit (9.8% grafts occluded) and caused transient renal insufficiency in 5.3% of patients [32]. Thus, treatment is needed with a spirin administered via a nasogastric tube within hours of operation.

In the Spanish study (GESIC) [35] all patients received dipyridamole 100 mg four times daily for 48 h before operation. Then randomized treatment was started 7 h after operation using low-dose aspirin (50 mg three

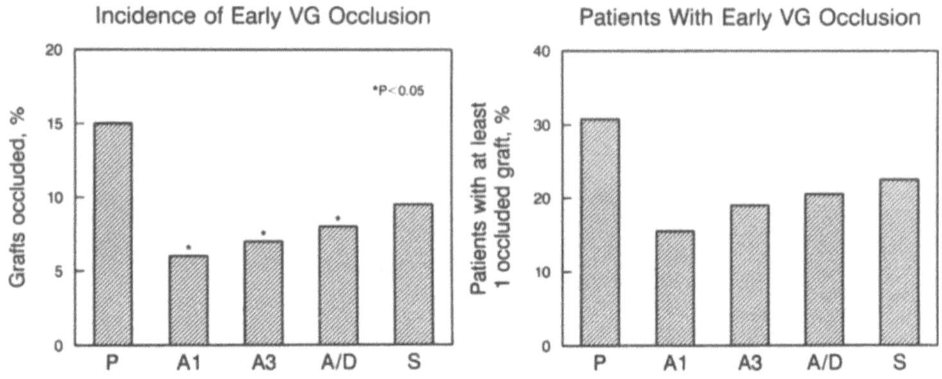

Fig. 4a,b. Early vein-graft (*VG*) occlusion. **a** Percentage of occluded grafts in each treatment group from Veterans Administration Trial (*P*, placebo; *A1*, aspirin once daily; *A3*, aspirin three times daily; *A/D*, aspirin/dipyridamole; *S*, sulfinpyrazone). *$p < 0.05$ refers to comparison between each treatment group and placebo by cluster analysis. The 95% confidence intervals (CI) of the differences are: A1 versus P, difference 8.4% (1.7, 15.0 CI); A3 versus P, difference 7.2% (0.5, 13.8 CI); A/D versus P, difference 6.8% (0.1, 13.4 CI); S versus P, difference 5.1% (−1.6, 11.8 CI). **b** Percentage of patients with at least one occluded graft (*P*, placebo; *A1*, aspirin once daily; *A3*, aspirin three times daily; *A/D*, aspirin/dipyridamole; *S*, sulfinpyrazone). The 95% CI of the differences are: A1 vs P, difference 13.4% (−0.2, 27.1 CI); A3 vs P, difference 11.2% (−2.5, 24.9 CI); A/D vs P, difference 9.2% (−4.5, 22.9 CI); S vs P, difference 8.1% (−5.5, 21.9 CI). (Reproduced from [32] with permission)

times daily) with placebo or dipyridamole 75 mg three times daily or double placebo. Of 1112 study patients 927 (83%) had vein graft angiography within 28 days of operation (mean 10 days). Aspirin plus dipyridamole significantly ($p = 0.017$) reduced the occlusion rate of distal anastomoses from 18% (placebo) to 12.9%. The occlusion rate in the aspirin group was 14%, which was of borderline significance compared to placebo ($p = 0.058$). Only aspirin plus dipyridamole significantly reduced ($p = 0.01$) the number of patients with occluded grafts (placebo 33%, aspirin 27%, aspirin plus dipyridamole 24%). Thus there was a trend favoring combined therapy.

Late Vein Graft Occlusion

New occlusion at 1 year after operation of all types of vein grafts which demonstrated angiographic patency within 30 days of operation is shown in the middle panel of Fig. 5. Repeat angiography was performed in 84% of patients at a median of 12 months (range 11–18 months) [3]. The percentage of patients with new occlusion was reduced from 27% in the placebo group to 16% in the treated group ($p = 0.038$; middle panel on right in Fig. 5). Overall at 1 year occlusion frequency was reduced from 25% of grafts in the placebo group to 11% in the treated group. These percentages corresponded

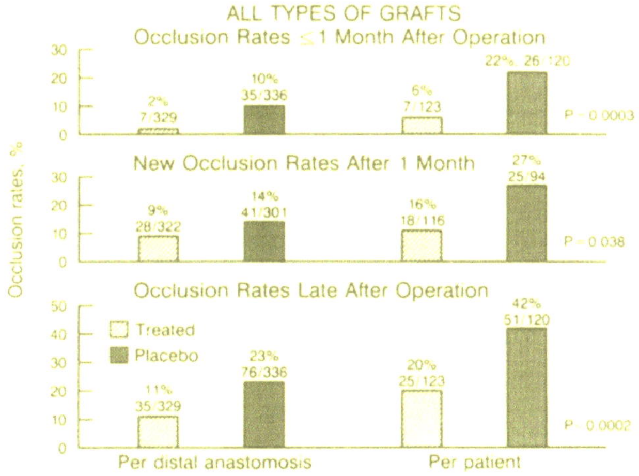

Fig. 5. Occlusion rates for all types of vein grafts. The rates are expressed per distal anastomosis and per patient (proportion with at least one occlusion). Occlusion is shown as events occurring within one month (95% confidence limits for the per patient difference, 8%–24%), as new events occurring beyond 1 month (in distal anastomoses and patients without occlusion within 1 month of operation) from angiography performed 1 year later (per patient, $p = 0.048$; 95% confidence limits for the difference, 9%–22%), and as events at a median of 1 year after operation (95% confidence limits for the per patient difference, 11%–34%). These subsets include only patients who had angiography within 1 month of operation and again 1 year later. Below each percentage is shown the ratio of distal anastomoses or patients with occlusion to total distal anastomoses or patients. (Reprinted with permission from [3])

to 47% of patients with one or more occlusions in the placebo group and 22% of patients with occlusion in the treated group which showed how marked the reduction was (95% confidence limits for the difference, 16%–35%). Thus, continuous antithrombotic therapy is necessary.

In a more recent trial of 249 patients randomized to aspirin 25 mg plus dipyridamole 200 mg twice daily or standard anticoagulant therapy and to either 3 months or 1 year of treatment, there was no difference in occlusion between the two active treatments within 2 weeks of operation (16% of patients with occlusion in the dipyridamole and aspirin group and 19% of patients with occlusion in the anticoagulant group), but after 9 more months, an additional vein graft occlusion was found in 22% of patients on extended active therapy and in 32% of the placebo group ($p = 0.08$). In addition, only 6% of individual vein grafts were occluded when antithrombotic therapy was continued for the last 9 months while occlusion was found in 13% of vein grafts in the placebo group ($p = 0.01$) [73]. Thus, continued antithrombotic therapy is necessary.

In the Veterans Administration Cooperative Study, angiography was performed late after operation in only 65% of patients at a median of 12 months (range 2–18 months). New occlusion of vein grafts from 9 days after

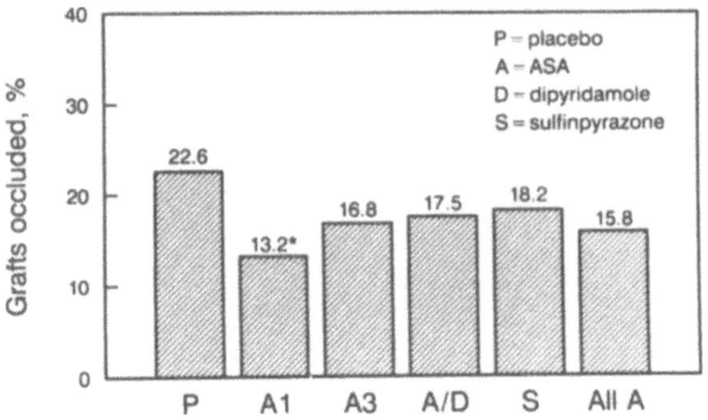

Fig. 6. Percentage of occluded graphs in each treatment group and overall for aspirin from the Veterans Administration Cooperative Study 1 year after operation (*P*, placebo; *A1*, aspirin once daily; *A3*, aspirin three times daily; *A/D*, aspirin/dipyridamole; *S*, sulfinpyrazone; A1 versus P, 9.4% difference 95% confidence intervals: 0.0, 18.7); A3 versus P, 5.8% difference (95% confidence intervals: −3.6, 15.2); A/D versus P, 5.1% difference (95% confidence intervals: −4.2, 14.5); S versus P, 4.6% difference (95% confidence intervals: −4.9, 13.8); all versus P, 6.8% difference ($p = 0.029$). (Reproduced with permission from [43])

operation to 1 year later occurred in 8.7% of aspirin-treated and 9.4% of placebo-treated grafts (p = NS). The proportion of grafts occluded at 1 year in the four treatment regimens compared with placebo for grafts in patients is shown in Fig. 6. The proportion of patients with one or more occlusions at 1 year was 44% in the placebo group (23% of grafts) compared with 35% in all treated groups ($p = 0.01$) or 16% of grafts in all aspirin-treated patients [43]. A possible explanation for the lack of continued treatment benefit over the next year in this study compared to the Mayo Clinic and the European studies may be the smaller number of patients at late risk and observed for a shorter period of time here (higher proportion of grafts occluded early – within 60 days – and "late" included patients studied between 2 and 11 months and 11–18 months, not just 11–18 months as in the Mayo Study), the smaller proportion of patients studied angiographically, the extent to which risk factors were modified (half of the Veterans Administration patients were current smokers), or patient compliance in taking therapy.

In a very recent trial in 948 patients from the Netherlands, aspirin alone (50 mg/day started at midnight after operation) and aspirin plus dipyridamole (5 mg/kg per 24 h intravenously for 28 h, started at 2000 hours on the day before operation until midnight after operation and continued orally in a slow-release form of 200 mg twice daily) were compared with oral anticoagulation (acenocoumarol 4 mg or phenprocoumon 6 mg started on the day before surgery and continued on the first postoperative day; doses were then adjusted from the second postoperative day to an international normalized ratio between 2.8 and 4.8). No early postoperative angiography was performed. It was calculated in advance that 292 patients per group were

Table 3. Frequency of vein-graft occlusion by type of graft and distal anastamosis, coronary artery lumen diameter, location of distal anastamosis, and endarterectomy (from [34])

	Occlusion by type of treatment					
	Aspirin + placebo		Asprin + dipyridamole		Oral anticoagulants	
	%	*n*	%	*n*	%	*n*
Single grafts	17	246	12	282	15	234
Lumen diameter (mm)						
≤1.0	26	7	18	62	26	94
1.1–1.5	17	441[a]	11	394[a]	13	398
1.6–2.0	9	192	8	224	9	209
>2.0	4	45	18	45	14	50
Location of distal anastomoses						
LAD	12	205	10	230	10	239
CX	16	322	11	316	12	329
RCA	16	230	11	218	18	229
Sequential grafts						
Grafts	23	194	20	179	22	214
Distal anastomoses	15	511	11	482	13	583
Distal anastomoses						
End to side	17	440	13	461	16	449
Side to side	11	317	9	303	9	348
Endarterectomy[b]	47	15	15	20	32	22

LAD, left anterior descending coronary artery; CX, circumflex coronary; RCA, right coronary artery.
[a] RR 0.66; 95% confidence interval 0.47–0.94.
[b] 13 vessels were classified as neither patent nor occluded.

required to demonstrate a 30% reduction in occlusion rate with a power of 80% at the 5% significance level. Repeat angiography was performed in 86% of patients ($n = 787$), which was 100 patients short of the number predicted to show a difference between groups. At angiography at 1 year, there was a strong trend toward reduced occlusion in the aspirin plus dipyridamole group compared with the groups treated either with aspirin alone or oral anticoagulants: for occlusion of distal anastomoses, it was 11%, 15%, and 13%, and for occlusion of vein grafts it was 15%, 20%, and 19%, respectively. Occlusion rates tended to be consistently lower in the aspirin plus dipyridamole group overall, throughout most subgroups, and especially in grafts placed into distal vessels with a lumen diameter ≤1.5 mm where differences were statistically significant (see Table 3).

Although clinical events were tabulated in 20%, 14%, and 17% in the aspirin plus dipyridamole, aspirin alone, and oral anticoagulant groups, respectively, this is not particularly meaningful because it included deep vein thrombosis and pulmonary embolism, which are not prevented or treated with antiplatelet therapy, as well as perioperative myocardial infarction, which is often related to the hemodynamics of the coronary disease rather than antithrombotic therapy.

Perioperative Bleeding

In the Mayo Clinic and Netherlands studies where dipyridamole was started before operation but aspirin started approximately 7 h after operation, there was no difference in chest tube blood loss, transfusion requirements for red cells, platelets, or fresh frozen plasma, or reoperation for bleeding (3%–5% of patients) [2, 34]. In the Veterans Administration Cooperative Study, preoperative aspirin was associated with a significant increase in chest tube blood loss, which was approximately 300 ml more in the worst aspirin group than in the placebo group. Reoperation for bleeding was 6.1% in the aspirin group compared with 1.9% of patients in the placebo and sulfinpyrazone groups [32].

Aspirin was administered before or 6 h after operation (325 mg/day) by the Veterans Administration Cooperative Group, and angiography was performed in 72% of patients an average of 8 days after operation. Vein graft occlusion was similar in both groups (7.4% versus 7.8% with and without preoperative aspirin, respectively). In the group taking aspirin before operation, none of the 22 distal anastomoses in y-grafts was occluded, while 7% of 43 distal anastomoses were occluded in the nonaspirin group; in addition, in the preoperative aspirin group, none of the 131 internal mammary artery grafts was occluded, while 2.4% in the 125 internal mammary grafts in the nonaspirin group. The latter results were of borderline significance and were retrospective observations which warrant a further prospective study. As expected, median blood loss 35 h after operation was 105 ml more in the preoperative than the postoperative aspirin group, red cell transfusion was 175 ml greater in the preoperative aspirin group, and the incidence of reoperation for bleeding was 6.3% in the preoperative aspirin group versus 2.4% in the postoperative aspirin group [82].

Very early administration of aspirin now appears warranted. Aspirin (325 mg/day) has been administered as early as 1 h after operation down the nasogastric tube and compared with placebo [83]. Angiography of vein grafts in 97% of patients a median of 7 days after operation showed occlusion in 1.6% of distal anastomoses in the aspirin group and 6.2% in the placebo group with no difference in chest tube blood loss or blood transfusion requirements between the groups. Reoperation for bleeding was performed in 4.8% of patients in the aspirin group and 1% of the placebo group.

Alternative Antithrombotic Therapy to Aspirin

In patients who are intolerant or allergic to aspirin, 250 mg ticlopidine twice daily may be started immediately after operation. In a study of 173 patients, this dosage was started 2 days after operation, and over 90% of patients were restudied by digital angiography at 10, 180, and 360 days after operation. The proportion of distal anastomoses occluded was reduced at 10 days from 13.4% in the placebo group to 7.1% in the treated group ($p < 0.05$), at 180 days from 24% to 15% ($p < 0.02$), and at 360 days from 26.1% to 15.9% ($p < 0.01$), in the placebo and treated groups, respectively [50]. Therapy could probably be started the evening before operation since ticlopidine has a delayed onset of action of at least 1–2 days and reaches a maximal affect at 3–5 days.

Oral anticoagulation significantly reduces aortocoronary vein graft occlusion, as shown initially when subcutaneous heparin and dipyridamole (in three divided doses) were administered three times daily for 7 days prior to starting oral anticoagulation versus no additional therapy after 7 days [84]. Eight weeks after operation, there was a significant reduction in the occlusion of distal anastomoses (from 15% in the placebo group to 10% in the oral anticoagulation group) and in the proportion of patients with one or more occlusions (33% of patients in the placebo group versus 19% in the oral anticoagulation group). As discussed above, oral anticoagulation started on the day before surgery at a fixed dose for two doses before adjusting to an international normalized ratio of 2.8–4.0 was nearly as effective as aspirin and dipyridamole and as effective as aspirin in reducing vein graft occlusion 1 year after operation. This study also showed the value of continuing therapy for at least a year after operation.

Current Recommendations

In patients with unstable angina heparin, aspirin, or both significantly reduce the incidence of myocardial infarction and death [85]. Furthermore, most patients presenting to hospital with acute coronary syndromes are on aspirin, which probably reduces the severity of their syndrome from a myocardial infarction to unstable angina or less severe infarction. Thus the benefits of reduced arterial thrombosis in these patients appear to outweigh the risks of a slightly greater risk of bleeding preoperatively after aortocoronary bypass graft surgery when they continue on aspirin up to the time of operation. Early withdrawal of antithrombotic therapy in patients with unstable angina increases the risk of recurrent ischemia and myocardial infarction to 13% of patients who are on heparin alone (within a median of 9 hours after withdrawal) and to 5% for patients who are also on aspirin alone [86]. Thus in patients with unstable angina who are awaiting aortocoronary bypass graft operation, optimal therapy would be the continuation of heparin and aspirin up to at least within 3–4h before operation (aPTT on heparin therapy approximately twice that of control). When used with heparin aspirin should be reduced to 80mg/day. Aspirin 160mg is the minimal loading dose when patients have not been on aspirin beforehand, and 80mg/day aspirin will maintain the antiplatelet effect with the lowest risk of side effects [12].

Aspirin alone is recommended as routine therapy. For patients not on aspirin before operation, it should be started 1h after operation down the nasogastric tube at a minimum dose of 160mg/day for loading and thereafter may be administered at 80–325mg/day and continued indefinitely.

From two studies, 225–400mg/day dipyridamole in addition to aspirin may be more effective than aspirin alone if 400mg/day dipyridamole is administered until 1–2h before operation and aspirin started within 7h after surgery, especially in patients who have vein grafts anastomosed to coronary arteries ≤1.5mm in diameter [34, 35]. The main benefit of dipyridamole may be in the perioperative period or perhaps during the first month.

Patients who are at high risk because of small coronary artery lumen diameters (≤1.5mm), low vein-graft blood flow (≤40ml/min), or distal coronary artery endarterectomy may be considered for combined therapy with oral anticoagulation (started on the day before operation) plus low-dose aspirin at 80–100mg/day [17]. In these high-risk patients, heparin may be administered at a relatively low dosage initially to maintain the aPTT at just above the upper limit of normal in the recovery room. The dosage may be increased to prolong the aPTT to 1.5 times that of control after the chest tubes are removed. This may then be switched to the oral anticoagulation maintaining the prothrombin time at an international normalized ratio of 3.0–4.0.

It is especially important to reduce all coronary risk factors including cessation of smoking, treatment of hypertension, optimal control of diabetes, and correction of lipid abnormalities. Progression of both aortocoronary vein-graft disease and native coronary artery disease may be significantly reduced with reduced low-density lipoprotein (LDL) cholesterol and increased high-density lipoprotein (HDL) cholesterol [87–90]. The only studies which showed a significant regression of vein-graft or coronary artery disease have been those where the HDL cholesterol has been increased with specific therapy, such as with niacin [89, 90].

Unless impossible from an anatomic, emergency, or technical standpoint, at least one internal mammary artery bypass graft should be included (usually to the largest and most significant coronary artery for myocardial blood supply, usually the left anterior descending coronary artery). No studies show a definite benefit of antiplatelet therapy in patients with internal mammary bypass grafts, but, as discussed above, one study showed a trend [82]. However, aspirin is indicated for patients with coronary artery disease and thus would be indicated in those who have internal mammary bypass grafts. Internal mammary artery bypass grafts appear responsible for reducing graft occlusion in retrospective and prospective studies [91–97] and improving survival in retrospective studies [91–96].

Prevention of Late Vein Graft Occlusion

The best prevention of late vein-graft occlusion is maximal reduction of all coronary risk factors and chronic aspirin therapy. This includes both a reduction in LDL cholesterol and an increase in HDL cholesterol since this appears to decrease the risk of atherosclerotic plaque disruption. This is suggested by the marked reduction in the number of coronary events by appropriately treating hyperlipidemia [89, 90]. In patients with incomplete correction of risk factors or those who already have one occluded vein graft or appear with new angina after coronary bypass surgery, consideration might be given to long-term anticoagulant therapy along with low-dose aspirin at 80 mg/day in order to prevent vein graft occlusion after atherosclerotic plaque disruption. Plaque disruption leads not only to local occlusion but also to potential occlusion of the entire vein graft proximal to the disrupted plaque, since vein grafts have no branches and thus are prone to long segments of occlusion. Thus large amounts of thrombus may accumulate in vein grafts which makes it very risky to perform percutaneous procedures such as atherectomy or balloon angioplasty. The role of chronic oral anticoagulation along with aspirin therapy is currently under study.

References

1. Fuster V, Dewanjee MK, Kaye MP, Josa M, Metke MP, Chesebro JH (1979) Nonınvasive radioisotopic technique for detection of platelet deposition in coronary artery bypass grafts in dogs and its reduction with platelet inhibition. Circulation 60:1508–1512
2. Chesebro JH, Clements I, Fuster V, Elveback LR, Smith HC, Bardsley WT, Frye RL, Holmes DR, Vliestra RE, Pluth JR, Wallacd RB, Puga FJ, Orszulak TA, Piehler JM, Schaff HV (1982) A platelet-inhibitor drug trial in coronary-artery bypass operations: benefit of perioperative dipyridamole and aspirin therapy on early postoperative vein-graft patency. N Engl J Med 307:73–78
3. Chesebro JH, Fuster V, Elveback LR, Clements I, Smith HC, Holmes DR, Bardsley WT, Pluth JR, Wallace RB, Orszulak TA, Piehler JM, Danielson GK, Schaff HV, Frye RL (1984) Effect of dipyridamole and aspirin on late vein-graft patency after coronary bypass operations. N Engl J Med 310:209–214
4. Pantely GA, Goodnight SH Jr, Rahimtoola SH, Rahimtoola SH, Harlan BJ, DeMots H, Calvin L, Rosch J (1979) Failure of antiplatelet and anticoagulant therapy to improve patency of grafts after coronary-artery bypass. N Engl J Med 301:962–966
5. Grundfest WS, Litvack F, Sherman T, Carroll R, Lee M, Chaux A, Kass R, Matloff J, Berci G, Swan JHC, Morganstern L, Forrester J (1985) Delineation of peripheral and coronary detail by intraoperative angioscopy. Ann Surg 202:394–400
6. Josa M, Lie JT, Bianco RL, Kaye MP (1981) Reduction of thrombosis in canine coronary bypass vein grafts with dipyridamole and aspirin. Am J Cardiol 47:1248–1254

7. Uni KK, Kottke BA, Titus JL, Frye RL, Wallace RB, Brown AL (1974) Pathologic changes in aortocoronary saphenous vein grafts. Am J Cardiol 34:526–532
8. Chesebro JH, Goldman S (1992) Coronary artery bypass surgery; antithrombotic therapy. In: Fuster V, Verstraete M (eds) Thrombosis and cardiovascular disorders. Saunders, Philadelphia, pp 375–388
9. Tschoop TB (1977) Aspirin inhibits platelet aggregation on, but not adhesion to, collagen fibrils: an assessment of platelet adhesion and deposited platelet mass by morphometry and ^{51}Cr-labeling. Thromb Res 11:619–632
10. Roth GL, Majerus PW (1975) The mechanism of the effect of aspirin on human platelets. I. Acetylation of a particulate fraction protein. J Clin Invest 56:624–632
11. Kyrle PA, Eichler HG, Jager U, Lechner K (1987) Inhibition of prostacyclin and thromboxane A_2 generation by low-dose aspirin at the site of plug formation in man in vivo. Circulation 75:1025–1029
12. Clarke RJ, Mayo G, Price P, Fitzgerald GA (1991) Suppression of thromboxane A_2 but not of systemic prostacyclin by controlled-release aspirin. N Engl J Med 325:1137–1141
13. Lam JYT, Chesebro JH, Steele PM, Heras M, Webster MWI, Badimon L, Fuster V (1991) Antithrombotic therapy for arterial injury by angioplasty: Efficacy of common platelet inhibitors versus thrombin inhibition in pigs. Circulation 84:814–820
14. Lewis HD, Davis JW, Archibald DG, Steinke WE, Smitherman TC, Doherty JE III, Schnaper HW, LeWinter MM, Linares E, Pouget JM, Sabharwal SC, Chesler E, DeMots H (1983) Protective effects of aspirin against acute myocardial infarction and death in men with unstable angina: results of a Veterans Administration cooperative study. N Engl J Med 309:396–403
15. UK-TIA Study Group (1988) United Kingdom Transient Ischaemic Attack (UK-TIA) Aspirin Trial: interim results. Br Med J 296:316–320
16. ISIS-2 (Second International Study of Infarct Survival) Collaborative Group (1988) Randomized trial of intravenous streptokinase, oral aspirin, both, or neither among 17 187 cases of suspected acute myocardial infarction: ISIS-2 Lancet 2:349–360
17. Turpie AGG, Gent M, Laupacis A, Latour Y, Gunstensen J, Basile F, Klimek M, Hirsh J (1993) A comparison of aspirin with placebo in patients treated with warfarin after heart-valve replacement. N Engl J Med 329:524–529
18. Graham DY, Smith LJ (1986) Aspirin and the stomach. Ann Intern Med 104:390–398
19. Cohen M, Parry G, Xiong J, Adams P, Chamberlain D, Fox K, Wieczorek I, McBride R, Chesebro J, Strain J, Fuster V, for ATACS (1993) Double blind randomized trial of a prostacyclin sparing aspirin formulation in rest angina and non-Q wave infarction (abstr). J Am Coll Cardiol 21:269A
20. Cohen M, Parry G, Xiong J, Adams P, Chamberlain D, Fox K, Wieczorek I, McBride R, Chesebro J, Strain J, Lancaster G, Fuster V, for ATACS (1993) Combination antithrombotic therapy reduces recurrent ischemia in unstable angina and non-Q wave infarction (abstr). J Am Coll Cardiol 21:270A
21. Roux S, Christeller S, Ludin E (1992) Effects of aspirin on coronary reocclusion and recurrent ischemia after thrombolysis: a meta-analysis. J Am Coll Cardiol 19:671–677
24. Chesebro JH, Badimon JJ, Badimon L, Fuster V (1993) Anticoagulant and antiplatelet therapy in acute coronary syndromes and atrial fibrillation. Cardiol Rev 1:167–176
24a. The GUSTO Angiographic Investigators (1993) The effects of tissue plasminogen activator, streptokinase, or both on coronary-artery patency, ventricular function, and survival after acute myocardial infarction. N Engl J Med 329:1615–1622
25. United States Pharmacopeial Convention (1993) Drug information for the health care professional, USP-DI-I, The United States Pharmacopeial Convention, Inc., Rockville, MD
26. Moncada S, Korbut R (1978) Dipyridamole and other phophodiesterase inhibitors act as antithrombotic agents by potentiating endogenous prostacyclin. Lancet 1:1286–1289

27. Crutchley DJ, Ryan US, Ryan JW (1980) Effects of aspirin and dipyridamole on the degradation of adenosine diphosphate by cultured cells derived from bovine pulmonary artery. J Clin Invest 66:29–35
28. FitzGerald GA (1987) Dipyridamole. N Engl J Med 316: 1247–1257
29. Hanson SR, Harker LA, Bjornsson TD (1985) Effect of platelet-modifying drugs on arterial thromboembolism in baboons: aspirin potentiates the antithrombotic actions of dipyridamole and sulfinpyrazone by mechanism(s) independent of platelet cyclooxygenase inhibition. J Clin Invest 75:1591–1599
30. The Persantine-Aspirin Reinfarction Study Group (1980) Persantine and aspirin in coronary heart disease. Circulation 62:449–461
31. Brown BG, Cukingnan RA, DeRouen T, Goeded LV, Wong M, Fee HJ, Roth JA, Carey JS (1985) Improved graft patency in patients treated with platelet-inhibiting therapy after coronary bypass surgery. Circulation 72:138–146
32. Goldman S, Copeland J, Moritz T, Henderson W, Zadina K, Ovitt T, Doherty J, Read R, Chesler E, Sako Y, Lancaster L, Emery R, Sharma GVRK, Josa M, Pacold I, Montoya A, Parikh D, Sethi G, Holt J, Kirklin J, Shabetai R, Moores W, Aldridge J, Masud Z, DeMots H, Floten S, Haakenson C, Harker L (1988) Improvement in early saphenous vein graft patency after coronary artery bypass surgery with antiplatelet therapy: results of a Veterans Administration cooperative study. Circulation 77:1324–1332
33. Ekeström SA, Gunnes S, Brodin UB (1990) Effect of dipyridamole (persantin) on blood flow and patency of aortocoronary vein bypass grafts. Scand J Thorac Cardiovasc Surg 96:332–341
34. van der Meer J, Hillege HL, Kootstra GJ, Ascoop CAP, Pfisterer M, van Glist WH, Lie KI, for the CABADAS research group of the Interuniversity Cardiology Institute of the Netherlands (1993) Prevention of one-year vein-graft occlusion after aortocoronary bypass surgery: a comparison of low-dose aspirin, low-dose aspirin plus dipyridamole, and oral anticoagulants. Lancet 324:257–264
35. Sanz G, Pajarón, Alegría, Coello I, Cardona M, Fournier JA, Gómez-Recio M, Ruano J, Hidalgo R, Medina A, Oller G, Coleman T, Malpartida F, Bosch X, and the Grupo Español para el Seguimiento del Injerto Coronario (GESIC) (1990) Prevention of early aortocoronary bypass occlusion by low-dose aspirin and dipyridamole. Circulation 82:765–773
36. Baumgartner HR (1979) Effects of acetylsalicylic acid, sulfinpyrazone, and dipyridamole on platelet adhesion and aggregation in flowing native and anticoagulated blood. Haemostasis 8:340–349
37. Kaegi A, Pineo GF, Shimizu A, Trivedi H, Hirsh J, Gent M (1974) Arteriovenous-shunt thrombosis: prevention by sulfinpyrazone. N Engl J Med 290:304–306
38. Steele PP, Rainwater J, Vogel R (1979) Platelet suppressant therapy in patients with prosthetic cardiac valves: relationship of clinical effectiveness to alterations of platelet survival time. Circulation 60: 910–913
39. Report from the Anturane Reinfarction Italian Study (1982) Sulfinpyrazone in post-myocardial infarction. Lancet 1:237–242
40. The Anturane Reinfarction Trial Research Group (1980) Sulfinpyrazone in the prevention of sudden death after myocardial infarction. N Engl J Med 302:250–256
41. Cairns JA, Gent M, Singer J, Finnie KJ, Froggatt GM, Holder DA, Jablonsky G, Kostuk WJ, Melendez LJ, Myers MG, Sackett DL, Sealey BJ, Tanser PH (1985) Aspirin, sulfinpyrazone, or both in unstable angina. N Engl J Med 313:1369–1375
42. Baur HR, Van Tassel RA, Pierach CA, Gobel RL (1982) Effects of sulfinpyrazone on early graft closure after myocardial infarction. Am J Cardiol 49:420–424
43. Goldman S, Copeland J, Moritz T, Henderson W, Zadina K, Ovitt T, Doherty J, Read R, Chesler E, Sako Y, Lancaster L, Emery R, Sharma GVRK, Josa M, Pacold I, Montoya A, Parikh D, Sethi G, Holt J, Kirklin J, Shabetai R, Moores W, Aldridge J, Masud Z,

DeMots (1989) Saphenous vein graft patency 1 year after coronary artery bypass surgery and effects of antiplatelet therapy: results of a Veterans Administration cooperative study. Circulation 80:1190–1197

44. Defreyn G, Bernat A, Delebassee D, Maffrand JP (1989) Pharmacology of ticlopidine: a review. Semin Thromb Hemost 15:159–166
45. O'Brien JR (1983) Ticlopidine, a promise for the prevention and treatment of thrombosis and its complications. Haemostasis 13:1–54
46. McTavish D, Faulds D, Goa KL (1990) Ticlopidine. An updated review of its pharmacology and therapeutic use in platelet-dependent disorders Drugs 40:238–259
47. Balsano F, Rizzon P, Violi F, Scrutinio D, Cimminiello C, Aguglia F, Pasotti C, Rudell G, Studio della ticlopida nell'Angina Instabile Group (1990) Antiplatelet treatment with ticlopidine in unstable angina. A controlled multicenter clinical trial. Circulation 82:17–26
48. Bertrand ME, Allain H, Lablanche JM (1990) Results of a randomized trial of ticlopidine versus placebo for prevention of acute closure and restenosis after coronary angioplasty. The TACT Study (abstr). Circulation [Suppl III] 82:–190
49. White CW, Knudson M, Schmidt D et al. (1987) Neither ticlopidine nor aspirin-dipyridamole prevents restenosis post PTCA: results from a randomized placebo-controlled multicenter trial (abstr). Circulation [Suppl IV] 76:–213
50. Limet R, David JL, Magotteaux P, Larock MP, Rigo P (1987) Prevention of aorta-coronary bypass graft occlusion. J Thorac Cardiovasc Surg 94:773–783
51. Markwardt F (1970) Hirudin as an inhibitor of thrombin. Methods Enzymol 19:924–932
52. Stone SR, Hofsteenge J (1986) Kinetics of the inhibition of thrombin by hirudin. Biochemistry 25:4622–4628
53. Markwardt F (1989) Development of hirudin as an antithrombotic agent. Sem Thromb Hemost 15:269–282
54. Glore GM, Sukumaran DK, Nilges M et al. (1987) The conformations of hirudin in solution: a study using nuclear magnetic resonance, distance geometry and restrained molecular dynamics. EMBO J 6:529–537
55. Haruyama H, Wuethrich K (1989) Conformation of recombinant desulfatohirudin in aqueous solution determined by nuclear magnetic resonance. Biochemistry 28:4301–4312
56. Rydel TJ, Ravichandran KG, Tulinsky A, Bode W, Huber R, Roitsch C, Fenton JWII (1990) The structure of a complex of recombinant hirudin and human alpha-thrombin. Science 249:277–280
57. Gruetter MG, Priestle JP, Rahuel J et al. (1990) Crystal structure of the thrombin-hirudin complex: a novel mode of serine protease inhibition. EMBO J 9:2361–2365
58. Heras M, Chesebro JH, Penny WJ, Bailey KR, Badimon L, Fuster V (1989) Effects of thrombin inhibition on the development of acute platelet-thrombus deposition during angioplasty in pigs: heparin versus recombinant hirudin, a specific thrombin inhibitor. Circulation 79:657–665
59. Heras M, Chesebro JH, Webster MWI, Mruk J, Grill DE, Penny WJ, Bowie EJW, Badimon L, Fuster V (1990) Hirudin, heparin, and placebo during deep arterial injury in the pig: The in vivo role of thrombin in platelet-mediated thrombosis. Circulation 82:1476–1484
60. Chesebro JH, Webster MWI, Zoldhelyi P, Roche PC, Badimon L, Badimon JJ (1992) Antithrombotic therapy in the progression of coronary artery disease. Circulation [Suppl III] 86:100–110
61. Markwardt F, Kaiser B, Novak G (1989) Studies on antithrombotic effects of recombinant hirudin. Thromb Res 54:377–388
62. Weitz JI, Hudoba M, Massel DR, Maranganori J, Hirsh J (1990) Clot-bound thrombin is protected from inhibition by heparin-antithrombin III but is susceptible to inactivation by antithrombin III-independent inhibitors. J Clin Invest 86:385–391
63. Zoldhelyi P, Chesebro JH, Mruk JS, Webster MWI, Grill DE, Fuster V (1992) Failure of aspirin compared with heparin or hirudin to enhance lysis by re-PA of platelet-rich thrombus after deep arterial injury in the pig. J Am Coll Cardiol [Suppl A] 19:91A

64. Cosgrove DM, Heric B, Lytle BW, Taylor PC, Novoa R, Golding LA, Stewart RW, McCarthy PM, Loop FD (1992) Aprotinin therapy for reoperative myocardial revascularization: a placebo-controlled study. Ann Thorac Surg 54:1031–1036
65. Zoldhelyi P, Webster MWI, Fuster V, Grill DE, Gaspar D, Edwards SJ, Cabot CF, Chesebro JH (1993) Recombinant hirudin in patients with chronic, stable coronary disease: safety, half-life, and effect on coagulation parameters. Circulation 88:2015–2022
66. Metke MP, Lie JT, Fuster V, Josa M, Kaye MP (1979) Reduction of intimal thickening in canine coronary bypass vein grafts with dipyridamole and aspirin. Am J Cardiol 43:1144–1148
67. Rajah SM, Salter MCP, Donaldson DR, Rao RS, Boyle RM, Partiridge JB, Watson DA (1985) Acetylsalicylic acid and dipyridamole improve the early patency of aorta-coronary bypass grafts: a double-blind, placebo-controlled, randomized trial. J Thorac Cardiovasc Surg 89:373–377
68. Mayer JE, Lindsay WG, Castaneda W, Nocoloff DM (1981) Influence of aspirin and dipyridamole on patency of coronary artery bypas grafts. Ann Thorac Surg 31:204–210
69. Lorenz RL, Schacky CV, Weber M, Meister W, Kotzur J, Reichardt B, Theisen K, Weber PC (1984) Improved aortocoronary bypass patency by low-dose aspirin (100 mg daily). Lancet 1:1261–1264
70. Brooks N, Wright J, Sturridge M, Pepper J, Magee P, Walesby R, Layton C, Honey M, Balcon R (1985) Randomized placebo controlled trial of aspirin and dipyridamole in the prevention of coronary vein graft occlusion. Br Heart J 53:201–207
71. McEnany MT, Salzman EW, Mundth ED et al. (1982) The effect of antithrombotic therapy on patency rate of saphenous vein coronary artery bypass grafts. J Thorac Cardiovasc Surg 83:81–89
72. Sharma GVRK, Khuri SF, Josa M, Folland ED, Parisi AF (1983) The effect of antiplatelet therapy on saphenous vein coronary artery bypass graft patency. Circulation 68 [Suppl II]:218–221
73. Pfisterer M, Burkart F, Jockers G, Meyer B, Regenass S, Burckhardt D, Schmitt HE, Muller-Brand J, Skarvan K, Stulz P (1989) Trial of low-dose aspirin plus dipyridamole vs. anticoagulants for prevention of aortocoronary vein graft occlusion. Lancet 2:1–7
74. Pumphrey CW, Fuster V, Dewanjee MK, Chesebro JH, Vlietstra RE, Kaye MP (1983) Comparison of the antithrombotic action of calcium antagonist drugs with dipyridamole in dogs. Am J Cardiol 51:591–595
75. Nuutinen LS, Pihlajaniemi R, Saarela E, Karkola P, Hollmen A (1977) The effect of dipyridamole on the thrombocyte count and bleeding tendency in open-heart surgery. J Thorac Cardiovasc Surg 74:295–298
76. Becker RM, Smith MR, Dobell ARC (1974) Effect of platelet inhibition on platelet phenomenon in cardiopulmonary bypass in pigs. Ann Surg 179:52–57
77. Teoh KH, Christakis GT, Weisel RD, Wong PV, Mee AV, Ivanov J, Madonik MM, Levitt DS, Reilly PA, Rosenfeld JM et al. (1988) Dipyridamole preserved platelets and reduced blood loss after cardiopulmonary bypass. J Thorac Cardiovasc Surg 96:332–341
78. Fuster V, Chesebro JH (1981) Current concepts of thrombogenesis: role of platelets. Mayo Clin Proc 56:102–112
79. Fuster V, Chesebro JH, Frye RL, Elveback LR (1981) Platelet survival and the development of coronary artery disease in the young: the effects of cigarette smoking, strong family history, and medical therapy. Circulation 63:546–551
80. Steele P, Rainwater J, Vogel R (1979) Platelet suppressant therapy in patients with prosthetic cardiac valves: relationship of clinical effectiveness to alteration of platelet survival time. Circulation 60:910–913
81. Donadio JV, Anderson CF, Mitchell JC, Holley KE, Illstrup DM, Fuster V, Chesebro JH (1984) Membrano-proliferative glomerulonephritis: a prospective clinical trail of platelet-inhibitor therapy. N Engl J Med 310:1421–1426
82. Goldman S, Copeland J, Moritz T, Henderson W, Zadina K, Ovitt T, Kern KB, Sethi G, Sharma GVRK, Khuri S, Richards K, Grover F, Morrison D, Whitman G, Chester E,

Sako Y, Pacold I, Montoya A, DeMots H, Floten S, Doherty J, Read R, Scott S, Spooner T, Masud Z (1991) Starting aspirin after operation: effects on early graft patency. Circulation 84:520–526
83. Gavaghan TP, Gebski V, Baron DW (1991) Immediate postoperative aspirin improves vein graft patency early and late after coronory artery bypass surgery. Circulation 83:1526–33
84. Gohlke H, Gohlke-Barwolf C, Sturzenhofecker P, Gornandt L, Ritter B, Reichelt M, Buchwalsky R, Schmuziger M, Roskamm H (1981) Improved graft patency with anticoagulant therapy after aortocoronary bypass surgery: a prospective randomized study. Circulation 64 [Suppl II]:22–27
85. Théroux P, Quimet H, McCans J, Latour J-G, Joly P, Lévy G, Pelletier E, Juneau M, Stasiak J, deGuise P, Pelletier G, Rinzler D, Waters DD (1988) Aspirin, heparin, or both to treat acute unstable angina. N Engl J Med 319:1105–1111
86. Theroux P, Waters D, Lam J, Juneau M, McCans J (1992) Reactivation of unstable angina after the discontinuation of heparin. N Engl J Med 327:141–145
87. Brensike FJ, Levy PR, Kelsey SF, Passamani ER, Richardson JM, Loh IK, Stone NJ, Aldrich RF, Battaglini JW, Morarty DJ, Fisher MR, Friedman L, Friedewald W, Detre KM, Epstein SE (1984) Effects of therapy with cholestyramine on progression of coronary arteriosclerosis: results of the NHLBI Type II Coronary Intervention Study. Circulation 69:313–324
88. Arntzenius AC, Kromhout D, Barth JD, Reiber JHC, Bruschke AVG, Buis B, van Gent CM (1985) Diet, lipoproteins, and the progression of coronary atherosclerosis. The Leiden Interventional Trial. N Engl J Med 312:805–811
89. Blankenhorn DH, Nessim SA, Johnson RL, Sanmarco ME, Azen SP, Cashin-Hemphill L (1987) Beneficial effects of combined colestipol-niacin therapy on coronary atherosclerosis and coronary venous bypass graft. JAMA 257:3233–3240
90. Brown G, Albers JJ, Fisher LD, Schaefer SM, Lin JT, Kaplan C, Zhao XQ (1990) Regression of coronary artery disease as a result of intensive lipid-lowering therapy in men with high levels of apolipoprotein B. N Engl J Med 323:1289–1298
91. Loop FD, Lytle BW, Cosgrove DM, Stewart RW, Goormastic M, Williams GW, Golding LAR, Gill CC, Taylor PC, Sheldon WC, Proudfit WL (1986) Influence of the internal-mammary-artery graft on 10-year survival and other cardiac events. N Engl J Med 314:1–6
92. Spencer FC (1986) The internal mammary artery: the ideal coronary bypass graft? N Engl J Med 314:50–51
93. Lytle BW, Loop FD, Cosgrove DM, Ratliff NB, Easley K, Taylor PC (1985) Long-term (5–12 years) serial studies of internal mammary artery and saphenous coronary bypass grafts. J Thorac Cardiovasc Surg 89:248–258
94. Barner HB, Swartz MT, Mudd JG, Tyras DH (1982) Late patency of the internal mammary artery as a coronary bypass conduit. Ann Thorac Surg 34:408–412
95. Tector AJ, Schmahl TM, Janson B, Kallies JR, Johnson G (1981) The internal mammary artery graft: its longevity after coronary bypass. JAMA 246:2181–2183
96. Grodin CM, Campaeau L, Lesperance J et al. (1984) Comparison of late changes in internal mammary artery and saphenous vein grafts in 2 consecutive series of patients 10 years after operation. Circulation 70 [Suppl I]:208–212
97. Sims FH (1983) A comparison of coronary and internal mammary arteries and implications of the results in etiology of arteriosclerosis. Am Heart J 105:560–566
98. Chesebro JH, Fuster V (1986) The pathogenesis and prevention of aortocoronary bypass graft occlusion and restenosis after arterial angioplasty: role of vascular injury and platelet-thrombus deposition. J Am Coll Cardiol 8:57B–66B

Anticoagulants and Antiplatelet Drugs to Prevent Aortocoronary Vein Graft Occlusion

M. Pfisterer

Introduction

Graft occlusion remains the most important adverse event after coronary artery bypass graft (CABG) surgery. Occlusion rates increase from 10%–15% per distal anastomosis in the first month to approximately 16%–26% at 1 year, averaging 37% at 5–7 years and 55% at 10–12 years [1, 2]. A recent study reported graft disease in 8% at 1 year, 38% at 5 years, and 75% at 10 years postoperatively [3]. The pathogenesis of vein graft occlusion appears to have some similarities with the development and progression of atherosclerosis, which is discussed by Jang and Fuster (this volume). Drug therapy should therefore be aimed at intervening in this pathogenesis. Since platelet deposition is an early factor in the occlusive process, platelet inhibitors play an important role here. Anticoagulants, on the other hand, are potent drugs to prevent arterial thrombus formation. These two groups of drugs have therefore been used during the past decade to prevent vein graft occlusion.

The present report summarizes and compares the clinical experiences with anticoagulant and antiplatelet drug therapies after CABG surgery with veins and indicates questions which need to be clarified in future research. For comparison of the different findings, occlusion rates per patient and per graft (distal anastomoses) were derived from all major prospective randomized clinical trials and related to the time since operation and the drug therapy administered. Treatment results are further subgrouped into those comparing active therapy to placebo and those comparing different active treatment regimens with each other. This enables the reader to assess the impact of each tested drug therapy by itself and in contrast to other treatment regimens.

Prevention of Early Graft Occlusion

Placebo-Controlled Studies

The effect of anticoagulants versus placebo was reported in 1981 by Gohlke et al. [4]. During the first 7 postoperative days subcutaneous heparin was

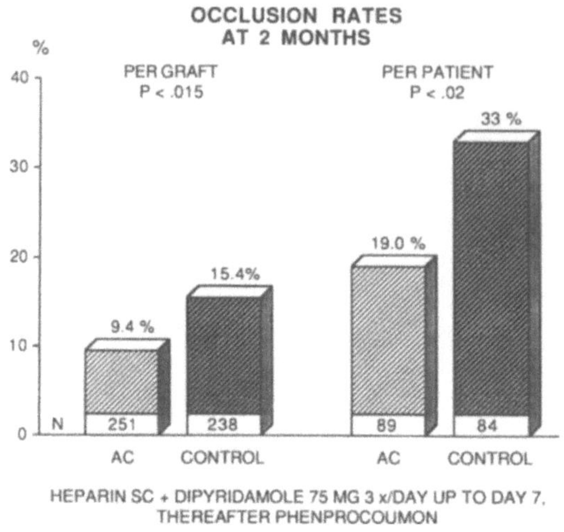

Fig. 1. Effect of anticoagulant (*AC*) versus placebo on occlusion rates at 2 months. (Adapted from [4])

combined with 3 × 75 mg dipyridamole per day followed by oral phenprocoumon, an anticoagulant, alone. Angiography performed in 173 patients after 2 months showed a significant reduction in occluded grafts per treated patient (19.0% versus 33.0% on placebo, $p < 0.02$) as well as per graft (9.4% versus 15.4%, $p < 0.01$; Fig. 1). This result is somewhat in contrast to an earlier small study ($n = 50$) which found no significant effect of warfarin therapy [5].

A positive effect of antiplatelet drugs to prevent bypass graft occlusion was first demonstrated by Chesebro et al. in 1982 [6]. Dipyridamole 3 × 75 mg per day was started 2 days before surgery and was combined with aspirin 3 × 325 mg/day beginning 7 hours after surgery. At the first angiographic control 1 month after surgery, only 6% of 123 treated patients had occluded grafts versus 22% of 120 patients receiving placebo ($p < 0.01$; Fig. 2). Occlusion rates per grafts were 3% and 10%, respectively ($p < 0.001$) in a total of 713 distal anastomoses. Similar results were found by Limet et al. with ticlopidine 2 × 250 mg per day starting on the second postoperative day [7]. In this study angiography was performed 10 days after surgery in 168 patients, and occlusion rates per patient were reduced from 33.3% (placebo) to 15.6% (ticlopidine, $p < 0.05$) and per graft from 13.4% to 7.1% in a total of 472 grafts (Fig. 3). Gavaghan and colleagues recently reported a significant reduction in occlusion rates at 1 week in 126 patients treated with 324 mg aspirin daily started within 1 h of CABG surgery: 4.0% versus 14.3% ($p < 0.003$) in 105 patients on placebo [8]. The corresponding occlusion rates per graft were 1.6% and 6.2% on aspirin and placebo, respectively (Fig. 4).

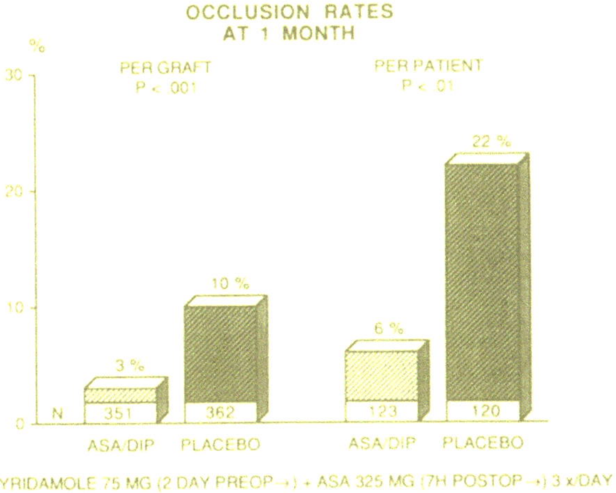

Fig. 2. Effect of aspirin plus dipyridamole (*ASA/DIP*) versus placebo on occlusion rates at 1 month. (Adapted from [6])

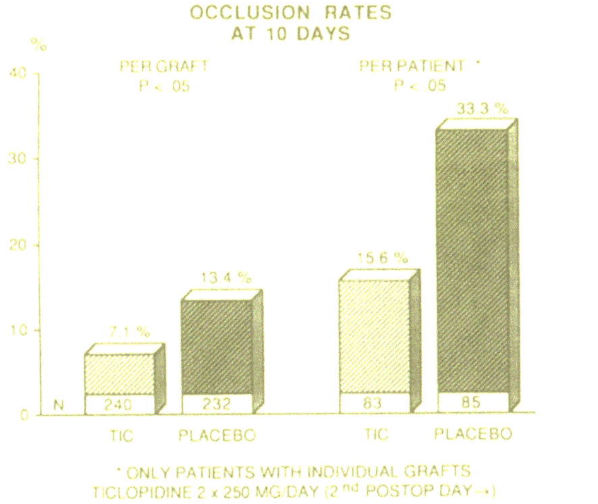

Fig. 3. Effect of ticlopidine (*TIC*) versus placebo on occlusion rates at 10 days. (Adapted from [7])

Comparative Drug Trials

A comparison between the effects of anticoagulants and those of combined aspirin/dipyridamole treatment was reported by our group in 1989 [9]. Oral anticoagulants were started on the first postoperative day in 125 patients, 2 × 200 mg dipyridamole per day 2 days preoperatively combined with a low

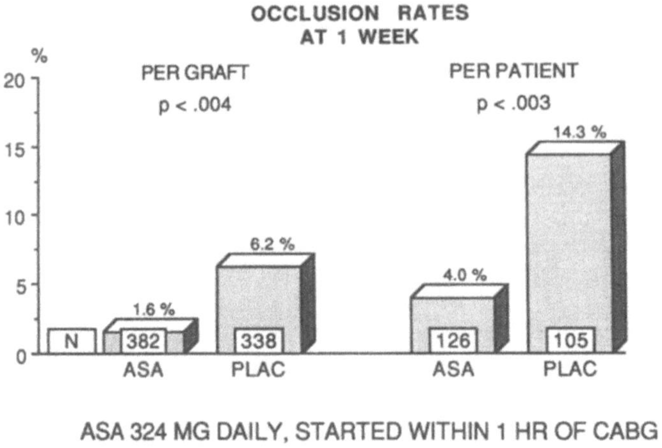

Fig. 4. Effect of aspirin versus placebo on occlusion rates at 1 week. (Adapted from [8])

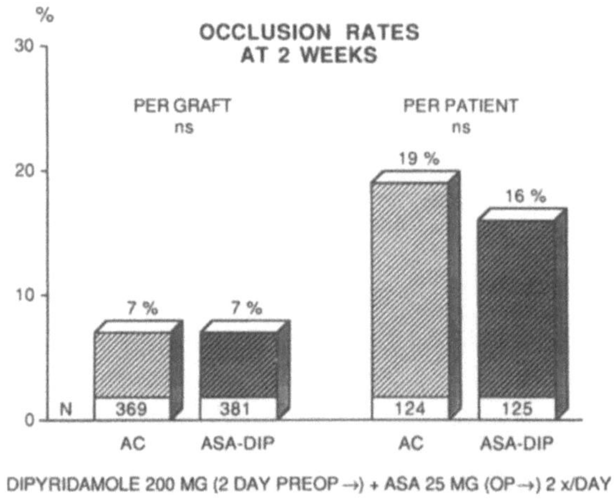

Fig. 5. Comparison of the effects of anticoagulants (*AC*) and aspirin plus dipyridamole (*ASA-DIP*) on occlusion rates at 2 weeks. (Adapted from [9])

dose of 2 × 25 mg aspirin per day starting in the morning of the operation, in 124 patients with a total of 750 grafts. There was no significant difference in occlusion rates at 2 weeks between the two treatment groups (Fig. 5). Similarly, Rothlin et al. found no significant difference in obstruction-free rates (<75% stenosis) at 3 months between 78 patients treated with ticlopidine (2 × 250 mg per day, starting the first postoperative day) and 71 patients treated with anticoagulants [10] (Fig. 6).

Four different antiplatelet regimens were compared by Goldman et al. in 1988 in a large group of 555 patients [11]: aspirin 325 mg once daily,

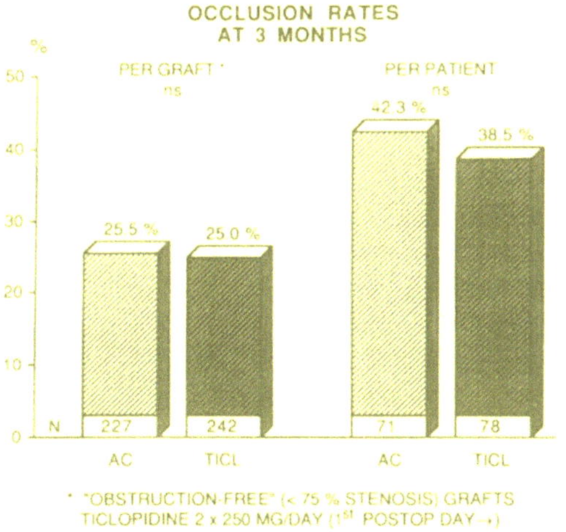

Fig. 6. Comparison of the effects of anticoagulants (*AC*) and ticlopidine (*TIC*) on occlusion rates at 3 months. (Adapted from [10])

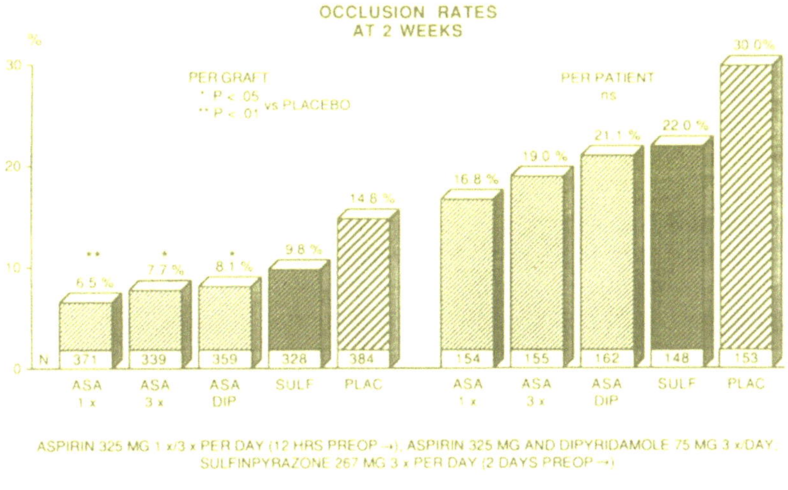

Fig. 7. Comparison of the effects of various antiplatelet drug regimens versus placebo on occlusion rates at 2 weeks. *ASA*, Aspirin; *DIP*, dipyridamole; *SULF*, sulfinpyrazone; *PLAC*, placebo. (Adapted from [11])

aspirin 325 mg t.i.d., aspirin combined with dipyridamole (325 mg and 75 mg respectively, t.i.d.), sulfinpyrazone 267 mg t.i.d., and placebo t.i.d. (Fig. 7). There were no significant differences in occlusion rates per patient, but there were significantly fewer occluded grafts in each of the three aspirin groups compared to placebo. It should be noted, however, that the addition of dipyridamole did not improve the results obtained by aspirin alone, that a

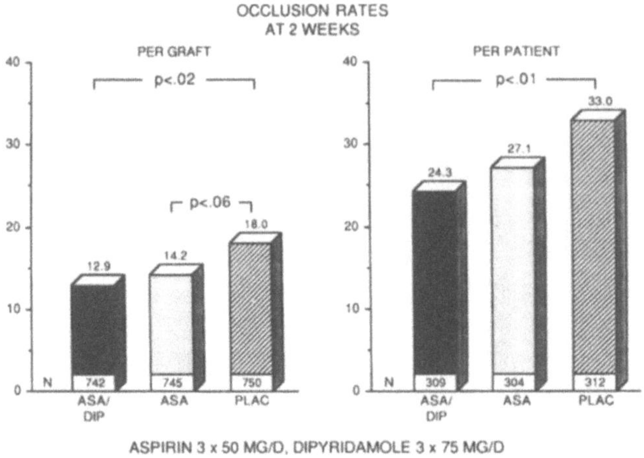

Fig. 8. Comparison of aspirin (*ASA*) and aspirin plus dipyrida-mole (*ASA/DIP*) versus placebo (*PLAC*) on occlusion rates at 2 weeks. (Adapted from [12]).

higher does of aspirin (3 × 325 mg) was not better than a lower does (1 × 325 mg), and that sulfinpyrazone had no significant effect on occlusion rates. These results are somewhat in contrast to the findings of a recent report by Sanz et al. who randomized 1112 patients to aspirin 3 × 50 mg per day, aspirin 50 mg combined with dipyridamole 75 mg t.i.d., and placebo [12]. In addition, all patients received dipyridamole 100 mg q.i.d. for 48 h before surgery. Angiography performed in 927 patients at 10 days postoperatively showed a significantly reduced number of patients with occluded grafts only for combined therapy (24.3% versus 33% on placebo, $p < 0.01$; versus 27.1% on aspirin alone, NS; Fig. 8). Occlusion rates per graft were reduced by aspirin alone ($p < 0.06$) and combined aspirin/dipyridamole ($p < 0.02$) as compared to placebo. On the other hand, there were no significant differences between the two active treatment regimens.

Thus, these studies lead to the following initial conclusion. The rate of early graft occlusion can be effectively reduced by antithrombotic treatment. Antiplatelet drug regimens seem to be as effective as anticoagulants, but it has been pointed out that early start of therapy (preferably before operation) is essential [1]. Thus, dipyridamole is usually started 24–48 h before surgery whereas there is some reluctance by surgeons for preoperative administration of aspirin due to an increased rate of diffuse postoperative bleeding [13]. By its vasodilating properties dipyridamole has a demonstrable beneficial effect on intraoperatively measured graft blood flow [9], its additional antithrombotic effect to that of aspirin to reduce the rate of graft occlusion, however, is still open to debate.

Prevention of Late Graft Occlusion

Placebo-Controlled Studies

There have been no large studies assessing the effects of anticoagulants versus placebo early and late after CABG surgery. In one study reported in 1982 there was a nonsignificant reduction in graft occlusion rates (17% versus 31% on placebo) on warfarin after 1 year, but it could not be resolved in that study whether this was an early or a late effect of drug therapy [14].

On the other hand, Chesebro et al. reported results of reassessment of occlusion rates of 210 of their initial 243 patients randomized to antiplatelet therapy and placebo [15]. New late grafts occlusions between the 1-month and the 1-year follow-up angiograms occurred in 27% of patients on placebo and in only 16% of patients on aspirin/dipyridamole ($p < 0.05$; Fig. 9). This late beneficial effect was also present for all distal anastomoses ($p < 0.05$) and was most pronounced for individual grafts (one proximal and one distal anastomosis; $p < 0.01$). These results were somewhat contradicted, however, by the 1-year follow-up report by Goldman et al. [16]. These authors found no difference in the rates of new late graft occlusion between all aspirin-treated patients (who had shown an early benefit) and placebo-treated patients between the 2-week and 1-year angiograms (Fig. 10). The discrepant results of these two studies could not be explained by the authors. The data of a further study by Gavaghan et al. [8] confirmed, however, the beneficial effect of prolonged treatment. New late graft occlusions occurred significantly less frequently on continued aspirin therapy (324 mg/day) than on placebo,

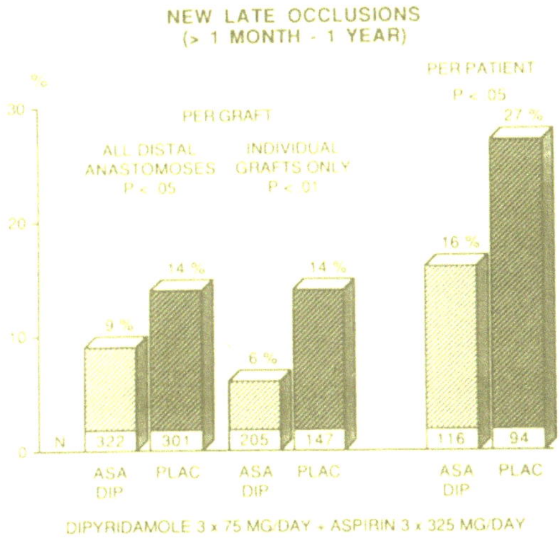

Fig. 9. Effect of aspirin plus dipyrdidamole (*ASA/DIP*) versus placebo (*PLAC*) on new late graft occlusion rates between 1 month and 1 year. (Adapted from [15])

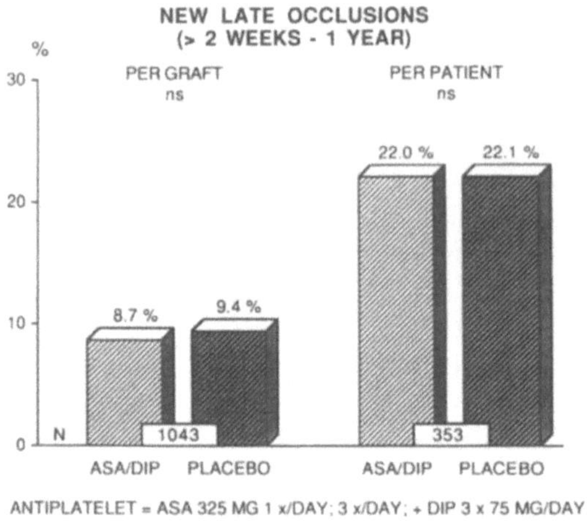

Fig. 10. Effect of different antiplatelet drug regimens based on dipyridamole (*DIP*) and/or aspirin (*ASA*) versus placebo on new late graft occlusions between 2 weeks and 1 year. (Adapted from [16])

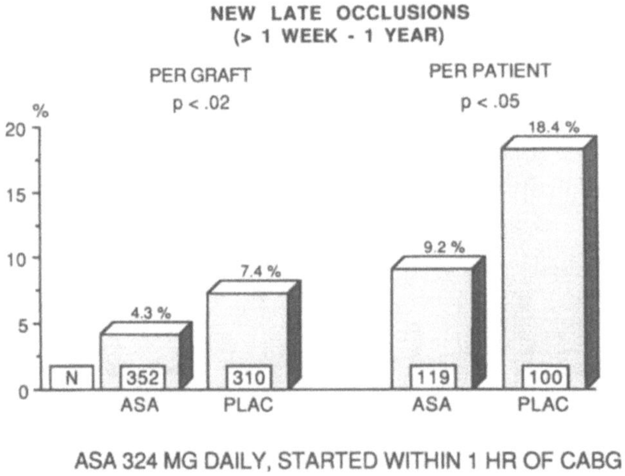

Fig. 11. Effect of aspirin versus placebo on new late graft occlusions between 1 week and 1 year. (Adapted from [8])

and this was true per patient (9.2% versus 18.4%, $p < 0.05$) and per graft (4.3% versus 7.4%, $p < 0.02$; Fig. 11).

In two additional studies the authors looked at late (1-year) angiograms only. Brown et al. reported a significantly lower occlusion rate at that time in a total of 127 patients treated with aspirin 3 × 325 mg per day or aspirin 3 × 325 mg plus dipyridamole 3 × 75 mg per day [17]. This treatment was started only 2–4 days after operation. Based on their findings these authors

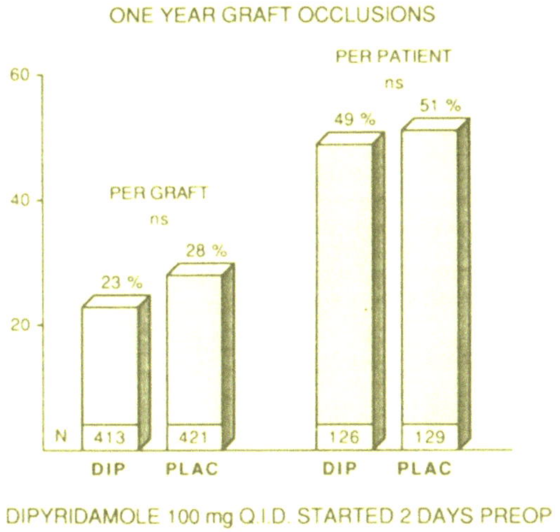

Fig. 12. Effect of dipyridamole versus placebo on one year graft occlusion rates. (Adapted from [18])

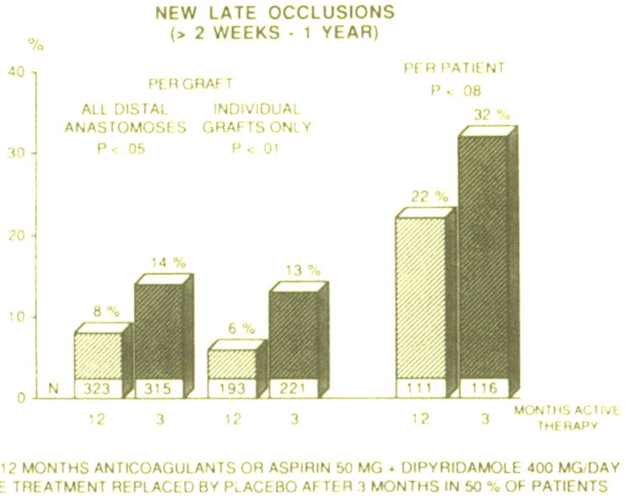

Fig. 13. Effect of withdrawal of antithrombotic therapy (anticoagulants or antiplatelet drugs) after 3 months and replacement by placebo in comparison with continued treatment for 12 months on new late graft occlusions between 2 weeks and 1 year. (Adapted from [9])

questioned the need for the addition of dipyridamole to aspirin, but the number in each group was in fact too small for such a conclusion. Ekeström and colleagues compared dipyridamole 100 mg q.i.d. started 2 days before surgery to placebo in 360 patients, 105 of whom had no follow-up angiogram (48 on dipyridamole and 57 on placebo) [18]. There were no significant differences in occlusion rates after 1 year regarding all patients (49% versus 53% on dipyridamole and placebo, respectively) nor regarding all distal anastomoses (23% versus 28%, NS; Fig. 12).

Comparative Studies

In a study by our group [9] half of the patients in each treatment group (aspirin/dipyridamol or anticoagulant) were randomized to placebo or to continued active treatment after 3 months. Follow-up angiography after 1 year showed a borderline significant reduction of patients with new graft occlusions between 2 weeks and 1 year (22% of treated patients versus 32% of placebo patients, $p < 0.08$; Fig. 13). The analysis per graft, however, revealed significantly fewer new graft occlusions in actively versus placebo-treated patients ($p < 0.05$). Similar to the findings by Chesebro et al. [15], this effect was most pronounced in individual grafts ($p < 0.01$). When these results are subdivided into subgroups who received anticoagulants or platelet inhibitors, the reduction in new late graft occlusions is very similar for both treatment regimens (Fig. 13). Due to the small numbers, however, the differences were only borderline significant for individual grafts. In one additional study reported by Guiteras in 1989 [19], comparing aspirin plus dipyridamole to triflusal (a new antiplatelet agent) plus dipyridamole and to placebo, new graft occlusion rates between 2 weeks and 6 months were significantly reduced by active treatment (12% on placebo, 7% on aspirin/dipyridamole, and 2.6% on triflusal/dipyridamole, $p < 0.06$). However, the analyses were based on a subgroup of those patients who had both follow-up angiograms (66% of all randomized patients), so that the possibility of bias cannot be excluded when interpreting these findings.

Taken together, these studies lead to a second conclusion. There is good evidence that continued anti thrombotic therapy up to 1 year is beneficial in patients after CABG surgery. Again, there does not seem to be a great difference between antiplatelet and anticoagulant therapy although there are only few data to support this statement. One large recently published study in Europe (Coronary Artery Bypass Aspirin Dipyridamole Anticoagulant Study) comparing low-dose (50 mg once daily) aspirin to aspirin plus dipyridamole (50 mg and 200 mg, respectively, per day) and to anticoagulants (started the day before operation) provides a more solid basis for such conclusions [20].

Predictors of Graft Occlusion and Side Effects of Therapy

Regarding predictors of early and late graft occlusions previous findings by Chesebro et al. [6, 15] and Brown et al. [17] were confirmed by our own results [9]. Irrespective of antithrombotic drug treatment early occlusions occurred more often in left circumflex and right coronary artery anastomoses than in left anterior descending and diagonal coronary artery grafts. Also, the occlusion rate was higher in multiple grafts (one proximal and at least two distal anastomoses), in grafts to endarterectomized vessels or to arteries with no or negligible anterograde runoff at preoperative angiography, and in grafts with a low blood flow and where the grafted artery diameter was less than 1.6 mm. Between 2 weeks and 1 year the same factors were associated with a higher occlusion rate as in the early postoperative period. Predictors of late graft occlusion in relation to duration of treatment indicated that all subgroups fared worse if active treatment was withdrawn. Grafts to the left anterior descending and diagonal coronary arteries, individual grafts, grafts with an acceptable preoperative angiographic runoff, and grafts to endarterectomized arteries showed the greatest benefit from continued therapy.

On the other hand, major side effects, especially bleeding complications after the immediate perioperative period, occurred significantly more often in patients treated with anticoagulants than in those treated with antiplatelet therapy in our comparative trial (11/124 versus 0/125 severe bleeding complications and 6/124 versus 1/125 mild bleedings, $p < 0.001$; Table 1) [9]. Mild side effects such as headache, dizziness, flush, and gastrointestinal symptoms, however, were significantly more frequent in patients treated with antiplatelet drugs than in those on anticoagulants (14/125 versus 6/124 patients, $p < 0.03$), although a quarter of these mild side effects occurred during the placebo phase of the study.

Conclusions and Implications

These additional observations lead to the following final conclusions and implications. Based on the results of a series of large prospective clinical trials there is no doubt that anticoagulants and different antiplatelet drug

Table 1. Prevention of aortocoronary vein graft occlusion: side effects of therapy with anticoagulants (AC) versus aspirin 50 mg + dipyridamole 400 mg (ASA-DIP; from [9])

	AC (n = 124)	ASA-DIP (n = 125)
Severe bleeding	11	0
Perioperative tamponade	3	2
Venous thromboembolism	0	4
Mild bleeding	6	1
Other mild side effects	6	14

regimens are able to reduce the rate of early and most likely also late bypass graft occlusion. Whereas anticoagulants seem to be as effective as antiplatelet drugs, severe bleeding complications are more frequent with anticoagulants, a finding which would favor the safer and easier platelet-inhibitory drug regimens. Antithrombotic therapy should most likely be continued for at least 1 year after CABG surgery, and subsets have been identified where this seems to be especially important.

Some questions, however, still remain to be solved. What is the optimal dose of aspirin given alone or in combination with dipyridamole? There is some evidence [9, 11, 12, 17] that a dose as low as 50 mg/day might be sufficient. But when should aspirin be started? Should it also be given several hours before surgery? And what is the exact role of dipyridamole? Although it has been shown in at least two studies [9, 18] that graft blood flow is significantly increased in patients treated with dipyridamole, this has not resulted in lower occlusion rates so far. Results of the recently published CABADAS (Coronary Artery Bypass Aspirin, Dipyridamole, Anticoagulant Study) in almost 1000 patients showed that aspirin, 50 mg per day, alone, is as effective as anticoagulants and that dipyridamole did not improve this result [20]. Finally, will the findings on the benefit of antithrombotic treatment, all obtained in patients with saphenous vein grafts, also prove applicable to internal mammary artery grafts?

The fact that these questions still remain unanswered, however, should in no way detract from the clear evidence of a benefit of antithrombotic therapy in prevention of CABG occlusion.

References

1. Verstraete M, Brown BG, Chesebro JH et al. (1986) Evaluation of antiplatelet agents in the prevention of aorto-coronary bypass occlution. Eur Heart J 7:4–13
2. Bourassa MG, Fisher LD, Campeau L, Gillespie MJ, McConney M, Lespérance J (1985) Long-term fate of bypass grafts: the Coronary Artery Surgery Study (CASS) and Montreal Heart Institute experiences. Circulation 72(V):71–78
3. Fitzgibbon GM, Leach AJ, Kafka HP, Keon WJ (1991) Coronary bypass graft fate: long-term angiographic study. JACC 17: 1075–1080.
4. Gohlke H, Gohlke-Bärwolf C, Stürzenhofecker P et al. (1981) Improved graft patency with oral anticoagulant therapy after aortocoronary bypass surgery: a prospective randomized study. Circulation 64 [Suppl 2]:22–27
5. Panteley GA, Goodnight SH, Rahimtoola S, Harlan BJ, DeMots H, Calvin L, Rosch J (1979) Failure of antiplatelet and anticoagulant therapy to improve patency of grafts after coronary-artery bypass. N Engl J Med 301:962–966
6. Chesebro JH, Clements IP, Fuster V et al. (1982) A platelet-inhibitor-drug trial in coronary-artery bypass operations. Benefit of perioperative dipyridamole and aspirin therapy on early postoperative vein-graft patency. N Engl J Med 307:73–78
7. Limet R, David JL, Magatteaux P, Larock MP, Rigo P (1987) Prevention of aorto-coronary bypass graft occlusion. Beneficial effect of ticlopidine on early and late patency rates of venous coronary bypass grafts: a double-blind study. J Thorac Cardiovasc Surg 94:773–783

8. Gavaghan TP, Gebshi V, Baron DW (1991) Immediate postoperative aspirin improves vein graft patency early and late after coronary artery bypass graft surgery. Circulation 83:1526–1533
9. Pfisterer M, Burkart F, Jockers G, Meyer B, Regenass S, Burckhardt D, Schmitt HE, Müller-Brand J, Skarvan K, Stulz P, Hasse J, Grädel E (1989) Trial of low-dose aspirin plus dipyridamole versus anticoagulants for prevention of aortocoronary vein graft occlusion. Lancet 1:1–7
10. Rothlin ME, Pfluger N, Speiser K et al. (1985) Platelet inhibitors versus anticoagulants for prevention of aortocoronary bypass graft occlusion. Eur Heart J 6:168–175
11. Goldman S, Copeland J, Moritz T et al. (1988) Improvement in early saphenous venin graft patency after coronary artery bypass surgery with antiplatelet therapy: results of a Veterans Administration cooperative study. Circulation 77: 1324–1332
12. Sanz G, Pajarón A, Alegría E, Coello I, Cardona M, Fournier JA, Gómez-Recio M, Ruano J, Hidalgo R, Medina A, Oller G, Colman T, Malpartida F, Bosch X, and the Grupe Español para el Seguimento del Infarto Coronario (GESIC) (1990) Prevention of early aortocoronary bypass occlusion by low-dose aspirin and dipyridamole. Circulation 82:765–773
13. Sethi GK, Copeland JG, Goldman S, Moritz T, Zadina K, Henderson WG (1990) Implications of preoperative administration of aspirin in patients undergoing coronary artery bypass grafting. J Am Coll Cardiol 15:15–20
14. McEnany MT, Salzman EW, Mundth ED, DeSanctis RW, Harthorne JW, Weintraub RM, Gates S, Austen WG (1982) The effect of antithrombotic therapy on patency rates of saphenous vein coronary artery bypass grafts. J Thorac Cardiovasc Surg 83:81–89
15. Chesebro JH, Fuster V, Elveback LR et al. (1984) Beneficial effect of dipyridamole and aspirin on late vein-graft patency after coronary bypass operations. N Engl J Med 310:209–214
16. Goldman S, Copeland J, Moritz T, Henderson W, Zadina K, Ovitt T, Doherty J, Read R, Chesler E, Sako Y, Lancaster L, Emery R, Sharma GVRK, Josa M, Pacold I, Montoya A, Parikh D, Sethi G, Holt J, Kirklin J, Shabetai R, Moores W, Aldridge J, Masud Z, DeMots H, Floten S, Haakenson C, Harker LA (1989) Saphenous vein graft patency 1 year after coronary artery bypass surgery and effects of antiplatelet therapy: results of a Veterans Administration cooperative study. Circulation 80:1190–1197
17. Brown BG, Cukingnan RA, DeRouen T, Goede LV, Wong M, Fee HJ, Roth Ja, Carey JS (1985) Improved graft patency in patients treated with platelet-inhibiting therapy after coronary bypass surgery. Circulation 72:138–146
18. Ekeström SA, Gunnes S, Brodin VB (1990) Effect of dipyridamole on blood flow and patency of aortocoronary vein bypass grafts. Scand J Thor Cardiovasc Surg 24:191–196
19. Guiteras P, Altimiras J, Aris A, Auge JM, Bassons T, Bonal J, Caralps JM, Catellarnau C, Crexells C, Masotti M, Oriol A, Pardo JM, Rutlant M (1989) Prevention of aortocoronary vein-graft attrition with low-dose aspirin and triflusal, both associated with dipyridamole: a randomized, double-blind, placebo-controlled trial. Eur Heart J 10:159–167
20. van der Meer J, Hillege H, Kootstra G, Ascoop C, Mulder B, Pfisterer M, van Gilst W, Lee K (1993) Prevention of one year graft occlusion after aortocoronary bypass surgery: a comparison of low dose aspirin (50 mg a day), low dose aspirin plus dipyridamole, and oral anticoagulants. Lancet 342:257–264

Calcium Antagonists in Patients Undergoing Coronary Artery Bypass Surgery

S.O. Gottlieb

Introduction

Calcium antagonists have demonstrated efficacy in cardiovascular medicine with clear antihypertensive, antiarrhythmic, and anti-ischemic properties. Due to the widespread use of calcium antagonists for patients with hypertension, arrhythmias, and ischemic heart disease, many patients who are undergoing coronary bypass surgery are often taking these medications. There are also several potential indications to initiate calcium antagonist therapy before, during, or after coronary bypass surgery and these will be addressed in this chapter under the following subheadings:

1. Antihypertensive therapy
2. Anti-arrhythmic therapy
3. Anti-ischemic therapy
4. Anti-atherosclerotic therapy

Calcium Antagonists for Postoperative Hypertension

Hypertension in the early postoperative period after coronary bypass surgery is a common problem, occurring in 50%–70% of patients. It is particularly common in patients who have received prior beta-blocker therapy, in patients with a history of hypertension, and after relief of ventricular outflow obstruction such as aortic stenosis. It is usually associated with increased systemic vascular resistance.

The antihypertensive properties of calcium antagonists are well-established and are due to direct peripheral vascular dilatation and reduction of systemic vascular resistance. While intravenous vasodilator infusions of sodium nitroprusside or nitroglycerin are commonly used after bypass surgery, recent studies suggest that dihydropyridine calcium antagonists may be particularly beneficial for control of postoperative hypertension. Dihydropyridine calcium antagonists may be preferable to verapamil or diltiazem type agents in this setting as the dihydropyridines have little or no effect on atrioventricular conduction, the intrinsic inotropic state, or left ventricular preload.

A randomized trial compared the intravenous administration of diltiazem, nifedipine, esmolol, and nitroprusside on hypertension after coronary artery bypass graft (CABG) [1]. All four treatments demonstrated comparable efficacy in reducing mean arterial pressure, however, heart rate decreased with both the betablocker esmolol and diltiazem, and one patient treated with diltiazem developed sinus arrest requiring atrioventricular (AV) pacing. An intermediate level of depression of left ventricular function was noted with diltiazem.

Several studies have examined the use of the dihydropyridine isradipine in post-CABG hypertension [2–5]. One study compared a titrated isradipine infusion to nitroprusside, and demonstrated a comparable reduction in blood pressure and systemic vascular resistance. The hemodynamic effects of isradipine are similar to those of intravenous nifedipine. Nitroprusside caused a reduction in pulmonary capillary wedge pressure and an increase in heart rate, with no significant change in the cardiac output. However, in comparison, pulmonary capillary wedge pressure was not significantly changed with isradipine and there was no accompanying tachycardia. These authors concluded that isradipine is a safe and effective agent with a preferable hemodynamic profile for patients in the early post-bypass state [4].

These observations were verified in another intravenous isradipine study demonstrating good control of postoperative hypertension, reduction of systemic vascular resistance, and increasing cardiac output without adverse effects [2]. While other dihydropyridine calcium blockers may have similar hemodynamic effects for the treatment of postoperative hypertension, some (i.e., nifedipine) are extremely light-sensitive and are, therefore, cumbersome for intravenous infusions. Isradipine appears to have an excellent pharmacodynamic profile for use in early postoperative hypertension and should be considered as an attractive alternative to other vasodilators.

Hypertensive patients may also require chronic oral therapy after coronary bypass surgery. In such patients, oral calcium antagonists may be considered to be effective antihypertensive agents. In patients who have recently undergone coronary bypass surgery, particular attention needs to be given to the status of the conduction system and left ventricular function when choosing an antihypertensive agent. In patients with left ventricular dysfunction, negative inotropic calcium blockers such as diltiazem or verapamil should be used with caution or avoided entirely, and dihydropyridine calcium blockers may be preferable. Use of once-daily dosing appears to be beneficial, and may also avoid reflex tachycardia which can be associated with short-acting forms of dihydropyridine calcium blockers. Long-acting preparations of nifedipine or amlodipine may be particularly useful for hypertension in this setting.

Use of Calcium Antagonists to Treat Arrhythmias After Bypass Surgery

Supraventricular arrhythmias, particularly atrial fibrillation and atrial flutter, are common after coronary bypass surgery. The therapeutic goal in such patients is initially to control the rate and then to resort sinus rhythm. While digoxin remains a mainstay therapy for this problem, calcium antagonists with negative chronotropic effects may also be useful.

For the prompt control of rapid atrial fibrillation or flutter, intravenous verapamil 5–10 mg is very effective. The blood pressure must be monitored closely, and this therapy may not be appropriate therapy for patients with borderline or low blood pressure. It is important to be certain that the arrhythmia is supraventricular in origin before infusing verapamil, particularly if the patient demonstrates a wide complex tachyarrhythmia. If atrial and ventricular wires are still present, the performance of an atrial electrocardiogram is particularly helpful in establishing the diagnosis of a supraventricular arrhythmia. If there is doubt or if the patient is hemodynamically compromised, immediate cardioversion is the treatment of choice.

Another recent alternative for the control of rapid atrial fibrillation in the postoperative setting is the use of intravenous diltiazem. This can be given by a bolus followed by an infusion and titrated to the desired rate control. Again, blood pressure should be carefully monitored with this therapy.

One study demonstrated that calcium antagonists given intraoperatively and postoperatively resulted in a reduced risk of ventricular arrhythmias in women after coronary bypass surgery [6]. Another study examining the predictors of postoperative ventricular dysrhythmias identified advanced age as the primary risk factor followed by preoperative use of calcium antagonists. It may be speculated that withdrawal of calcium antagonists ocurring with bypass surgery may result in increased ventricular instability or predispose to coronary vasoconstriction [7]. However, there is little clinical evidence to support the presence of a calcium antagonist rebound phenomenon [8].

Use of Calcium Antagonists to Treat Perioperative Myocardial Ischemia

Based on the established anti-ischemic efficacy of calcium antagonists and the known ischemic stress experienced by patients undergoing bypass surgery, it is reasonable to postulate that calcium antagonists may reduce the incidence of ischemia and postoperative myocardial infarction. One randomized blinded study examined the efficacy of intravenous infusion of diltiazem (0.15 mg/kg bolus followed by 2 mcg/kg/min) during anesthesia and surgery before institution of cardiopulmonary bypass [9]. This demonstrated a significant reduction in the determinants of myocardial oxygen consumption when used in conjunction with fentanyl and benzodiazipine anesthesia. The favorable hemodynamic effects were associated with a trend towards a reduction in perioperative ischemic events. However, insufficient data are available with regard to the potential for reduction of postoperative myocardial infarction with such therapy.

Another randomized study compared the effect of the infusion of nifedipine versus intravenous nitroglycerin on the incidence of perioperative myocardial ischemia and infarction in patients undergoing coronary bypass surgery [10]. Three-channel continuous electrocardiographic monitoring was used to identify ischemia, and cardiac enzymes were analyzed for evidence of myocardial necrosis. The infusion of intravenous nifedipine resulted in fewer transient ischemic events (6% treatment versus 18% placebo; $p > 0.01$), fewer myocardial infarctions (4% treatment versus 12% placebo; $p >$

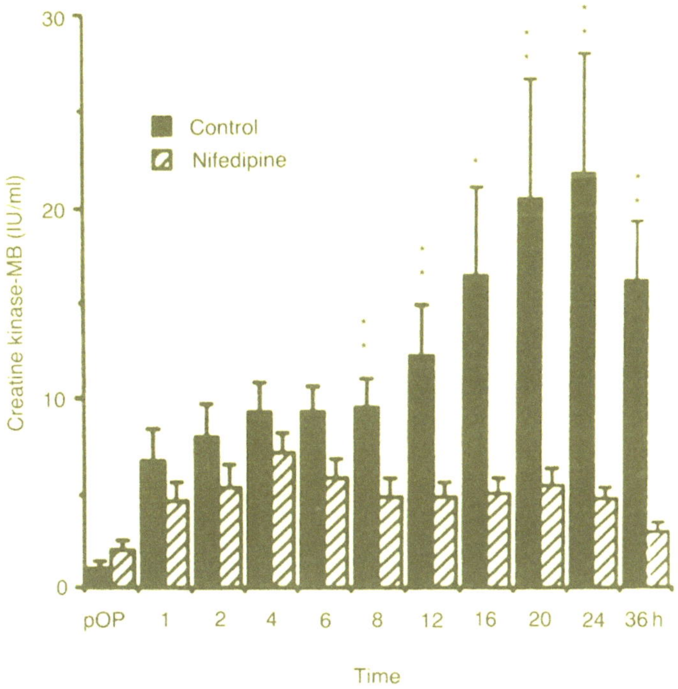

Fig. 1. Serum creatine kinase-MB levels before surgery (*pOP*) and for 36 h after opening of the aortic cross clamp. *MB*, MB-isoenzyme of creatine kinase; control, nitroglycerin group ($n = 50$); nifedipine, nifedipine group ($n = 53$). Data are given as mean ± SEM; ** value differs significantly from that for nifedipine group ($p < 0.01$). Reproduced with permission from [10]

0.001) and a lower postoperative peak value of creatine kinase and creatine kinase MB elevations (Fig. 1). It is of interest that the placebo group received intravenous nitroglycerin, and the addition of a calcium blocker resulted in clinical benefits beyond those seen with intravenous nitroglycerin. The incidence of premature complexes or ventricular arrhythmias was not significantly different between the two groups.

A previous study did not show significant benefit of nifedipine on the incidence of postoperative ischemia, perhaps because of the fact that the infusion was started 2h after the onset of the reperfusion [11]. The benefit noted in this study starting at the time of extracorporeal circulation emphasizes the potential importance of the early reperfusion period in the development of ischemia. The most likely pathophysiologic explanation for the benefit of nifedipine in this study is a direct effect on the coronary vasculative bed increasing myocardial flow in the subendocardial layers. There were no significant differences between the nifedipine and nitroglycerin groups with regard to major hemodynamic measurements such as blood pressure and heart rate. In addition, nifedipine may be a functional antagonist of alpha-2-receptor-mediated sympathetic coronary vasoconstriction, which has been suggested to be an important mediator of ischemia during anesthesia. Nifedipine has also been demonstrated to be a weak antiplatelet agent. However, it is unlikely that its major anti-ischemic effect is due to an antithrombotic mechanism.

Some concern has arisen about a potential association between preoperative use of calcium antagonists and postoperative low output state [12]. However, this is not a clearly recognized syndrome. In addition, due to the weak antiplatelet effects of some calcium antagonists, there was initial concern about the potential for postoperative bleeding in patients on therapy [13]. Randomized trials, however, have not supported these concerns and no excess risk of bleeding has been documented [8].

Use of Calcium Antagonists as Antiatherosclerotic Agents

A number of studies in different animal models of atherosclerosis have demonstrated that atherosclerosis can be significantly retarded with the use of calcium antagonists [14–25]. The precise mechanism responsible for these observations remains in debate, but is apparently not simply a reflection of antihypertensive effects of the calcium antagonists. There may be a number of interactive mechanisms, but the observations are also apparently independent of the effects on the plasma lipid levels. The process of atherogenesis includes a number of steps which are calcium dependent and could potentially be modified by the use of calcium antagonists (Fig. 2). These include the migration and proliferation of smooth muscle cells, growth factors, and chemotaxis. In addition, calcium antagonists may inhibit platelet function,

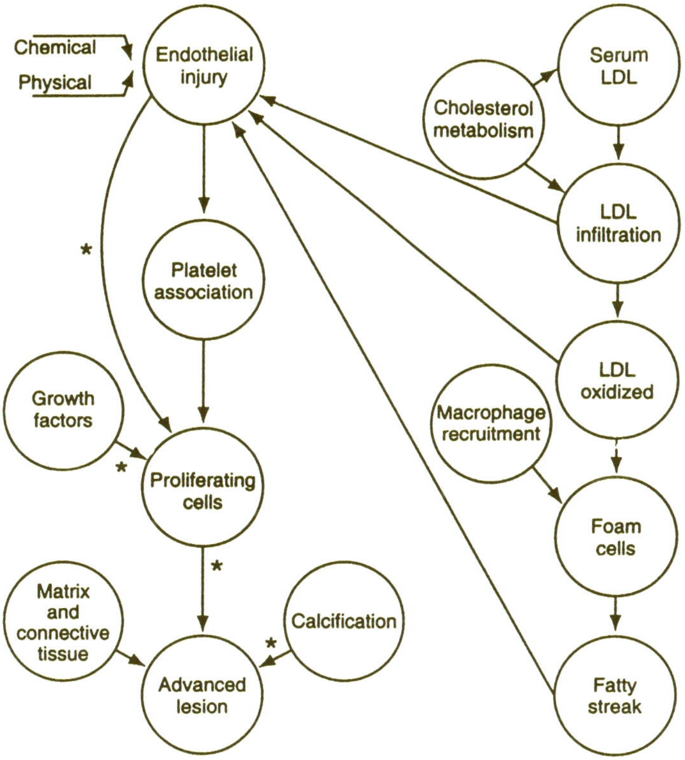

Fig. 2. The "atherogenic cascade" – the sequence of events that lead or contribute to atherosclerosis. Steps known or believed to be sensitive to calcium-channel antagonists at cardiovascular concentrations are marked with an asterisk. Reproduced with permission from [26]

insert antioxidant properties, up-regulate the low-density lipoprotein (LDL) receptors, and facilitate the metabolism of cholesterol esters [26].

Several clinical trials have examined the efficacy of calcium antagonists on the progression of human atherosclerosis [27–31]. The INTACT study examined the effect of nifedipine versus placebo on the progression of disease in the native coronary artery bed in 425 patients with mild coronary artery disease [31]. Using quantitative coronary angiographic techniques and 3-year arteriographic follow-up in 82% of the population, nifedipine therapy demonstrated no significant effect on the progression or regression of *pre-existing* coronary lesions over the 3-year period. However, the formation of *new* coronary lesions per patient was reduced by 28%. There was no significant effect of nifedipine on plasma lipoprotein values. Due to the apparent effect of therapy on the development on new coronary lesions, the authors postulated that the calcium antagonists may have an effect on early lipid-related lesions, possibly preferentially affecting the early stages of

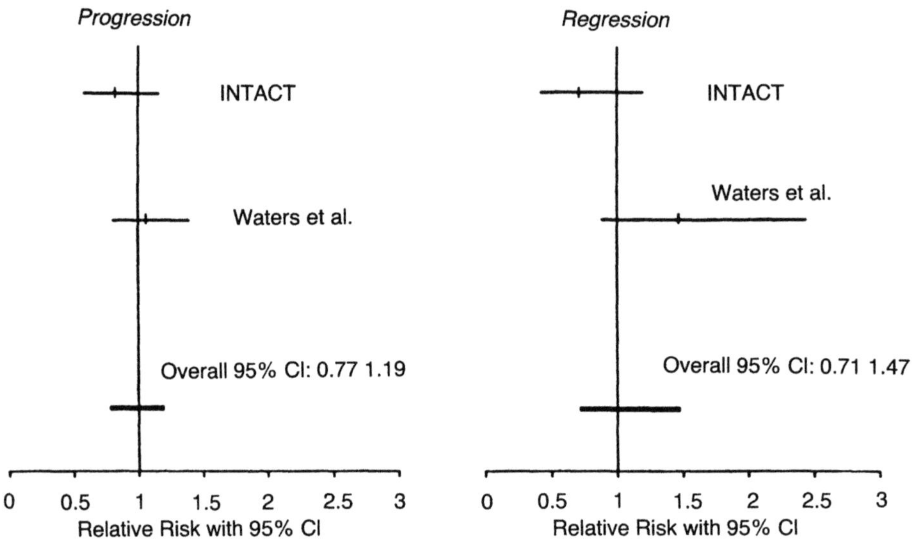

Fig. 3. Relative risks for angiographic progression and regression of coronary artery disease for both calcium antagonist trials and the overall relative risk. The horizontal bars indicate the 95% confidence interval. For progression the portion left to the line of unity indicates a beneficial effect (reduction in progression); for regression the portion right to the line of unity indicates a beneficial effect (increase in regression). Reproduced with permission from [25]

atherogenesis such as the accumulation of macrophage-derived foam cells and proliferating smooth muscle cells [31].

Another study examined the effects of nifedipine, propranolol, and isosorbide dinitrate on patients with coronary disease on the progression or regression of atherosclerosis in native coronary arteries [28]. This study demonstrated a reduced rate of progression with nifedipine, but not with the beta blocker and nitrate therapy. The effects of the dihydropyridine calcium antagonist, nicardipine on native coronary atherosclerosis were assessed in 383 patients [27]. This study, like the INTACT study, found no significant difference in the rate of progression of existing lesions between the nicardipine and placebo groups (Fig. 3). However, the rate of progression of minimal lesions (20% or less) over the 2-year follow-up was significantly reduced by nicardipine (15% nicardipine versus 27% placebo; $p > 0.05$). Using stepwise logistic regression analysis, baseline systolic blood pressure, and a change in blood pressure was correlated with progression of minimal lesions, suggesting that the antihypertensive effect of the calcium blocker may have played a role.

Pathologic studies of aortocoronary saphenous vein bypass grafts have suggested that the early development of intimal proliferation and atherosclerotic debris make these grafts a human model of accelerated atherosclerosis [32]. A 10-year follow-up study has indentified risk factors for the development of atherosclerosis in saphenous vein grafts [33]. The plasma lipid values particularly elevated LDL, LDL apoprotein B, and decreased high-density lipoprotein (HDL) levels were associated with a higher rate of graft occlusion (see chapter by Drexel and Amann, this volume).

Findings from the Cholesterol-lowering Atherosclerosis Study (CLAS) demonstrated that progressive reduction of total cholesterol, LDL cholesterol and elevation of HDL cholesterol with pharmacologic therapy (niacin and colestipol in combination) resulted in a reduction of disease progression in bypass grafts [34]. Further analyses from this study suggest that dietary changes principally designed at lowering fat intake was associated with a reduction in the rate of disease progression. Other studies examining the rate of disease progression in bypass grafts principally focused on the use of antiplatelet agents. A large randomized trial in 407 patients examined the effects of a combination of dipyridamole and aspirin, demonstrating a significant reduction in the incidence of vein graft occlusion with antiplatelet therapy (11% versus 25% placebo) [35–37].

Given this background knowledge on the early rate of progression of disease in the coronary bypass grafts, and with the assumption that factors affecting the development of new atherosclerotic lesions are at work in the production of bypass graft disease, a randomized trial examining the potential antiatherosclerotic effects of calcium antagonist nifedipine in coronary bypass grafts was performed [29]. Patients eligible for this trial included patients undergoing bypass surgery at Johns Hopkins Hospital who were at high risk for the development of bypass graft disease, i.e., who had two or more major coronary risk factors including active smoking, hyperlipidemia, hypertension, or premature coronary disease (age less than

Table 1. Exercise treadmill data (from [29] with permission)

	Placebo (n = 72)		Nifedipine (n = 72)	
	n	%	n	%
2-month ETT performed	61	85	52	72
Angina	4	7	3	6
ST depression	16	26	6	12*
Exercise duration (s) (mean ± SEM)	622 ± 28		649 ± 33	
12-month ETT performed	52	72	40	56
Angina	7	13	3	8
ST depression	16	31	10	25
Thallium positive	17	33	15	38
Exercise duration (s) (mean ± SEM)	703 ± 41		786 ± 40	

*p = 0.05.

50 years). Patients were randomized to nifedipine 60 mg daily or placebo beginning 5–7 days after bypass surgery, and followed for 12 months. They underwent a 2-month exercise evaluation and 1-year angiography. All patients received concomitant aspirin and dipyridamole, and beta blockers and nitrates were used as needed to control hypertension and postoperative ischemia. A total of 144 patients were randomized, and repeat angiography was performed within 1 year in 64 patients. At 2 months, the number of patients with positive exercise stress tests was reduced in the nifedipine group (12% versus 26% placebo; $p = 0.05$) (Table 1). At follow-up angiography, a total of 136 grafts were examined in the placebo group and 93 grafts in the nifedipine group. The percentage of grafts free of disease was 52% in the placebo group versus 67% in the nifedipine group ($p = 0.04$) (Figs. 4, 5, 6). Multivariate analysis demonstrated the presence of prior

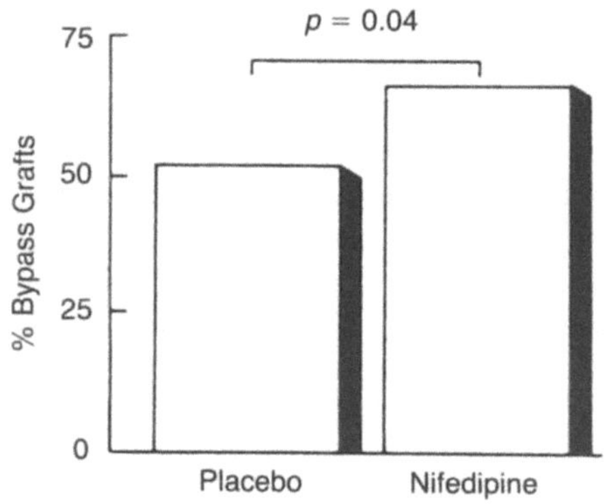

Fig. 4. Percentage of bypass grafts with no lesion. Reproduced with permission from [29]

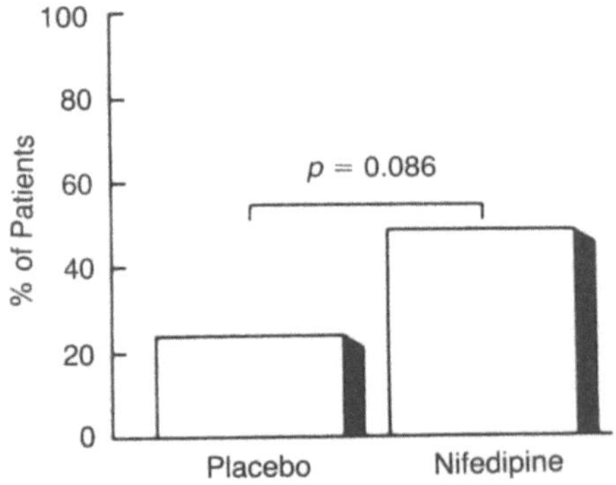

Fig. 5. Percentage of patients with no lesions in bypass grafts. Reproduced with permission from [29]

Table 2. Multivariate analysis of the probability of bypass graft lesions in patients with and without prior myocardial infarction (MI) (data from [29] with permission)

	Variable tested	p Value	Predicted probability
Variables related to number of bypass grafts with any lesion (multiple logit analysis)	Family history of premature coronary artery disease	0.006	–
	Number of vessels >70% lesion	0.003	–
	Nifedipine/placebo group	0.006	–
	Prior MI	0.16	–
Identification of patients with any bypass graft lesion [multivariate (logistic regression) analysis]	Prior MI	0.004	–
	Group	0.37	–
Predicted probability in patients with bypass graft lesion	Nifedipine, no prior MI	–	0.296
	Placebo, no prior MI	–	0.589
	Nifedipine, no prior MI	–	0.695
	Placebo, prior MI	–	0.885

Patients with no prior MI who were treated with nifedipine had the lowest predicted probability of bypass graft lesions (30%) and patients with prior MI who were treated with placebo and the highest probability of lesions (89%).

myocardial infarction and placebo treatment to be important predictors of patients who would develop bypass graft disease (Table 2). This study suggests that calcium antagonist therapy with nifedipine in the postoperative period may reduce the development of bypass graft disease, and further studies performed in conjunction with lipid-lowering therapy are indicated.

Another study evaluated the effects of the addition of diltiazem or placebo to antiplatelet therapy in 112 patients undergoing bypass surgery [38]. Coronary angiography at one year showed a nonsignificant trend toward a higher rate of graft occlusion associated with diltiazem than with placebo (15% versus 7.5%).

The suggestion of a beneficial effect of a calcium antagonist on the development of new coronary lesions in trials examining native coronary arteries, together with the observations noted in the one trial of the bypass graft patients, suggests that calcium antagonists may exert a beneficial effect in the development of new atherosclerotic lesions. Further studies are needed to examine the role of the independent contributions of calcium antagonists, together with lipid-lowering therapy, antioxidant therapy, and other behavior modifications to establish the clinical relevance of these observations. Available studies suggest that intra- and postoperative use of calcium antagonists may significantly reduce the incidence of myocardial ischemia and infarction in the early postoperative period and the later development of vein graft disease.

Summary

In summary, calcium antagonists are clearly established agents in the treatment of hypertension, arrhythmias, and myocardial ischemia. They may also have the potential for retarding the development of atherosclerosis. They have a clear clinical role for the treatment of patients before, during, and after coronary bypass surgery for the treatment of hypertension, arrhythmias, ischemia, and possibly retarding the development of atherosclerosis.

References

1. Boylan JF, O'Leary G, Weisel RD et al (1990) A comparison of diltiazem, esmolol, nifedipine and nitroprusside therapy of post-CABG hypertension. Can J Anesth 6:S156 (abstract)
2. Lawrence CJ, Lestrade A, deLange S (1991) Isradipine, a calcium antagonist, in the control of hypertension following coronary artery-bypass surgery. Am J Hypertens 4:207S–209S
3. Brister NW, Barnette RE, Schartel SA et al (1991) Isradipine for treatment of acute hypertension after myocardial revascularization. Crit Care Med 19:334–338
4. Underwood SM, Feneck RO, Davies SW et al (1989) Use of isradipine in hypertension following coronary artery bypass surgery. Am J Med 86:81–87
5. Colson P, Medioni P, Saussine M et al (1992) Hemodynamic effect of calcium channel blockade during anesthesia for coronary artery surgery. J Cardiothorac Anesth 6:424–4428
6. Hicks GL, Salley RK, DeWeese JA (1984) Calcium channel blockers: an intraoperative and postoperative trial in women. Ann Thorac Surg 37:319–322
7. Ferraris VA, Ferraris SP, Gilliam HS et al (1991) Predictors of postoperative ventricular dysrhythmias: a multivariate study. J Cardiovasc Surg 32:12–20
8. Gottlieb SO, Ouyang P, Achuff SC et al (1984) Acute nifedipine withdrawal: Consequences of preoperative and late cessation of therapy in patients with prior unstable angina. J Am Coll Cardiol 4:382–388
9. Colson P, Medioni P, Saussine M et al (1992) Hemodynamic effect of calcium channel blockade during anesthesia for coronary artery surgery. J Cardiothorac Vasc Anesth 6(4): 424–428
10. Seitelberger R, Zwolfer W, Huber S et al (1991) Nifedipine reduces the incidence of myocardial infarction and transient ischemia in patients undergoing coronary bypass grafting. Circulation 83:460–468
11. Seitelberger R, Zwolfer W, Binder TM (1990) Infusion of nifedipine following coronary artery bypass grafting decreases the incidence of early postoperative myocardial ischemia. Ann Thorac Surg 49:61–68
12. Myles PS, Olenikov I, Bujor MA et al (1993) ACE-inhibitors, calcium antagonists and low systemic vascular resistance following cardiopulmonary bypass. A case-control study. Med J Aust 158:675–677
13. Becker RC, Alpert JS (1990) The impact of medical therapy on hemorrhagic complications following coronary artery bypass grafting. Arch Int Med 150:2016–2021
14. Henry PD, Bentley KI (1981) Suppression of atherogenesis in cholesterol-fed rabbit treated with nifedipine. J Clin Invest 68:1366–1369
15. Henry PD (1990) Anti-atherogenic effects of calcium channel blockers: possible mechanisms of action. Cardiovasc Drugs Ther 4:1015–1020

16. Weinstein DB, Helder JG (1987) Antiatherogenic properties of calcium antagonists. Am J Cardiol 59:163B–172B
17. Henry P (1990) Calcium antagonists as anti-atherosclerotic agents. Arteriosclerosis 10:963–965
18. Kober G, Schneider W, Kaltenbach M (1989) Can the progression of coronary sclerosis be influenced by calcium antagonists? J Cardiovasc Pharmacol 13:S2–S6
19. Holzgreve H, Burkle B (1993) Anti-atherosclerotic effects of calcium antagonists. J Hypertens 11:555–559
20. Ginsburg R, Davis K, Bristow MR et al (1983) Calcium antagonists suppress atherogenesis in aorta but not in the intramural coronary arteris of cholesterol-fed rabbits. Lab Invest 49:154–158
21. Rouleau JL, Parmley WW, Stevens J et al (1983) Verapamil suppresses atherosclerosis in cholesterol-fed rabbits. J Am Coll Cardiol 1:1453–1460
22. Willis AL, Nagel B, Churchill V et al (1985) Antiatherosclerotic effects of nicardipine and nifedipine in cholesterol-fed rabbits. Arteriosclerosis 5:250–255
23. Parmley WW (1990) Vascular protection from atherosclerosis: potential of calcium antagonists. Am J Cardiol 66:16I–22I
24. Nayler WG, Panagiotopoulos S (1993) The antiatherosclerotic effect of the calcium antagonists and their implications in hypertension. Am Heart J 125:626–629
25. Vos J, DeFeyter PJ, Simoons ML et al (1993) Retardation and arrest of progression or regression of coronary artery disease: a review. Prog Cardiovasc Dis 35:435–454
26. Triggle DJ (1992) Calcium-channel antagonists: mechanisms of action, vascular selectivities, and clinical relevance. Cleve Clin J Med 59:617–627
27. Waters D, Lesperance J, Francetich M et al (1990) A controlled clinical trial to assess the effect of a calcium channel blocker on the progression of coronary atherosclerosis. Circ 82:1940–1953
28. Loaldi A, Polese A, Montorsi P et al (1989) Comparison of nifedipine, propranolol and isosorbide dinitrate on angiographic progressoin and regression of coronary arterial narrowings in angina pectoris. Am J Cardiol 64:433–439
29. Gottlieb SO, Brinker JA, Mellits ED et al (1989) Effect of nifedipine on the development of coronary bypass graft stenoses in high-risk patients: a randomized, double-blind, placebo-controlled trial. Circulation 80:II228 (abstract)
30. Borhani NO, Brugger SB, Byington RP (1990) Multicenter study with isradipine and diuretics against atherosclerosis. J Cardiovasc Pharmacol 15:S23–S29
31. Lichtlen PR, Hugenholtz PG, Rafflenbeul W et al (1990) Retardation of angiographic progression of coronary artery disease by nifedipine. Lancet 335:1109–1113
32. Unni KK, Kottke BA, Titus JL et al (1974) Pathologic changes in aortocoronary saphenous vein grafts. Am J Cardiol 34:526–532
33. Campeau L, Enjalbert M, Lesperance J et al (1984) Risk factors relative to atherosclerosis in saphenous vein bypass grafts and native vessels: a 10-year followup study. N Engl J Med 311:1329–1332
34. Blankenhorn DH, Nessim SA, Johnson RL et al (1987) Beneficial effects of combined colestipol-niacin therapy on coronary atherosclerosis and coronary venous bypass grafts. JAMA 257:3233–3240
35. Chesebro JH, Fuster V, Elveback LR et al (1984) Effect of dipyridamole and aspirin on late vein-graft patency after coronary bypass operations. N Engl J Med 310:209–214
36. Brown BG, Cukingnan RA, DeRouen T et al (1985) Improved graft patency in patients treated with platelet-inhibiting therapy after coronary bypass surgery. Circulation 72:138–146
37. Chesebro JH, Webster MWI, Smith HC et al (1989) Antiplatelet therapy in coronary disease progression: reduced infarction and new lesion formation. Circulation 80:II266 (abstract)
38. McCallister BD, Giorgi LV, Ligon R et al (1989) Effectiveness of aortocoronary bypass: a one year angiographic study using diltiazem and antiplatelet therapy. Circulation 80:II392

Revascularization Strategies

Percutaneous Transluminal Coronary Angioplasty in Patients with Failed Bypass Graft Surgery

J. Hollman

Introduction

The problem of patients with recurrent anginal pain following successful coronary bypass graft surgery is a growing one with important consequences. Coronary bypass surgery is now being performed on approximately 200 000 patients per year in the United States, a fairly constant number over the past 5–7 years [1]. Over this period the age of patients receiving primary operations has steadily risen. The mean age of patients undergoing primary operation has increased from 53 in the early 1970s to 58 in the early 1980s and continues to rise [2]. Thus, many patients with failed bypass graft surgery due to vein graft atherosclerosis are now in their late 60s or 70s. Because of the increased risk and diminished efficacy of repeat bypass surgery and the diminished efficacy of percutaneous transluminal coronary angioplasty (PTCA) in patients with old vein grafts, elderly patients with prior bypass surgery are subjected to aggressive medical therapy. With increased use of PTCA in younger patients with symptomatic angina, it has been the older patient with failed surgery who has supplied the clinical material for young cardiologists to learn the value of medical therapy.

To understand effectively the indications and use of PTCA in patients who have undergone bypass surgery one must understand the problem of second coronary revascularization procedures. Reoperation is technically more difficult than primary operation because of adhesions, inadequate cardioplegia, risk of embolism from atherosclerotic grafts, and risk of interrupting patent functioning bypass conduits (see chapter of von Segesser and Turina, this volume).

Adhesions increase the risk of vascular injury and prolong the anesthesia time. During opening and exposure the right ventricle or caval structures may be inadvertently entered, with resultant large blood loss. Because myocardial disease is more diffuse and extensive in reoperation cases, the ability to deliver antegrade cardioplegia adequately is impaired, with resultant greater myocardial injury. This has been lessened by the use of retrograde cardioplegia, but nonetheless myocardial infarction rate is four to seven times higher in reoperations. This higher infarction rate is also due to vein graft embolism, a problem that cannot be helped by more effective cardioplegia. Finally, disastrous consequences can occur when a patent internal mammary artery is transsected prior to cannulation for bypass surgery. This may leave the entire heart ischemia without the protection of cardiopulmonary bypass. Concern over such disasters has led many surgeons to use femoral-femoral bypass, established either percutaneously or by cut-down prior to opening the chest.

These inherent problems in surgical technique also make emergency back-up surgery difficult for PTCA patients who have previously undergone coronary artery bypass graft surgery (CABG).

Despite these limitations the incidence of repeat CABG is growing, and it is estimated that in 1995, 55 000 patients will undergo reoperations in the United States [3]. The cumulative incidence of reoperations is 3% at 5 years, 12% at 10 years, 17% at 12 years, and 38% at 15 years [4]. The major reason for reoperation is vein graft atherosclerosis. Patients are more likely to require reoperation if they receive vein graft only with the initial operation, continue to smoke, or have hyperlipidemia. The younger the patient at the time of initial operation, the more likely it is that the patient will require reoperation in the first 10 years following primary surgery. Finally, it must be recognized that about 50% of all ungrafted vessels will develop significant coronary obstruction during the first 10 years following CABG.

Patient Selection

Patients most likely to benefit from angioplasty are those who have recently had surgery with early bypass graft failure or patients with progressive disease, patent grafts, or disease approachable through the native vessels. The patients least likely to benefit from PTCA following failed CABG are patients with vein graft atherosclerosis 3 or more years following bypass graft surgery.

Principle 1: Do Native Vessel if Possible. Webb et al. have reported on the results in the San Francisco Heart Institute [5]. They found in 422 post-CABG patients that although native vessel PTCA and vein graft PTCA had equal initial success rates, the risk of late events (i.e., infarction 11% versus 4% and reoperation 19% versus 10%) was higher in vein graft dilation compared to native vessel dilation. This underscores the importance of dilating the native vessel whenever patent and suitable for PTCA.

Principle 2: PTCA Is Best in Young Vein Grafts. The age of the vein graft has been shown in Cleveland Clinic data to effect the initial results and the long term results following PTCA. In patients less than 36 months post-CABG the complication rate and actuarial event-free survival rate (free of symptom recurrence, myocardial infarction, repeat PTCA, bypass surgery or death) was 0% and 67%. Similar figures for patients more than 36 months after

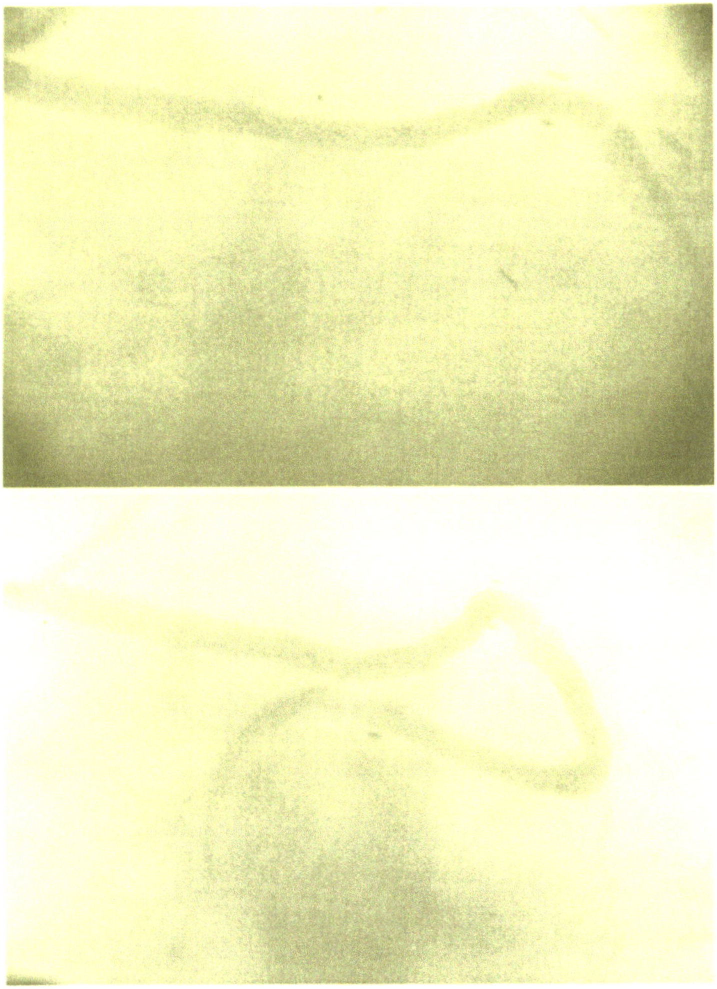

a b

Fig. 1a,b. Unusual case of "touch-up" angioplasty in the first few months following CABG. This patient experienced a perioperative myocardial infarction in the anterior descending distribution. Postoperatively the patient continued to experience angina pectoris. Cardiac catheterization 2 months after surgery demonstrated a discrete stenosis most likely from a venous valve due to failure to reverse the saphenous vein. This lesion responded well to coronary angioplasty, and the patient experienced good anginal relief and had a good angiographic result 6 months later. **a** Before PTCA; very discrete lesion with slow antegrade. **b** Study 6 months later demonstrates good continued success

surgery were 14.9% and 36% [7]. Thus, PTCA in old vein grafts carries a higher initial cost for a lower long-term benefit. Webb and the group from San Francisco confirmed these results, showing lower initial success and more late events in patients with vein graft PTCA longer than 1 year after surgery. This does constitute an important principle in the follow-up of a

b

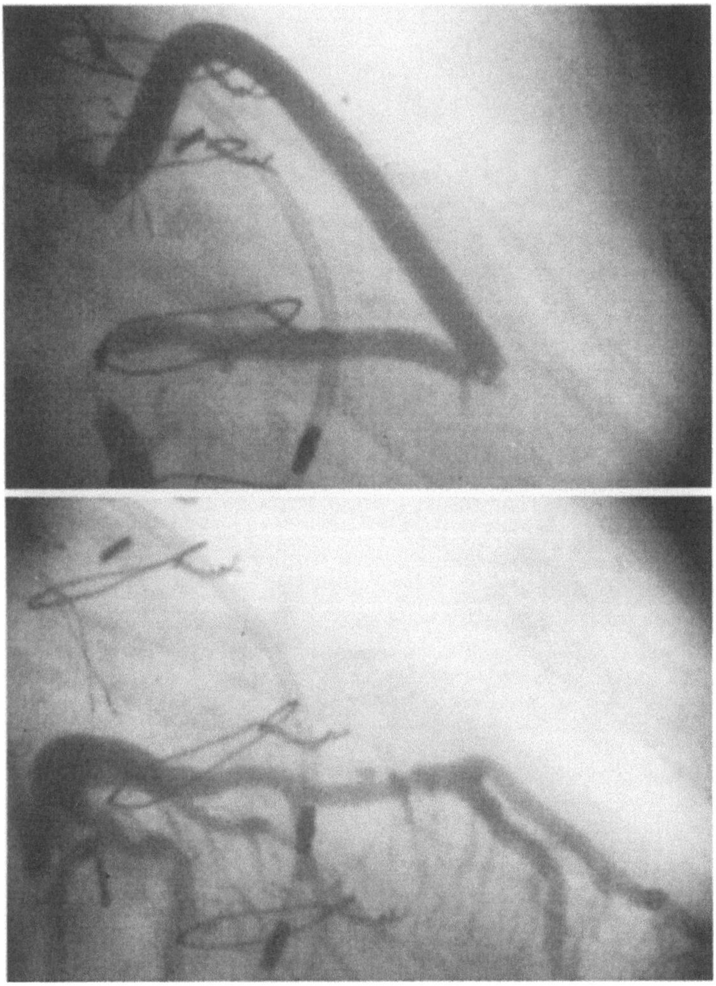

Fig. 2a,b. A case in which the saphenous graft was anastomosed to the anterior cardiac vein rather than the left anterior descending coronary artery (LAD). Angioplasty of the ulcerative lesions in the LAD successfully relieved the ischemia that coronary surgery failed to relieve. **a** Before PTCA. **b** After PTCA

patients after CABG. Patients with early symptoms following successful CABG are often ideal candidates for PTCA. Vein graft stenosis is due to initimal hyperplasia at this time and often responds well, with good long-term results, to PTCA. This is one place where PTCA can "touch up" the initial results obtained by CABG. (See Figs. 1, 2 for unusual cases of "touch up" following CABG.)

Principle 3: Distal Anastomotic Sites Are the Best Location for PTCA. Douglas et al. were the first to report that distal anastomotic sites have the best long-term results following vein graft PTCA, and that proximal anastomoses have a higher recurrence rate [6, 7]. These authors found 20% recurrent stenosis in distal sites (n = 51), 62% in middle sites (n = 65), and 79% in proximal sites (n = 14). The high recurrence rate at the proximal anastomosis has been confirmed by others [5, 8]. In fact, however, it is still worthwhile to attempt PTCA in early vein graft stenosis with proximal anastomotic lesions since the complication rate is low compared to repeat surgery. Patients who develop recurrent stenosis may well respond to second angioplasty.

While the above three principles in patient selection are germane, they do not solve the problem in every patient. Reoperation at Cleveland Clinic [11] entailed 6.8% mortality in patients over the age of 60 years. Clearly one would be hesitant to recommend reoperation for mild angina if the anatomy is not associated with a poor long-term survival. The Milwaukee group [20] reported a 12% mortality with three or more operations; again, one would be hesitant to recommend a third bypass unless the angina is severe, or the anatomy predicts a poor long-term survival. Angioplasty, however, has lower mortality in post-CABG patients (see Table 1) if the patient has lesions that are ideal for PTCA (short, concentric, focal disease). Then PTCA should be offered to the patient even though he might not be considered a candidate for elective reoperation. Patients with severe symptoms and unfavorable anatomy for PTCA or repeat CABG are a particularly difficult group. One such patient whom we have described was having rest

Table 1. Risks of revascularization in post-CABG patients

Reference	Location	n	Mortality	MI	CVA	E-CABG	5-year survival
CABG center							
Lytle [11]	Cleveland Clinic	1500	3.4%	7.2%	2.1%	N/A	87%
Brenowitz [23]	Milwaukee[a]	150	12.0%	4.7%	2.0%	N/A	76%
Foster [3]	CASS	283	5.3%	6.4%	0%	N/A	–
Reul [4]	Texas Heart	1000	4.8%	4.0%		N/A	
Verheul [24]	Amsterdam	200	7.5%			N/A	84%
PTCA center							
Douglas [8]	Emory	116	0%	0.8%		2.6%	–
Dorros [10]	Milwaukee	61	3.3%	4.9%		1.6%	–
Corbelli [25]	Cleveland Clinic	94	1.1%	3.2%		4.3%	–
Pinkerton [26]	Indiana	236	0.4%	3.0%		3.0	–
Webb [6]	San Francisco	422	0.2%	3.1%		3.1	89%
Serruys [18]	Netherlands[b]	454	0.7%	2.8%		1.3%	74%
Plako [7]	Cleveland Clinic[b]	101	2.0%	–		2%	–

MI, Myocardial infarction; CVA, cerebrovascular accident; E-CABG, emergency coronary artery bypass grafting.

[a] Includes only patients bypassed for the third time or more.

[b] Includes patients vein-graft dilation only. Other studies are in postoperative patients having dilation of either the bypass graft or native vessels.

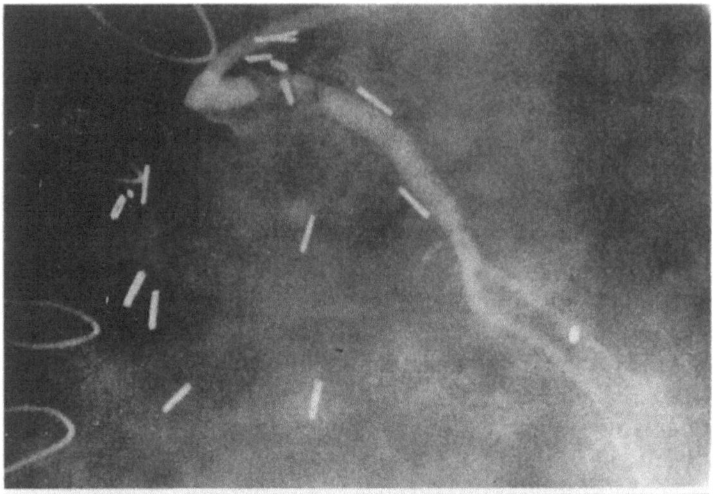

a

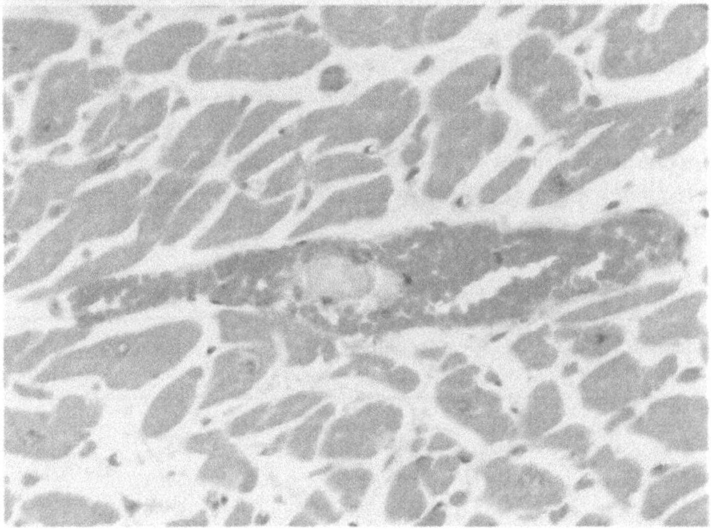

b

Fig. 3a,b. Atherosclerotic embolism from old saphenous vein bypass grafts. **a** The 6-year-old vein graft before PTCA in a patient considered to be a nonoperative candidate. **b** Atherosclerotic embolism in a branch of the circumflex artery surrounded by red cell thrombus

angina [12]. His two previous surgeries and severe left ventricular impairment were cause for two surgeons at our Clinic to refuse to offer him a third operation. Angioplasty of a 6-year vein graft resulted in multiple atheromatous emboli and microinfarctions of his myocardium. Despite support measures including intra-aortic balloon pumping, he died. At postmortem multiple atherosclerotic particles were seen in the small coronary vessels (Fig. 3). The infarctions predated the PTCA, implying that a portion of his unstable angina was due to spontaneous atheroembolism.

Liu has utilized the database at Emory University to identify 22 patients with atherosclerotic emboli during vein graft angioplasty. Comparing these patients to patients not manifesting embolism, he identified four risk factors for embolism: thrombus, diffuse disease, eccentricity, and ulceration [13]. In a separate study the Emory group has shown that a lesion on a bend in the midportion of old vein graft is more likely to progress to total occlusion than a lesion not on a bend (45% versus 20%) [14]. From these studies and observations one can conclude that when PTCA is contemplated in late vein graft stenosis, lesions that are discrete, concentric, without ulceration, located in a straight portion of the graft, and free of thrombus are the best to attempt. If multiple risk factors for poor outcome are present, it is best to reconsider repeat CABG.

Technical Aspects

The most important factor in performing vein graft angioplasty is obtaining a stable guiding catheter position. I have used almost exclusively multipurpose type or E1 Gamal type catheters for vein graft angioplasty. These catheters once in place and "cross-braced" allow for the passage of most balloons and other devices (Fig. 4).

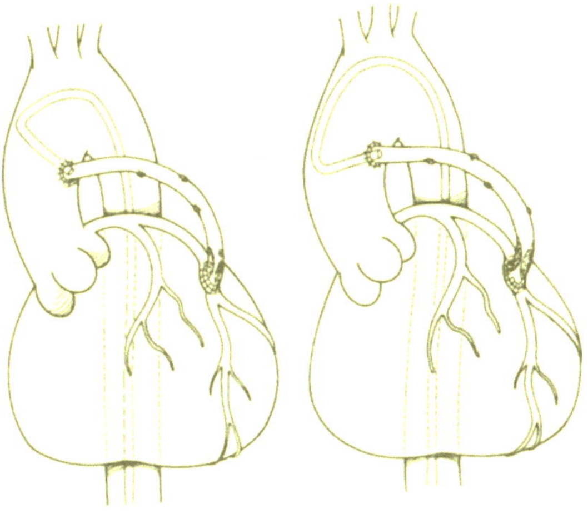

Fig. 4. Illustration of the cross-bracing procedure. *Left*, the multipurpose type of catheter is advanced to the ascending aorta and then rotated in a clockwise or counterclockwise direction until it engages the ostium of vein graft to be dilated. *Right*, after engagement the catheter is gently advanced until the tip points upward and parallel to the graft take-off. This gives maximal power to the operator when trying to push a balloon or other device down the graft and across the lesion

The newer bypass graft catheters are useful at times but do not readily cross-brace. There are separate ones for left- and right-sided bypass grafts. They require less technical skill to engage them and are also useful in situations in which the multiple purpose catheter does not engage the ostium of the graft.

Patients with one surgery usually have the left-sided grafts on the lower left side of the ascending aorta with the circumflex grafts above the left anterior descending and diagonal graft. Grafts to the right coronary artery are usually on the lower right side of the ascending aorta. Patients with multiple bypass surgeries sometimes have the grafts located in unusual positions on the ascending aorta and can be technically more challenging.

It should be remembered that the ascending aorta can be diseased with friable atherosclerotic material. Prior to the advent of soft-tipped catheters, two relatively young patients of mine each experienced a cerebral vascular accident during PTCA of their bypass grafts, a phenomena that I attributed to guiding catheter manipulation in the ascending aorta [15]. I have not observed this since the availability of soft-tipped catheters; however, it is still wise to be cautious and use a minimal amount of catheter manipulation in the ascending aorta.

Internal Mammary Angioplasty

Internal mammary angioplasty is usually required within a few months of surgery. The site of PTCA is nearly always the distal anastomosis. Using standard internal mammary artery (IMA), catheters from the transfemoral approach may be tried, particularly if the IMA is relatively straight. I personally prefer a percutaneous brachial approach to right IMAs because of the difficulties encountered in selectively catheterizing the right IMA from the groin. If the percutaneous brachial approach is used, either a right Judkin's type guiding catheter or an IMA catheter can be used to deliver the balloon catheter to the ostium of the IMA.

The length of the artery from the tip of the guiding catheter to the distal anastomosis is 20–30 cm depending on the tortuosity of the IMA. Anticipating this problem, Dr. Gruentzig had special, long (140-cm) balloon catheters made for his first IMA attempt. Although this attempt was not successful, the standard length for PTCA balloons became 140 cm after this problem was appreciated.

The length and tortuosity separating the guiding catheter from the lesion makes the guiding catheter less important. The balloon catheter must be flexible and soft to traverse the vessel and low profile to cross the lesion. Very little force can be applied from the guiding catheter. Before balloons were of such low profile, I had tried to force balloons down IMA grafts and thereby caused dissection with the guiding catheter proximally or with the balloon catheter when trying to force the balloon over a wire and around a sharp bend in the IMA.

Current catheters have made IMA angioplasties less technically challenging. My first choice currently is either an ACE balloon on a wire from Scimed or the 10s system from Advanced Catheter Systems.

New Devices

At the time of this writing the only two commercially available new devices are the Simpson Athercath and the Eximer laser. The technical aspects of passing these devices are still to be worked out, but guiding catheter position is much more important than it is for routine PTCA. Stenting of old vein grafts appears to be promising, but long-term data are still not available.

Thrombolysis of Vein Grafts

Hartmann et al. [16] has described the use of urokinase to open a thrombosed vein graft. This technique involves the use of the SOS infusion wire and the prolonged infusion of urokinase at 50000–100000 units per hour. These infusions require the guiding catheter to remain in the aorta for 16h–3 days. These infusions must be monitored periodically and the infusion catheter's position readjusted. This technique is an adaptation of the technique of opening peripheral arteries using direct infusion of thrombolytic agents.

Clinical Results

Initial success is expected with most PTCA procedures using current techniques. The complication rate with PTCA in post-CABG patients is similar to that in nonoperated patients, and the Mid-American Heart group have found that previous bypass surgery protects from major complications and especially death. It is postulated that this might happen because of an often greater number of conduits to supply the heart (assuming some bypass grafts patient). The Emory group analyzed their experience in 1263 patients with prior CABG undergoing PTCA. They had 46 patients (3.6%) who underwent surgery following failed PTCA. The 33 patients who had acute ischemia showed a significantly higher mortality and Q wave myocardial infarction rate compared to the 13 patients without ischemia [17].

Fewer long-term results are available, but data from the San Fancisco Heart Institute demonstrate 89% 5-year survival, with over 70% of patients free of death, myocardial infarction or late CABG. Predictions of late death or myocardial infarction include increased number of diseased vessels, unstable angina, and/or ejection fraction below 25% [5].

Dutch researchers have published a preliminary report on 454 patients undergoing saphenous vein PTCA, in whom they observed 0.7% mortality, 2.8% procedure-related infarctions, and 1.3% emergency CABG. Their actuarial survival at 5 years was 74%; event-free survival at 5 years (alive, no myocardial infarction, no repeat PTCA or CABG) was relatively low at 26%. This was heavily dependent on the length of time between CABG and PTCA. In patients within 1 year after CABG event-free survival was 45%, in those 1–5 years thereafter 25%, and in those longer than 5 years only 19% [18]. This is in keeping with the Cleveland Clinic findings (F.D. Loop, unpublished data).

IMA angioplasty has been reported by several centers; however, the two largest reports are those from the Mid-American Heart Institute (n = 45) [19], and the Cleveland Clinic (n = 31) [20]. Mammary artery graft body disease is rare, but nearly 25% of the Kansas City group had disease in the body of the graft. In most reported cases the disease is at the anastomosis with the native artery or in the artery distal to the anastomosis. The expected success rate is 85%–90%, with failure more likely when increased tortuosity is present. Complications include dissection of the IMA graft.

Vein graft rupture following balloon angioplasty is an unusual complication but should be more benign than native vessel rupture in patients who have not undergone bypass surgery, where pericardial tamponade is a frequent complication. Following bypass graft surgery pericardial adhesions often surround the bypass grafts, limiting the amount of extravasation of blood. The benign course of an elective graft body dilation and rupture has been described [21].

Clinical Implications

Angioplasty following CABG is a useful tool. Over the years suspicions that vein graft PTCA is less valuable than native vessel PTCA have been confirmed. It is also apparent that the older the vein graft is, the less likely that PTCA will be beneficial.

The initial complications of PTCA after CABG appear to differ little from those of PTCA in patients without prior CABG. If the patient becomes ischemic by the PTCA procedure, the risk of surgery and the risk of infarction are probably greater than in the patient who had not received a bypass. Methods to stabilize these patients using perfusion catheters, temporary and/or permanent stents and percutaneous bypass might well also reduce the complications.

Future Directions

It is important to establish new means of stabilizing patients. This is being evaluated at present using permanent stents and thermal catheters. These devices should reduce the need for acute bypass surgery to about 10% of the current emergency rate, or about 0.3%.

Effective measures to reduce recurrent stenosis are of utmost importance. The newer devices might reduce the recurrence rate compared to balloon angioplsty, but the basic vascular biology is unchanged. Thus it is expected that old bypass grafts will continue to be associated with a higher initial complication rate and a higher recurrence rate. Recurrent stenosis lesions in vein grafts have a high recurrence rate (50%) following directional atherectomy [22]. New devices may be of value where coronary balloon angioplasty is particularly poor, such as the proximal stenosis of vein grafts (see Fig. 5).

Old vein grafts with diffuse friable atherosclerotic disease might never be safely approached using percutaneous techniques. It may be wiser to find effective means of recannalizing the native vessels. Certainly this also would be challenging and the recurrent rate high, but the potential for healing might still be better in a recannalized native vessel.

Altering the rate of bypass graft failure is a national goal. Cardiac surgeons are doing their part by using more IMA grafts. Hyperlipidemia is a clear risk factor for vein graft failure. Continued cigarette smoking is a risk factor for events following successful CABG. It makes no sense to continue to pursue only the high-technology portion of the equation. Interventional cardiology must also be involved in lipid lowering and risk factor modifica-

a

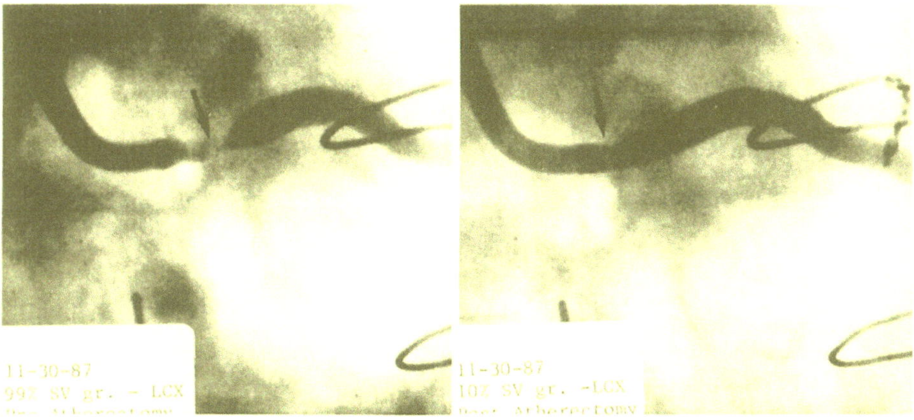

b

Fig. 5a,b. This patient was the third in the world to undergo coronary atherectomy. The initial result was sustained in clinic follow-up. Ostial stenosis following balloon angioplasty has up to a 70% recurrence rate tion following bypass surgery. The level to which lipids should be lowered, however, has not been determined. The ongoing multicenter trial sponsored by the NHLBI for lipid lowering to prevent late vein graft attrition may provide insight into this problem.

References

1. Hartzler GO (1990) PTCA in evolution: why is it so popular. Cleve Clin J Med 57:121–124
2. Cosgrove DM, Loop FD, Lytle BW et al. (1984) Primary myocardial revascularization – trends in surgical mortality. J Thorac Cardiovasc Surg 88:673–684
3. Cosgrove DM (1993) Is coronary reoperation without the pump an advantage? Ann Thorac Surg 55:329
4. Reul GL, Cooley DA, Ott DA et al. (1979) Reoperation for recurrent coronary artery disease. Arch Surg 114:1269
5. Loop FD, Lytle BW, Gill CC et al. (1983) Trends in selection and results of coronary artery reoperations. Ann Thorac Surg 36:380
6. Webb JG, Myler RK, Shaw RE et al. (1990) Coronary angioplasty after coronary bypass surgery: initial results and late outcome in 422 patients. JACC 16:812–820
7. Platko WP, Hollman J, Whitlow P, Franco I (1989) Percutaneous transluminal angioplasty of saphenous vein graft stenoses: long-term follow-up. JACC 14:1645–1650
8. Douglas JS Jr, Gruentzig AR, King SB III et al. (1983) Percutaneous transluminal coronary angioplasty in patients with prior coronary bypass surgery. JACC 2:745–754
9. Douglas J, King S, Roubin G, Schlunpf M (1986) Percutaneous angioplasty of venous aortocoronary graft stenosis: late angiographic and clinical outcome. Circulation 74:II–221
10. Dorros G, Johnson WD, Tector AJ et al. (1984) Percutaneous transluminal coronary angioplasty in patients with prior coronary artery bypass grafting. J Thorac Cardiovasc Surg 87:17–26
11. Lytle BW, Loop FD, Cosgrove DM et al. (1987) Fifteen hundred coronary reoperations. J Thorac Cardiovasc Surg 93:847–859
12. Trono R, Sutton C, Hollman J, Suit P, Ratliff NB (1989) Multiple myocardial infarctions associated with atheromatous emboli following percutaneous transluminal angioplasty of saphenous vein grafts – a clinico-pathologic correlation. Cleve Clin Med J 56:581–584
13. Liu MV, Douglas JS, King SB III (1989) Angiographic predictors of coronary embolization in PTCA of vein graft lesions (abstract). Circulation 80 [Suppl II]:II-172
14. Ba'alkaki HA, Weintraub WS, Ghazzal ZMB et al. (1990) Restenosis after angioplasty of mid-saphenous vein grafts: is lesion morphology important? Circulation 82 [Suppl III]: III-679
15. Galbreath C, Salgado ED, Furlan AJ, Hollman J (1986) Central nervous system complications of percutaneous coronary angioplasty. Stroke 71:616–619
16. Hartmann J, McKeever L, Teran J et al. (1988) Prolonged infusion of urokinase for recanalization of chronically occlused aortocoronary bypass grafts. Am J Cardiol 61:189–191
17. Weintraub WS, Cohen CL, Curling PE et al. (1990) Results of coronary surgery after failed elective coronary angioplasty in patients with prior coronary surgery. JACC 16:1341–1347
18. Serruys PW, Meester H, Thijs, Plokker HW (1990) Long-term follow-up after attempted angioplasty of saphenous vein bypass grafts: the Dutch experience 1980–1989. Circulation 82 [Suppl III]:III-678
19. Shimshak TM, Giorgi LV, Johnson WL et al. (1988) Application of percutaneous transluminal coronary angioplasty to the internal mammary artery graft. JACC 12:1205–1214
20. Dimas AP, Arora RR, Whitlow PL et al. (1991) Percutaneous transluminal angioplasty involving internal mammary artery grafts. Am Heart J 122:423–442

21. Drummer E, Furey K, Hollman J (1987) Rupture of saphenous vein bypass graft during coronary angioplasty. Br Heart J 78–81
22. US Directional Coronary Atherectomy Investigation Group (1990) Restenosis following directional coronary atherectomy in a multicenter experience. Circulation 82:III-679
23. Brenowitz JB, Johnson WD, Kayser KL et al. (1988) Coronary artery bypass grafting for the third time or more. Circulation 78 [Suppl I] I:166–170
24. Verheul HA, Moulijn AC, Hondema S et al. (1991) Late results of 200 repeat coronary artery bypass operations. Am J Cardiol 67:24–30
25. Corbelli J, Franco I, Hollman J et al. (1985) Percutaneous transluminal coronary angioplasty after previous coronary artery bypass surgery. Am J Cardiol 56:398–403
26. Pinkerton CA, Slack JD, Orr CM, VarTassel JW, Smith ML (1988) Percutaneous transluminal angioplasty in patients with prior myocardial revascularization. Am J Cardiol 61:156–226

Intraluminal Stents in Coronary Bypass Grafts

P. Urban and B. Meier

Background

The number of patients undergoing coronary artery bypass grafting has increased dramatically over the past 15 years in the United States and in Europe [1], and in Switzerland alone over 3600 bypass operations were performed in 1990 [2]. Angiographically, 11%–25% of vein grafts are occluded at 1 year [3, 4]; 11 years after surgery 40% of vein grafts are occluded, and 46% have severe atherosclerosis [5]. As a consequence, symptoms reccur in 7% of patients annually [6], and such patients constitute a sizable proportion of any cardiology practice. There are, however, only few data on what constitutes optimal management for them, and the relative merits of medical treatment, transluminal angioplasty, and repeat surgery have not been established unequivocally [5].

Percutaneous balloon angioplasty has become a well-established approach for selected cases, and its simplicity, speed, and rapid availability make it an attractive option. It is associated with high initial success and low complication rates [7, 8]. Medium-term results, however, have shown a higher incidence of restenosis in vein grafts than in native coronary arteries, with unsatisfactory angiographic results at 6 months in 40%–60% of cases [9]. Furthermore, despite the increasing use of thromboplasty, associating balloon angioplasty with prolonged local administration of thrombolytic agents [10], grafts that are totally occluded or very diffusely diseased are often not suitable targets for a conventional percutaneous approach [11].

The Stent Concept

Although balloon angioplasty has proven to be a highly effective technique for relieving stenosis and occlusion of coronary arteries, its main limitations remain those of abrupt closure, complicating about 5% of procedures [12], and restenosis that occurs in about a third of the dilated native vessels within the first 6 months following the procedure [13]. Because of the anatomical and rheological aspects that are central to both these problems, several

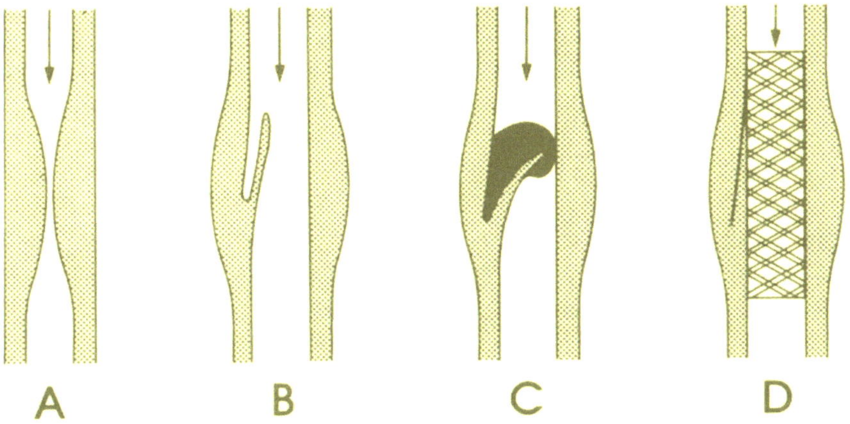

Fig. 1A–D. Diagram of stent implantation for treatment of abrupt occlusion. **A** Coronary stenosis before balloon angioplasty. **B** After balloon angioplasty, streching of the arterial wall has been induced together with plaque rupture. **C** An intimal flap forms with superimposed thrombus, and this acutely occludes the lumen. **D** Stent implantation "tacks down" the flap and prevents elastic recoil of the dilated segment. (Reprinted with permission from [64])

adjuncts to balloon coronary angioplasty (atherectomy devices, lasers, stents) have recently received considerable attention in an attempt to overcome some of the limitations of the technique while maintaining the advantage of a percutaneous access. A complete review is beyond the scope of this chapter, and discussion here is limited to the use of intravascular stents.

Stent implantation allows the operator to "tack down" the plaque and intimal flaps created by the initial balloon angioplasty and thus prevent embolization of disrupted plaque, improve rheology and immediate angiographic appearance, abolish residual transstenotic gradient [14, 15], and prevent elastic recoil of the dilated segment (Fig. 1).

Ideally, an implantable stenting device should satisfy the following criteria: (a) exert sufficient radial force to effectively support the vessel and maintain an appropriate lumen diameter without inducing pressure necrosis, (b) be flexible enough along its long axis to adapt to tortuous coronary anatomy, (c) remain stable once positioned, (d) be implantable percutaneously through standard angioplasty guiding catheters with a simple introducing device, (e) be biologically inert so as not to induce a foreign body reaction, (f) be nonthrombogenic, and (g) be rapidly covered by neoendothelium.

Historical Development

In 1912 Carrel [16] reported the experimental use of surgically implanted intravascular stents to treat aortic aneurysm and dissection. Over half a century later, Dotter was the first to describe percutaneous intravascular stenting, using both plastic tubing and stainless steel coil spring prostheses [17]. Several different metal coil designs, made either of stainless steel or nitinol (a temperature-dependent, shape-memory nickel and titanium alloy) were used in the experimental animal by Dotter and others [18, 19]. Maass et al. [20] in Zurich described the experimental use of several different self-expanding stents that could be elongated by torsion onto an ad hoc introducing device and then released into the vascular lumen where they expanded due to their elastic properties. However, the design required a bulky introducing system and was thus unsuitable for small arteries. Positioning of such prostheses could be achieved without inducing pressure necrosis, and endothelial covering in previously normal arteries was complete within 6 weeks. A combination of parietal intimal proliferation and microthrombi was observed more frequently in veins than in arteries. Gianturco's group [21, 22] described a spring-loaded stainless steel stent with a zigzag pattern that was implanted into large vessels, but stent migration was observed in some cases, and prosthesis stability appeared to be suboptimal. The stent's design also restricted its use to the covering of short vascular segments.

Currently Available Stent Types

Self-Expanding Stent. Many of the initial problems of self-expanding stents were solved when the coil concept was further developed and led to the use of a mesh design with several interwoven strands (Fig. 2). Such a device (Schneider-Medinvent) was the first stent to be used for clinical purposes. The stent consists of multiple (16–24) stainless steel strands of 0.06 or 0.08 mm diameter arranged in a self-expanding mesh design. The stent is flexible along its long axis, and for coronary implants its length varies between 15 and 30 mm and its diameter between 3.0 and 6.5 mm in the fully expanded state. For any given lesion a stent is selected so that its fully expanded diameter is somewhat larger than the estimated normal lumen of the recipient vessel; it is then stable once positioned and exerts a residual radial pressure on the arterial wall. For implantation (Fig. 3), the stent is compressed and thereby elongated on a delivery system. This is introduced via a standard 8-F guiding catheter over an exchange guide wire after completion of the initial balloon angioplasty.

Balloon-Expandable Stents. Several types of metallic stents mounted on angioplasty balloons have been developed more recently [23–30]. The two stent types with which most experience has been gained are made of stainless steel and are expanded to the desired diameter in situ by inflation of the balloon on which they are mounted. The Palmaz-Schatz stent (Johnson and Johnson) is a 15-mm-long stainless steel tubular structure that consists of two articulated sections (Fig. 4). The Gianturco-Roubin stent (Cook) is a longitudinally flexible stainless steel coil system that features a par-

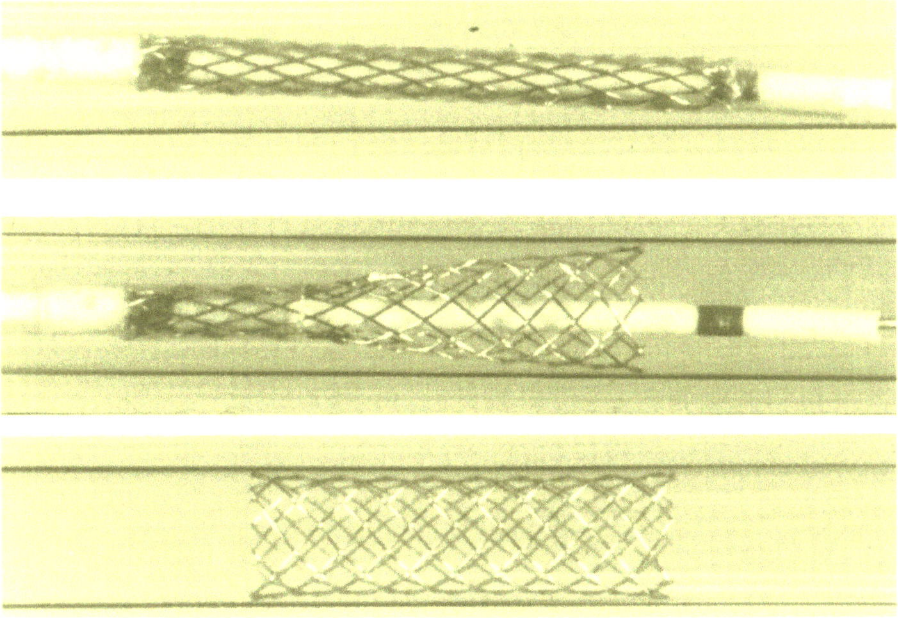

Fig. 2. Self-expanding Wallstent (Schneider-Medinvent). *Top*, stent on introducer, elongated by constraining membrane; *center*, membrane partially pulled back, stent expanding; *bottom*, stent released in definitive position

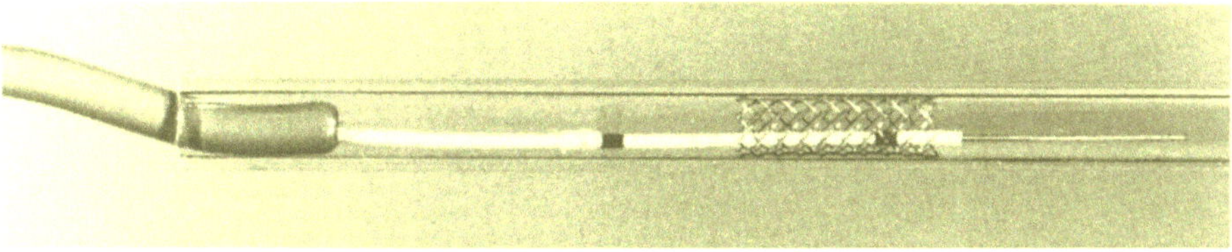

Fig. 3. Introducer and released self-expanding stent through an 8-F guiding catheter, over an exchange guidewire. (Reprinted with permission from [64])

ticularly low stent/endoluminal surface ratio (Fig. 5). Other metallic balloon-expandable stents have been developed more recently, but clinical experience with them is still rather limited. The Wiktor stent (Medtronic) [31, 32] has the advantage of being made of tantalum and is thus well visible on fluoroscopy and X-ray film, a quality not shared by stainless steel stents. The Strecker stent (Boston Scientific) [33] is also made of tantalum and has a "knitted" structure with excellent stability on the delivery balloon and good flexibility for negotiating curves. It is manufactured in several lengths

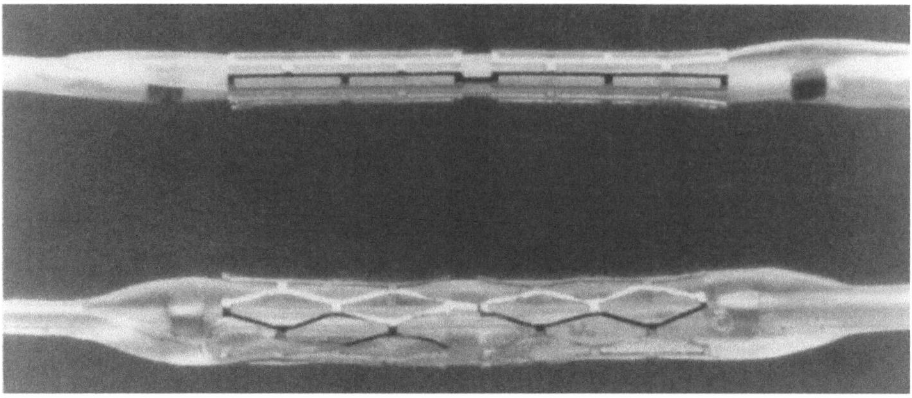

Fig. 4. Palmaz-Schatz articulated balloon expandable stent. (Reprinted with permission from [65])

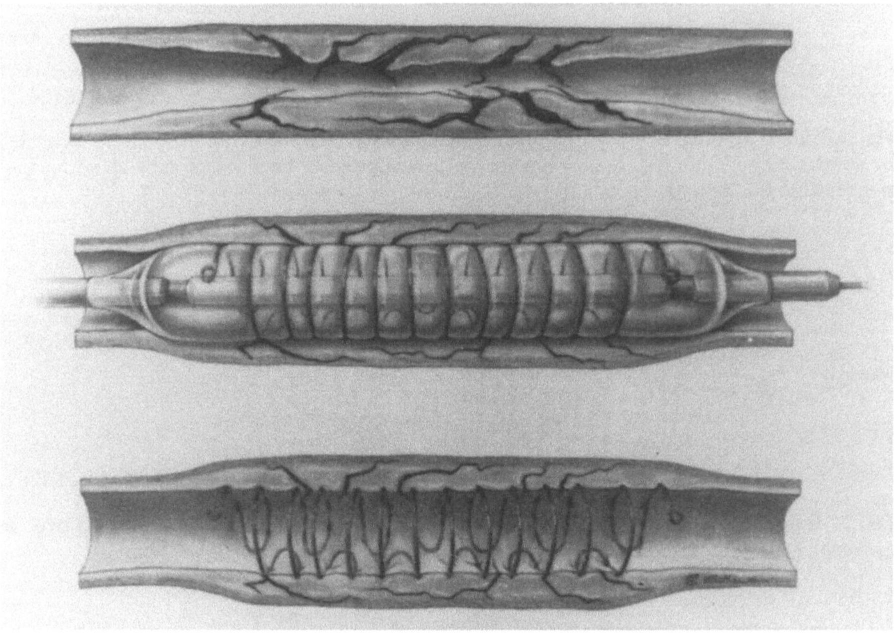

Fig. 5. Diagramatic representation of the Gianturco-Roubin balloon-expandable stent. (Courtesy of Dr. G.S. Roubin, University of Alabama, Birmingham, AL)

(from 20 to 45 mm), a feature that is shared by the self-expanding and the Gianturco-Roubin stents, and may be of importance for stenting of saphenous bypass grafts. As with the self-expanding device, all these systems require anticoagulant and antiplatelet treatment to prevent early thrombosis.

Histology

Experimental evidence in dogs, pigs, and rabbits shows that a thin fibrin and platelet layer is deposited over the stent within minutes following implantation [26, 34–37]. The stent then gradually becomes embedded in thickened intima, and the endoluminal surface is entirely covered by neoendothelium. The neoendothelial covering is completed within 1–3 weeks, depending on the type of stent and the species studied. Using a balloon expandable stent in the rabbit model, Palmaz et al. [25] observed an immature endothelial cover with a "crazy-paving" aspect after 1 week, and this was replaced by normal-appearing endothelium with flat, elongated cells at 8 weeks. The rapidity of the endothelial coating is due to the mesh design allowing islands of endothelium to grow between the stainless steel strands and eventually coalesce. With the Palmaz-Schatz stent, for example, the metal-covered surface represents only 15% of the total stented area. At 6 months there is no significant change, and the thickness of the neointima usually varies between 50 and 500 μm (Fig. 6). No pressure necrosis is seen, but thinning and slight fibrosis of the underlying media are usually observed with all stent devices [25, 26].

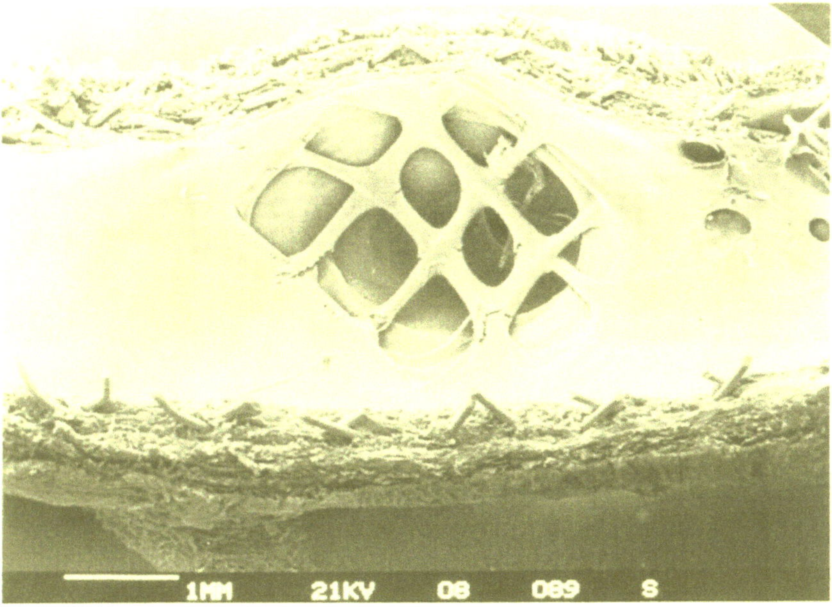

Fig. 6. Scanning electron micrograph 9 months after implantation of a self-expanding stent in a canine femoral artery. There is complete endothelial coating. A side branch orifice is covered by the stent and has remained patent. (Reprinted with permission from [34])

Data from clinical specimens are scarce [38, 39], but they essentially confirm the experimental findings: the stented segments are reendotheliazed 3–24 weeks after implantation, tissue overlying the stent wires consists primarily of smooth muscle cells, and there is minimal inflammatory reaction to the stent wires.

Clinical Use of Coronary Stents

Technique

Self-Expanding Stent. For elective stenting procedures, angioplasty of the target lesion is first carried out according to current practice, and the balloon catheter is then withdrawn leaving a long exchange guidewire (300 cm) across the lesion. The diameter of the stent is chosen so that it is about 15%–20% (0.5–1 mm) larger in its fully expanded state than the measured normal diameter of the target segment. The introducing system is advanced across the lesion over the guidewire (Fig. 7), the constraining membrane is inflated and then pulled back slowly under fluoroscopic guidance. This releases the stent into the vascular lumen, and the introducing system can be retrieved. The balloon catheter is reintroduced into the stented segment over the guidewire, and a final inflation is performed to

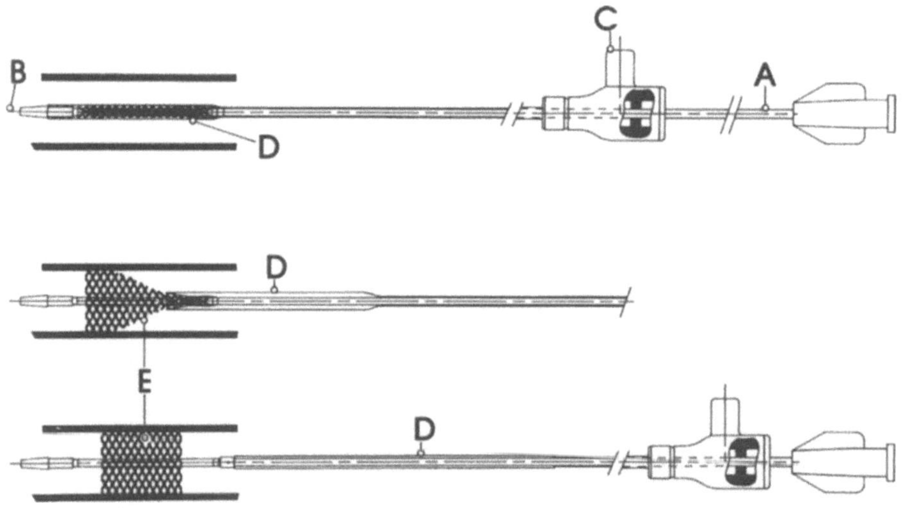

Fig. 7. Self-expanding stent and introducing system. Schematic representation. *A*, Central shaft; *B*, exchange guidewire; *C*, inflation port; *D*, constraining membrane; *E*, stent. For implantation, the constraining membrane *D* is inflated, and pulled back over the central shaft *A*. This gradually releases the stent *E*. (Reprinted with permission from [64])

"smooth" any remaining irregularities. The angiographic appearance is consistently improved compared to the immediate results of angioplasty alone, and this is confirmed both by gradient measurements [14] and by quantitative angiography [15, 40]. The technical limitations of the system are few. Distal locations in tortuous vessels can be negotiated without difficulty, and large diameter arteries or vein grafts can be treated with the same small-diameter introducing catheter (1.57 mm) since the expansion ratio of the stent is excellent (maximum unconstrained diameter available, 6.5 mm). Stability is good, and embolization, migration, or premature stent release has not been observed. However, because of poor visibility on X-ray, precise placement of the device is sometimes difficult, in particular for the less experienced operator, since the shortening of the stent and relative movements of the stent and introducing system must be correctly estimated. A margin of error of 2–5 mm should usually be allowed for.

Balloon-Expanded Stent. Most stents are premounted on standard angioplasty balloon, and the system can be exchanged after completion of the initial balloon angioplasty over a long exchange wire. Inflation of the balloon in situ expands the stent into its definitive position, and the deflated balloon is then retrieved. Using the Palmaz-Schatz model, a simple and effective alternative consists in crimping the naked stent onto the previously used angioplasty balloon to deliver it to the target site. Whatever method is used, precise positioning of balloon-expanded stents is easier than with the self-expanding type, and diameter matching of the stent and artery is reliably achieved using higher inflation pressures or a larger balloon when necessary. Immediate recoil of Palmaz-Schatz stents is minimal, although some concern has been expressed regarding the later occurrence of this during follow-up in stents implanted in vein grafts. With Strecker and Gianturco-Roubin stents a 10%–15% immediate recoil must be allowed for and the delivery balloon sized accordingly [33, 41].

Adjunct Medication

Early experimental evidence shows that heparin significantly decreases the rate of acute thrombotic occlusion when given perioperatively for stenting of normal canine arteries [34]. Other workers [26], using balloon-expandable stents, also gave heparin in the experimental setting and showed that aspirin is superior to warfarin in preventing subsequent stent thrombosis. Although the use of low molecular weight dextran remains controversial, there is some experimental evidence [36] favoring its use during the implantation procedure together with aspirin, dipyridamole, and heparin.

The drug regimen that we currently use clinically is largely empirical, and is usually prescribed for 3–6 months. It requires a high degree of patient compliance, and its importance with the current stent models available cannot be overstated. Before the procedure the patient receives aspirin in addition to his usual medication. In the catheterization laboratory intravenous heparin is administered with or without a simultaneous dextran infusion. After the procedure is completed, heparin is continued until oral anticoagulation is effective, and this is combined with aspirin and dipyridamole.

Indications

Abrupt Postangioplasty Occlusion. Sigwart et al. [34, 42] were the first to report the use of self-expanding stents to treat abrupt postangioplasty occlusion in a small group of 11 patients. There were no deaths, two patients has non-Q wave myocardial infarction, and one developed stent thrombosis 3 months after implantation. De Feyter et al. [43] also used the self-expanding device for 15 patients after angioplasty failure. There were three subacute stent occlusions, and eight patients underwent early elective surgery within 48 h after stent implantation. More recently, Roubin et al. [41] reported the use of balloon-expandable stents (Gianturco-Roubin) to treat established or threatened acute closure after angioplasty in 115 patients. Stenting was associated with a 2% in-hospital mortality, a 4% need for CABG, and a 7% occurrence of Q wave infarction. Twelve of 119 lesions (10%) were in saphenous vein grafts, but results were not reported specifically for this subgroup. Our own experience in Geneva now covers 49 patients treated for failed angioplasty with self-expanding (n = 20) or Palmaz-Schatz balloon-expandable stents (n = 41). Hospital mortality has been 4%, the need for emergent CABG 4%, and Q wave infarction has occurred in 10% of procedures. Four patients (8%) underwent semielective CABG during the same hospital stay.

Prevention of Restenosis. Initial hopes were high that stents would abolish restenosis [34], but quantitative angiographic evaluation of the early multicenter experience (elective and emergent stent procedures) with the self-expanding device has clearly demonstrated that this is not the case [44], with restenosis rates of 14% or more depending on the chosen method of evaluation. Furthermore, the same series documented a high incidence of early complications, related both to subacute stent thrombosis and bleeding because of anticoagulant treatment. The long-term follow-up (24–43 months) of the first 56 patients treated in Lausanne (59% emergent implants) was reviewed by Goy et al. [45]. Overall mortality was high, with seven deaths (12%), most of which were cardiac, but not all appeared directly stent related; stent occlusion was documented in eight cases (14%), and restenosis developed within the stent in five (9%). Schatz et al. [39] reported the use of elective stent implantation with a balloon-expandable system in 226 patients; the early stent thrombosis rate was 3.5%, major complication rate with optimized anticoagulation was only 0.6%, and 92% of patients were asymptomatic 3 months after stenting. Elective stent implantation is clearly a safer procedure than "bail-out" treatment in terms of early complications, but because of the significant risk of bleeding and/or stent thrombosis, together with the obvious fact that restenosis can be a persistent problem despite stent implantation, preliminary data of several randomized studies (BENESTENT, RENT, STRESS) suggest that stenting indeed does have an positive effect in the prevention of restenosis at least in native coronary arteries [45a].

Stenting of Venous Bypass Grafts

Specifics of Venous Grafts as Stent Recipients

In several ways, saphenous vein grafts are ideal targets for stent implantation. (a) Their diameter is usually larger than that of native coronary arteries, and this should contribute to decreasing the incidence of both acute complications [41, 46] and hemodynamically significant restenosis [44]. (b) Except for the distal anastomotic site, there are no side branches, and this makes implantation technically easier and does not jeopardize future interventions. (c) Conventional balloon angioplasty is limited by an increased risk of embolic complications and a high rate of restenosis; both of these may be partially controlled by stent implantation. (d) Several years after surgery bypass grafts are often diffusely diseased, and they thus make poor targets for PTCA. In selected cases, implantation of several stents or one single long stent may render a percutaneous approach feasible (Figs. 8, 9).

Results of Clinical Trials

Self-Expanding Stent. The first report on saphenous vein stenting was from the Lausanne group with the self-expanding device, and results were favorable [47]. Thirteen patients (14 grafts) were treated with 20 stents. Implantation was successful in all cases, and there were no major in-hospital complications. During a median follow-up of 7 months, three patients required repeat PTCA to the same graft outside the stent, and two had restenosis within the stent also treated by PTCA. There was one death from progressive congestive heart failure 7 months after stenting. The early multicenter experience with the Schneider-Medinvent self-expanding stent in venous bypass grafts up to December 1989 comprised the implantation of 146 devices to treat 109 lesions in 76 patients (Medinvent, personal communication). All procedures were technically successful. Thrombotic complications occurred in six cases (8%), one of which was successfully

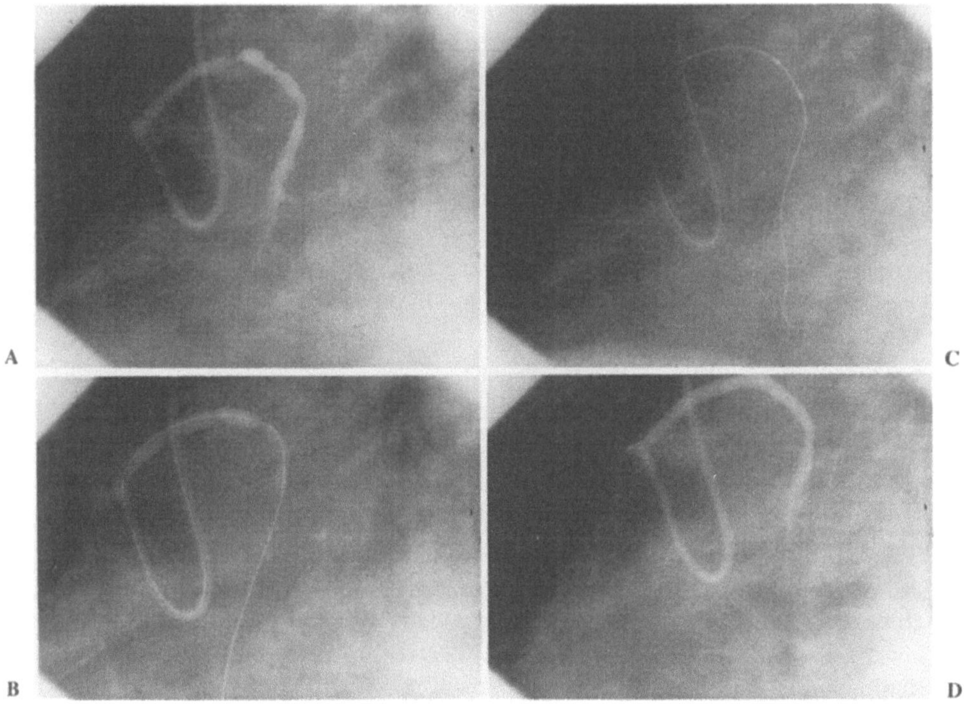

Fig. 8A–D. A 70-year-old male patient with recurrent exercise-induced angina 7 years after bypass surgery and 3 years after a first balloon angioplasty procedure to the same site. **A** Left anterior oblique projection showing a tight restenosis in the body of the venous graft to the left anterior descending coronary artery. **B** The initial indentation on the 3.5-mm balloon during angioplasty. **C** The constrained stent on its delivery system is placed across the lesion. **D** After implantation of a single 4 × 26 mm stent no residual stenosis is visible. The result was maintained at follow-up angiography 6 months later

recanalized. There were six cases of myocardial infarction (8%) and one in-hospital death. Five other patients died during follow-up, but only one of these from a cardiac cause. There were thus two cardiac deaths (3%) altogether. Overall, these results are better than those obtained in native coronary vessels in terms of acute complications [44, 45]; this is probably due mostly to the larger diameter of vein grafts and perhaps also to the lack of vasomotor tone and generally higher compliance of the grafts. Late restenosis in vein grafts has been evaluated by quantitative coronary angiography [48] of 82 follow-up films (6 months or more). Using the criterion of a greater than 50% stenosis, 15 patients were shown to have developed restenosis, a rate of 18%.

Balloon-Expandable Stents. Strumpf et al. [49] have reported the elective use of stents to treat 30 de novo and restenotic lesions in saphenous bypass grafts of 26 patients at a mean of 8.8 years following surgery. Early success

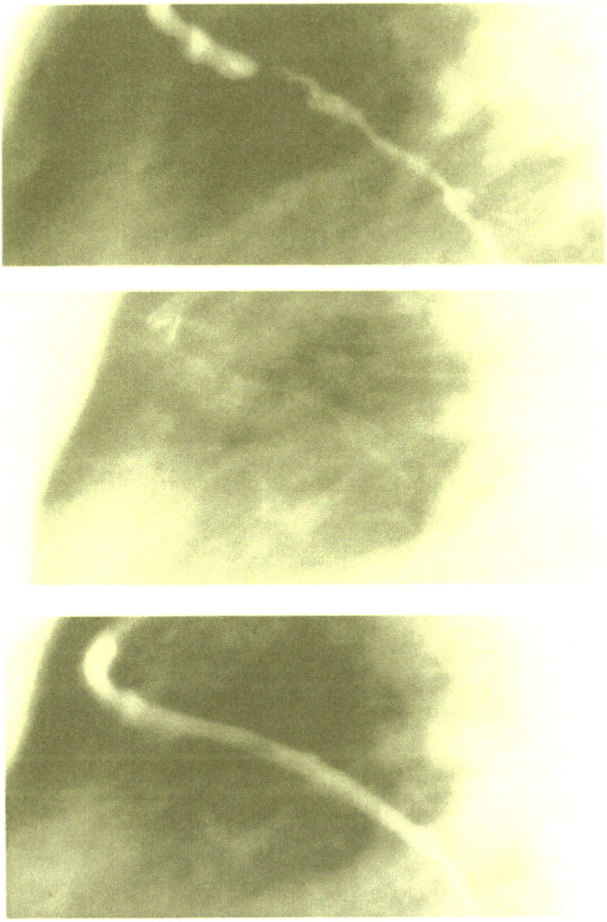

Fig. 9. *Top*, left lateral view of a diffusely diseased venous graft to a marginal branch in a 68-year-old patient with recurrent angina 8 years after bypass surgery. *Center*, after implantation three sequential self-expanding stents are visible without contrast injection. *Bottom*, the final result shows an improved lumen, with some residual irregularities

was obtained in 92% of procedures. There were two cases of distal stent embolization that were treated by a combination of thrombolytic therapy, repeat stenting, and balloon angioplasty. Two deaths occurred during follow-up, but neither of them was stent related. At follow-up 14 patients underwent control angiography, and the restenosis rate was 13%. Leon et al. [50] found a 98% technical success rate in a multicenter evaluation of Palmaz-Schatz stents in 220 saphenous vein grafts of 192 patients. Subacute thrombosis occurred in 1%, embolism in 3%, myocardial infarction in 1%, emergency bypass was required in 4%, and in-hospital mortality was 2%. The long-term restenosis rate was 28% for 99 stents with follow-up an-

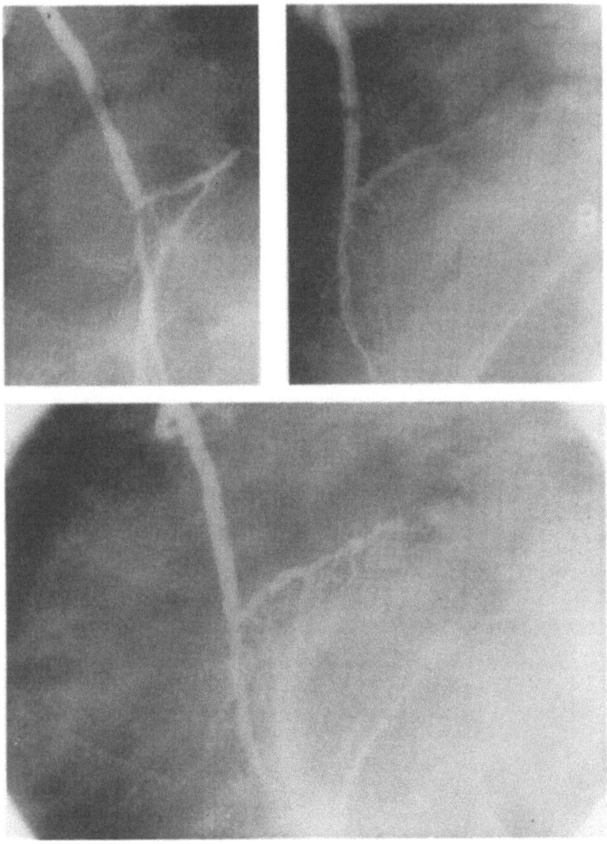

Fig. 10. 69-year-old male patient with bypass surgery 8 years previously. *Top left*, in the left lateral projection, a tight stenosis in visible in the body of the saphenous vein graft to the left anterior descending coronary artery, as well as a second lesion in the native vessel, immediately distal to the anastomosis. *Top right*, after balloon angioplasty of both sites, the result to the native vessel lesion is excellent, but a subocclusive dissection has developped in the body of the graft. The 0.014" wire is still in place. *Bottom*, final result after a single Palmaz-Schatz stent has been implanted in the body of the graft with the previoulsy used 4.0 mm monorail balloon. No residual stenosis is visible

giographic control. In addition to elective stenting, "bail-out" stenting has also been used in venous grafts: 12 of the 115 patients (10%) treated by Roubin et al. [41] for failed angioplasty had saphenous vein graft disease, and Mehl et al. [51] reported the successful use of a Palmaz-Schatz device to treat abrupt postangioplasty closure in a bypass graft. Our own experience in this indication has also been encouraging (Fig. 10).

Limitations

Thrombosis

As discussed above, the potential for stent thrombosis is quite clearly the main limitation of the current devices. It makes a short-term combined anticoagulant and antiplatelet regimen mandatory, and it creates an unstable period of up to 3 weeks during which abrupt thrombotic occlusion may occur without warning symptoms despite continued medication. This is in contrast to balloon angioplasty where acute complications are very rare beyond 24 h after the procedure. With increasing experience, several risk factors for acute stent thrombosis have become apparent.

Vessel and Stent Diameter. Small diameter stents carry a greater risk of thrombosis than do large ones [41, 52, 53], and this probably explains the lower acute and subacute occlusion rates observed in vein grafts. It is thus not recommended to stent arteries that have been treated with angioplasty balloons smaller than 3.0 mm.

Flow. Systemic hypotension, poor distal runoff, untreated stenosis proximal, and well-developed collaterals can all contribute to decreased flow through the stent and potentiate thrombus formation. It has also been our observation and that of other workers that complete coverage of the dissection is of major importance. Significant unstented inflow and outflow irregularities should probably prompt further intervention whenever possible to optimize flow.

Indication. When stenting is elective (with an appropriate vessel and stenosis morphology), the acute and subacute thrombosis rates are markedly lower than with emergent stenting following postangioplasty occlusion [54].

Stent and Vessel Mismatch. With the self-expanding stent, a diameter mismatch (ratio > 1.5) between stent and recipient vessel has been shown to be associated with thrombotic occlusion in the experimental animal. Although this degree of mismatch has not been seen in clinical practice, it may be that when the stent is somewhat large the turbulent flow at the stent extremities contributes to thrombus formation. This makes optimal sizing an important factor, especially since good impaction of the stent struts into the vessel wall is probably equally important to limit thrombus deposition [55].

Multiple Stent Implantation. Multiple stent implantation has been associated with an increased early complication rate with the Palmaz-Schatz stent [39], and this is ascribed to the overlap between the stents. This important observation concerns mainly native vessels; whether it also applies to the same degree in diffusely diseased large diameter vein grafts is not known.

Thrombocytosis. Leon et al. [53] have shown that thrombosis occurs more frequently with balloon-expandable stents when the platelet count is high.

Compliance with Drug Regimen. The drug treatment used during and after stenting has been developed empirically and is not identical in all centers, but a combination of anticoagulants and antiplatelet drugs is now regularly used by all groups. Noncompliance has been associated with an increased incidence of thrombotic complications [39, 53, 56]

Learning Curve. With increasing experience and better patient selection, acute thrombotic events have become less frequent. Provided a catheterization laboratory is immediately available, acute stent thrombosis can often be treated effectively by balloon angioplasty and thrombolytic agents [46]. When it is promptly reversible, it does not appear to compromise the long-term results.

Bleeding

Complications of bleeding from the femoral puncture site are more frequent than after angioplasty alone since the anticoagulant treatment is generally not interrupted to remove the arterial sheath. In our experience 8% of patients have required either blood transfusion or surgical revision of the femoral artery or both before leaving hospital. Recently, two different sealing devices have been developed to close the arterial puncture site after percutaneous procedures, and these will probably contribute significantly to decrease the local bleeding complications. We have used the Vasoseal collagen plug (Datascope) [57] in ten patients after coronary stenting and found that although bleeding from the puncture site still occasionally occurs, it is not severe enough to require surgery or blood transfusion.

Misplacement/Embolization

An early problem with the balloon-expandable stents was misplacement/embolization, but this has now been largely overcome. It can still be a problem with tortuous anatomy and is compounded by poor stent visibility for the stainless steel devices.

Duration of Hospital Stay and Cost

Because of the necessity to adjust the anticoagulation regimen, the hospital stay is longer than with a standard PTCA procedure and typically ranges from 3 to 6 days for an uncomplicated case. This is the major reason for the higher cost of the procedure [58], and some authors have suggested beginning warfarin therapy prior to the stenting procedure to shorten the hospital stay [59].

New Stents

Retrievable Metallic Stents. Muhlestein et al. From Duke University [60] have described the use of a tantalum single wire stent implanted percutaneously in peripheral arteries of dogs. After implantation and complete release, this can be straightened and retrieved percutaneously using a modified bioptome catheter. Such an approach could theoretically obviate the need for long-term anticoagulation. A different, basketlike device has been used by Gaspard et al. [61] to temporarily stent human coronary arteries in the clinical setting.

Biodegradabhle Devices. Use of a bioresorbable polymer has been invesigated in vitro [62] with the hope that a temporary nonmetallic support may also decrease thrombus formation and reduce the need for anticoagulant therapy.

Cellular Stent Seeding. Seeding of metallic stents with endothelial cells can be achieved in vitro, and such stents can then be implanted in the experimental animal [63]. Whether such a complex approach will contribute to decreased thrombosis and/or restenosis within the stent remains to be determined. Dichek et al. from the National Institutes of Health [63] have taken the cellular seeding concept one step further and reported the use of genetically engineered cells to markedly enhance the local secretion of tissue-type plasminogen activator after they are fixed to the stent prior to implantation. This elegant intervention is one of the ways in which drugs may be delivered locally to the stent environment. Not only may this perhaps represent a better means of ensuring antithrombotic protection than oral systemic therapy, but the day may come when stents will be used as a support for local drug delivery to a specific local or downstream target.

Conclusions

The concept of percutaneous arterial stenting was introduced over 23 years ago, but it was not until it was realized that stents can be used to address some of the limitations and complications of coronary balloon angioplasty that major interest in the technique appeared. Now, after 6 years of clinical use, although several important problems remain, coronary stenting has given us reason for optimism. The procedure has essentially lived up to initial expectations in terms of technical feasibility and reliability. It is simple to implement and constitutes the best current alternative to emergency surgery for abrupt postangioplasty closure that does not respond to conventional management. The available data also suggest that restenosis may be favorably influenced by stent implantation in selected subgroups, and several randomized studies are underway to confirm this.

However, the Achilles heel of coronary stenting obviously remains the problem of acute or subacute thrombosis. Although its incidence appears to be decreasing as the learning curve progresses, it still makes a complex drug regimen mandatory and thereby induces bleeding complications at the vascular access site. It also creates a prolonged unstable period of several weeks after implantation during which acute thrombotic occlusion may occur without warning symptoms.

Given the fact that conventional balloon angioplasty alone in vein grafts is hampered by a high risk of early embolic complications and late restenosis, stent implantation can often be a useful adjunct to a percutaneous interventional approach. Thrombotic complications also appear to be less frequent after stenting of vein grafts, probably because of their often large diameter and absence of side branches. If improvements can be made to stent design and adjunct medication so that thrombotic complications are abolished, indications for stenting of vein grafts and native coronaries will widen. With currently available devices, stents should probably be used in vein grafts for specific indications only: (a) poor angioplasty results with established or threatening occlusion, (b) selected cases of diffuse disease with a high likelihood of embolic complications following balloon angioplasty alone, and (c) restenosis after previous balloon angioplasty. The use of primary stenting to prevent subsequent restenosis, although conceptually attractive, is still only supported by preliminary data of randomized trials suggesting a beneficial effect in native coronary arteries.

References

1. Feinleib M, Havlik RJ, Gillum RF, Pkras R, McCarthy E, Moien M (1989) Coronary heart disease and related procedures: National Hospital Discharge Survey data. Circulation 79 [Suppl I]:13–8
2. Meier B, Pfisterer H, Bertel O (1992) Interventions cardiaques en Suisse. Schweiz Med Wochenschr 122:432–440
3. Chesebro JH, Fuster V, Elveback LR et al. (1984) Effect of dipyridamole and aspirin on late vein-graft patency after coronary bypass operation. N Engl J Med 310:209–214
4. Pfisterer M, Burkart F, Jockers G et al. (1989) Trial of low-dose aspirin plus dipyridamole versus anticoagulants for prevention of aortocoronary vein graft occlusion. Lancet 2:1–6
5. Bourassa MG, Fisher LD, Campeau L, Gillespie MJ, McConney M, Lesperance J (1985) Long-term fate of bypass grafts: the Coronary Artery Surgery Study (CASS) and Montréal Heart Institute experiences. Circulation 73 [Suppl V]:71–78

6. Schweiger MJ, Roccario E, Weil T (1992) Treatment of patients following bypass surgery: a dilemma for the 1990s. Am Heart J 123:268–271
7. Plokker HWT, Meester H, Serruys PW (1991) The Dutch experience in percutaneous transluminal coronary angioplasty of narrowed saphenous veins used for aortocoronary arterial bypass. Am J Cardiol 67:361–366
8. Côté G, Myler RK, Stertzer SH et al. (1987) Percutaneous transluminal angioplasty of stenotic coronary artery grafts: 5 years' experience. J Am Coll Cardiol 9:8–17
9. Douglas J, Gruentzig A, King SB, Hollman J, Ischinger T, Meier B (1983) Percutaneous transluminal angioplasty in patients with prior coronary bypass surgery. J Am Coll Cardiol 2:745–754
10. Hartmann JR, McKeever LS, Stomato NJ et al. (1991) Recanalization of chronically occluded aortocoronary saphenous vein bypass grafts by extended infusion of urokinase: initial results and short-term clinical follow-up. J Am Coll Cardiol 18:1517–1523
11. De Feyter PJ, Serruys PW, van den Brand M, Meester H, Beatt K, Suryapranata H (1989) Percutaneous transluminal angioplasty of a totally occluded venous bypass graft: a challenge that should be resisted. Am J Cardiol 64:88–90
12. Simpfendorfer C, Belardi J, Bellamy G, Galan K, Franco I, Hollman J (1987) Frequency, management and follow-up of patients with acute coronary occlusions after percutaneous transluminal coronary angioplasty. Am J Cardiol 59:267–269
13. Meier B (1988) Restenosis after coronary angioplasty: review of the literature. Eur Heart J 9 [Suppl C]:1–6
14. Sigwart U, Kaufmann U, Goy JJ, Kappenberger L (1987) Suppression of residual trans-stenotic pressure gradient after PTCA by implantation of self expanding stents (abstract). Circulation 76 [Suppl IV]:IV-186
15. Puel J, Juillière Y, Bertrand M, Rickards A, Sigwart U, Serruys PW (1988) Early and late assessment in stenosis geometry after coronary arterial stenting. Am J Cardiol 61:546–553
16. Carrel A (1912) Results of the permanent intubation of the thoracic aorta. Surg Gynecol Obstet 15:245–248
17. Dotter CT (1969) Transluminally-placed coilspring endarterial tube grafts. Invest Radiol 4:329–332
18. Dotter CT, Buschmann RW, McKinney MK, Roesch J (1983) Transluminal expandable nitinol stent grafting: preliminary report. Radiology 147:259–260
19. Cragg A, Lund G, Rysavy J, Castaneda F, Castaneda-Zuniga W, Amplatz K (1983) Nonsurgical placement of arterial endoprostheses: a new technique using nitinol wire. Radiology 147:261–263
20. Maass D, Demierre D, Deaton D, Largiader F, Senning A (1983) Transluminal implantation of self-adjusting expandable prostheses: principles, techniques and results. Prog Artif Org 27:979–987
21. Wright KC, Wallace S, Charnsangavej C, Carrasco CH, Gianturco C (1985) Percutaneous endovascular stents: an experimental evaluation. Radiology 156:69–72
22. Charnsangavej C, Carrasco CH, Wallace S et al. (1986) Stenosis of the vena cava: preliminary assessment of treatment with expandable metallic stents. Radiology 161:295–298
23. Palmaz JC, Sibbitt RR, Reuter SR, Tio SO, Rice WJ (1985) Expandable intraluminal graft: a preliminary study. Radiology 156:73–77
24. Palmaz JC, Sibbitt RR, Tio FO, Reuter SR, Peters JE, Garcia F (1986) Expandable intraluminal vascular graft: a feasibility study. Surgery 99:199–205
25. Palmaz JC, Windeler SA, Garcia F, Tio FO, Sibbitt RR, Reuter SR (1986) Atherosclerotic rabbit aortas: expandable intraluminal grafting. Radiology 160:723–726
26. Roubin GS, Robinson KA, King SB et al. (1987) Early and late results of intracoronary arterial stenting after coronary angioplasty in dogs. Circulation 76:891–897
27. Schatz RA, Tio FO, Palmaz JC (1987) Balloon expandable intravascular stents in diseased human cadaver coronary arteries (abstract). Circulation 76 [Suppl IV]:IV-26
28. Schatz RA (1989) A view of vascular stents. Circulation 79:445–457

29. Schatz RA, Palmaz JC, Penn IM, Levine SL (1989) Balloon expandable intravascular stent (BEIS) in human coronary arteries: a follow-up report (abstract). J Am Coll Cardiol 13:106A.
30. Roubin GS, Douglas JS, Lembo NJ, Black AJ, King SB (1989) Intracoronary stenting for acute closure following percutaneous transluminal coronary angioplasty (abstract). Circulation 78 [Suppl II]:II-407
31. White CJ, Ramee SR, Ross TC et al. (1988) A new percutaneous balloon expandable stent (abstract). Circulation 78 [Suppl II]:II-409
32. Van der Giessen WJ, Van Woerkens LJ, Beatt KJ, Serruys PW, Verdouw PD (1989) Coronary stenting with a radiopaque athrombogenic, balloon-expandable stent (abstract). Circulation 80 [Suppl II]:II-173
33. Hamm CW, Beythien C, Sievert H et al. (1991) First clinical experience with the Strecker-stent for acute coronary occlusion after PTCA (abstract). Circulation 84 [Suppl II]:II-198
34. Sigwart U, Puel J, Mirkovitch V, Joffre F, Kappenberger L (1987) Intravascular stents to prevent occlusion and restenosis after transluminal angioplasty. N Engl J Med 316:701–706
35. Rousseau H, Puel J, Joffre F, Sigwart U, Duboucher C, Imbert C et al. (1987) Self-expanding endovascular prosthesis: an experimental study. Radiology 164:709–714
36. Palmaz JC, Garcia OJ, Kopp DT, Schatz RA, Tio FO, Ciaravino V (1987) Balloon expandable intra-arterial stents: effect of anticoagulation on thrombus formation (abstract). Circulation76 [Suppl IV]:IV-45
37. Schatz RA, Palmaz JC, Tio FO, Garcia F, Garcia O, Reuter SR (1987) Balloon-expandable intracoronary stents in the adult dog. Circulation 76:450–457
38. Anderson P, Bajaj RK, Baxley WA, Roubin GS (1992) Vascular pathology of balloon-expandable flexible coil stents in humans. J Am Coll Cardiol 19:372–381
39. Schatz RA, Baim DS, Leon M, Ellis SG, Goldberg S, Hishfeld JW et al. (1991) Clinical experience with the Palmaz-Schatz coronary stent. Circulation 83:148–161
40. Serruys PW, Juillière Y, Bertrand M, Puel J, Rickards AF, Sigwart U (1988) Additional improvement of stenosis geometry in human coronary arteries by stenting after balloon dilatation. Am J Cardiol 61:71–6G
41. Roubin GS, Cannon AD, Agrawal SK et al. (1992) Intracoronary stenting for acute and threatened closure complicating percutaneous transluminal coronary angioplasty. Circulation 85:916–927
42. Sigwart U, Urban P, Golf S et al. (1988) Emergency stenting for acute occlusion following coronary balloon angioplasty. Circulation 78:1121–1127
43. de Feyter P, DeScheerder I, van den Brand M, Laarman G, Suryapranata H, Serruys PW (1990) Emergency stenting for refractory acute coronary occlusion during coronary angioplasty. Am J Cardiol 66:1147–1150
44. Serruys PW, Strauss BH, Beatt KJ et al. (1991) Angiographic follow-up after placement of self-expanding coronary artery stent. N Engl J Med 324:13–17
45. Goy JJ, Sigwart U, Vogt P et al. (1991) Long-term follow-up of the first 56 patients treated with intracoronary self-expanding stents (the Lausanne experience). Am J Cardiol 67:569–572
45a. Fergusen JJ (1994) Meeting highlights. Circulation 89:950
46. Sigwart U, Urban P, Sadeghi H, Kappenberger L (1989) Implantation of 100 intracoronary stents. Learning curve effect on the occurrence of acute complications (abstract). J Am Coll Cardiol 13:107A
47. Urban P, Sigwart U, Golf S, Kaufmann U, Sadeghi H, Kappenberger L (1989) Intravascular stenting for stenosis of aorto-coronary venous bypass grafts. J Am Coll Cardiol 13:1085–1091
48. Serruys PW, Reiber JH, Wijns et al. (1984) Assessment of percutaneous transluminal coronary angioplasty by quantitative coronary angiography: diameter versus densitometric area measurements. Am J Cardiol 54:482–488

49. Strumpf RK, Mehta SS, Ponder R, Heuser RR (1992) Palmaz-Schatz stent implantation in stenosed saphenous vein grafts: clinical and angiographic follow-up. Am Heart J 123:1329–1336
50. Leon MB, Ellis SG, Pichard AD, Baim DS, Heuser RR, Schatz RA (1991) Stents may be the preferred treatment for focal aortocornary vein graft disease (abstract). Circulation 84:II-249
51. Mehl JK, Schieman G, Dittrich H, Buchbinder M (1990) Emergent saphenous vein graft stenting for acute occlusion during percutaneous transluminal coronary angioplasty. Cathet Cardiovasc Diagn 21:266–270
52. Sigwart U, Kaufmann U, Golf S et al. (1988) L'incidence et le traitement de la resténose coronarienne malgré l'implantation d'une endoprothèse. Schweiz Med Wochenschr 118: 1715–1718
53. Leon MB, Almagor Y, Erbel R, Teirstein PS, Perez J, Schatz RA (1989) Subacute thrombotic events after coronary stent placement: clinical spectrum and predictive factors (abstract). Circulation 80 [Suppl II]:II-174
54. Fajadet J, Marco J, Cassagneau B, Robert G, Vandormael M (1991) Clinical and angiographic follow-up in patients recieving a Palmaz-Schatz stent for prevention or treatment of abrupt closure after coronary angioplasty (abstract). Eur Heart J 12 [Suppl]:165
55. Neville RF, Almagor Y, Bartorelli AL, Virmani R, Perlman MW, Leon MB (1989) Slotted and tubular balloon expandable stents across vein graft anastomotic sites (abstract). Circulation 80 [Suppl II]:II-259
56. Puel J, Joffre F, Rousseau H, Guermonprez B, Lancelin MC, Morice MC et al. (1987) Endo-prothèses coronariennes auto-expansives dans la prévention des resténoses après angioplastie transluminale, Arch Mal Coeur 8:1311–1312
57. Ernst J, Kloos R, Schrader R, Kaltenbach M, Sigwart U, Sanborn T (1991) Immediate sealing of arterial puncture sites after catheterization and PTCA using a vascular hemostasis device with collagen: an international registry (abstract). Circulation 84 [Suppl II]:II-68
58. Dick RJ, Popma J, Muller DWM, Burek KA, Topol E (1991) In-hospital costs associated with new percutaneous coronary devices. Am J Cardiol 68:879–885
59. Rosenschein U, Ellis SG (1992) Preprocedure warfarinization and brachial approach for elective coronary stent placement – a possible strategy to decrease cost and duration of hospitalization. Cathet Cardiovasc Diagn 25:290–292
60. Muhlestein JB, Quigley PJ, Mikat EM, MacGregor DC, de Coriolis P, Stack RS (1989) Percutaneous removal of endovascular stents: initial experimental results (abstract). Circulation 80 [Suppl II]:II-259
61. Gaspard PE, Didier BP, Delsanti GL (1990) The temporary stent catheter: a non operative treatment for acute occlusion during coronary angioplasty (abstract). J Am Coll Cardiol 15:118A
62. Slepian MJ, Schindler A (1988) Polymeric endoluminal paving/sealing: a biodegradable alternative to intracoronary stenting (abstract). Circulation 78 [Suppl II]: II-409
63. Dichek DA, Neville RF, Zweibel JA, Freeman SM, Leon MB, Anderson WF (1989) Seeding of intravascular stents with genetically engineered endothelial cells. Circulation 80:1347–1353
64. Sigwart U, Urban P (1989) Use of coronary stents following balloon angioplasty. In: Brannwald E (ed) Heart disease, vol 5 (update 1989). Saunders, Philadelphia, p 111
65. Ellis SG (1990) The Palmaz-Schatz stent: ptential coronary applications. In: Topol E (ed) Textbook of interventional carduology. Saunders, Philadelphia, p 625

Reoperation: Techniques and Choice of Conduits

L.K. von Segesser and M.I. Turina

Introduction

Successful primary coronary artery revascularization results not only in relief of pain but also prolongation of life. The Coronary Artery Surgery Study (CASS) showed significantly lower rate of fatal myocardial infarctions in patients with surgical coronary artery revascularization than in those with medical treatment [25]. However, longer follow-up periods brought up an increasing number of patients with recurrent angina pectoris. Recurrent myocardial ischemia after surgical coronary artery revascularization can be due to various causes, including inadequate patient selection, technical errors, incomplete primary revascularization, graft to coronary artery mismatch, graft failure, progression of coronary artery disease, and all sorts of combinations. Compilation of late patency rates (Fig. 1) for saphenous vein grafts and internal thoracic artery grafts reported in 26 studies summarizing the results of far more than 10000 coronary artery revascularization procedures showed a long-term patency rate at 10-year follow-up of 72% ± 20% for internal thoracic artery grafts compared to 55% ± 21% for saphenous vein graft ([38]; see chapter by Loop, this volume).

Obviously, one of the most predominant factors responsible for recurrent myocardial ischemia is the so-called vein graft disease. An angiography of a vein graft performed in a patient with recurrent angina during late follow-up is depicted in Fig. 2. The fact that the macroscopic appearance of angiographically diseased vein grafts is in most cases worse (Fig. 3) than expected is a common finding. Finally, the microscopic analysis shows the atheromatous nature of the lesions detected in the diseased vein graft (Fig. 4). Sergeant et al. [30] reported the return of angina within a period of 15–20 years after surgery in most patients. Fox et al. [11] estimated that as many as 7% of patients who have had an aortocoronary bypass operation will require a second bypass procedure within 10–12 years. Cosgrove et al. [7] found an annual incidence of reoperation of 12% at 5 years and 3.9% at 12 years.

The exact mechanism of venous graft disease is still not fully understood. A number of contributing mechanisms have been described, including hydraulic problems related to the important disparity of diameters for saphenous vein grafts and coronary arteries, difficulties in maintaining the

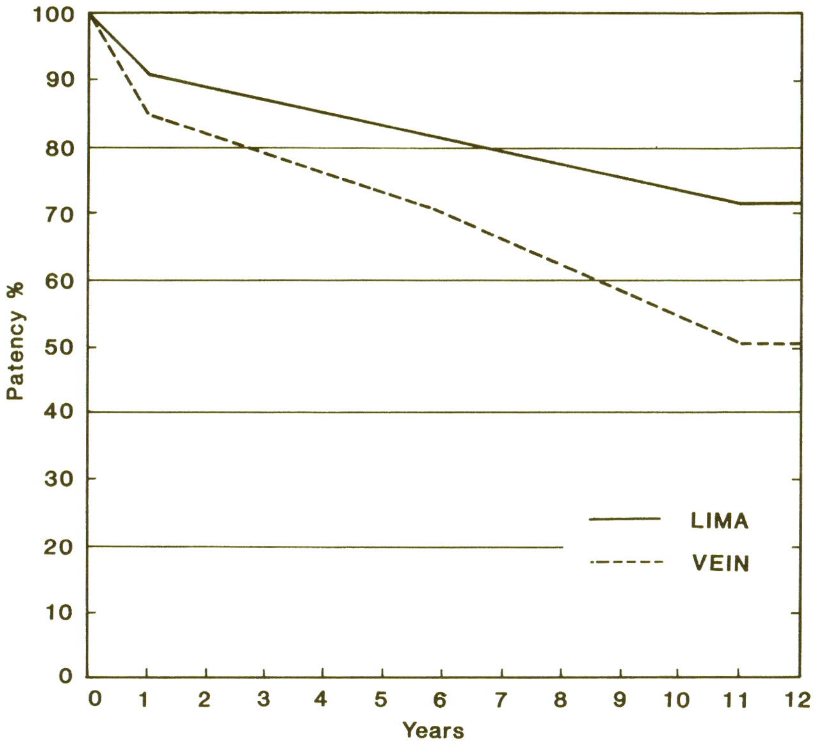

Fig. 1. Patency rates of left internal thoracic artery grafts onto the left anterior descending coronary artery (*continuous line*) in comparison to saphenous vein grafts (*dashed line*). (*Data compiled by von Segesser [38] from 26 studies reported in the literature*)

endothelial cell lining in venous grafts during harvesting [16], less pronounced vasomotor activity of saphenous vein grafts [18], more marked smooth muscle cell proliferation due to pulsatile stretch observed for saphenous vein grafts [27], and others. However, bypass attrition can occur even if coronary artery revascularization is by the means of the internal thoracic artery. Lytle et al. [19] reported stenoses of the internal thoracic artery in as many as 9% of patients within 22 months. Furthermore, deterioration of saphenous vein grafts implanted for complementary revascularization as well as progression of coronary artery disease of the distal coronary bed may lead to repeat coronary artery revascularization even if the internal thoracic artery is functioning perfectly well.

Indications of Reoperation

Although the indications for repeat coronary artery revascularizations are similar to those for primary procedures in theory, and include proven

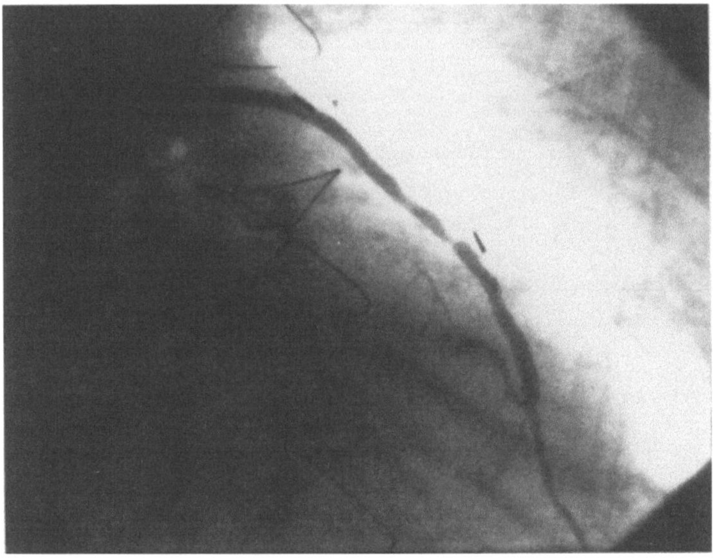

Fig. 2. Coronary artery angiogram. Direct injection of an aortocoronary artery saphenous vein graft established 4 years earlier. A significant stenosis is clearly visible

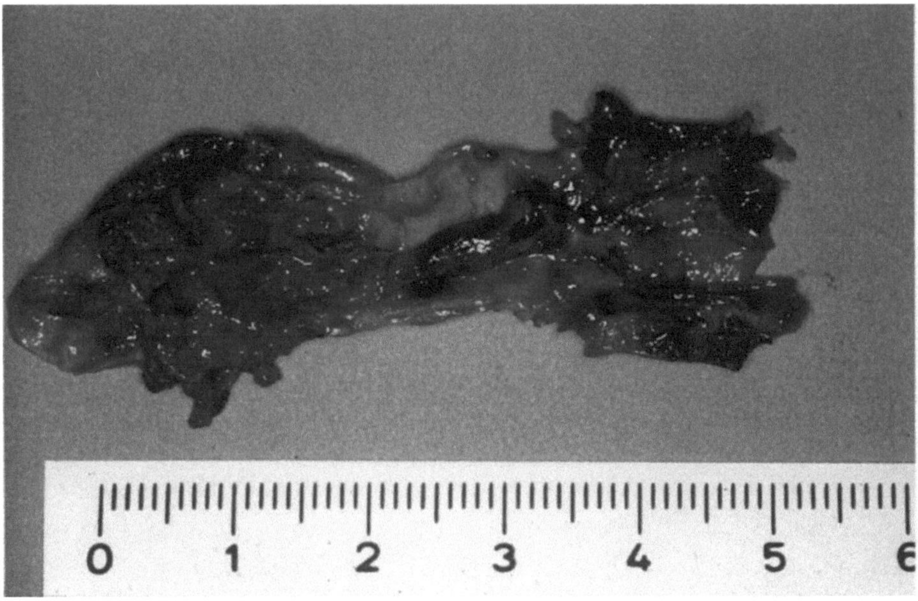

Fig. 3. Macroscopic view of a saphenous vein graft removed during reoperation because of significant vein graft disease. As usual, the macroscopic view is very impressive

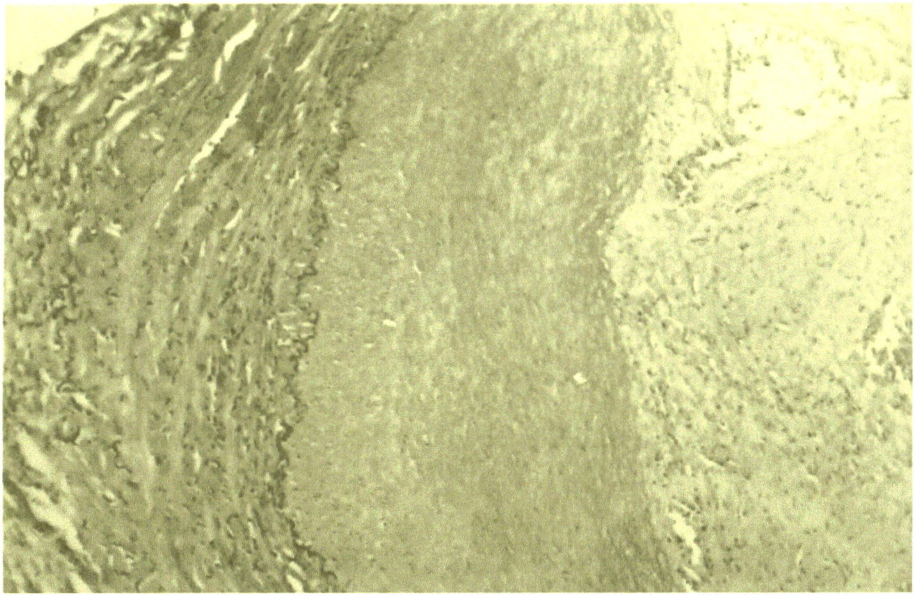

Fig. 4. Microscopic view of a venous aortocoronary bypass with significant graft disease

ischemia, favorable coronary artery anatomy, adequate graft material, sufficient ventricular function, and acceptable general condition, practically repeat procedures are performed mainly for symptomatic purposes as prognostic indications rarely apply. This is due to the fact that repeat procedures carry higher morbidity and mortality rates than primary procedures [1]. Hence, thorough individual evaluation of each case is mandatory, as a specific function of clinical presentation, myocardial mass at risk, anatomy of native coronary arteries and other conduits, potentially available bypass material and its quality, and required associated procedures. The benefit of possible repeat procedure must be carefully balanced against its potential risk.

Choice of Conduits in Repeat Revascularization Procedures

The choice of conduits for repeat coronary artery proceduers is somewhat different from that for primary operations. By definition, part of the theoretically available graft material has already been harvested for the primary procedure and is no longer available. Some potential conduits may also have been damaged despite the fact that they had not been used for revascularization. In the past, unplanned ligation of the internal thoracic artery occurred quite often if large peristernal bands made from stainless steel (or synthetic materials) were used for sternal closure. In other cases the internal thoracic artery has been ligated deliberately because of bleeding complications. Another problem specific to repeat procedures is the evaluation of grafts with respect to the potential graft flow. This is of prime importance if patent venous grafts must be replaced. To avoid potential mismatch between a new graft and the coronary artery bed to be revascularized, the dependent myocardial mass must be carefully evaluated and the new conduit be selected accordingly.

The internal thoracic artery is the best graft available for coronary revascularisation [2, 5, 9, 19, 38, 44]. This is true not only for primary revascularizations but also for secondary procedures [6, 20]. As mentioned above, the superiority of the internal thoracic artery with regard to patency is not fully understood, and many potential mechanisms have been suggested. Obviously the internal thoracic artery even in situ is less prone to develop atheromatous lesions than the coronary arteries [15]. The fact that the wall of internal thoracic arteries is mainly of the elastic type may play a role (Fig. 5). However, other factors are also involved, including the reduced number of anastomoses in pedicled grafts, similar size as coronary arteries resulting in low Reynolds numbers at the anastomoses, intact endothelial lining [16] with potential antithrombotic prostacyclin secretion [24], responsiveness to vasoactive mediators [31], endothelium-dependant relaxation [18] due to nitric oxide [32], and the resistance to pulsatile stretch [27]. On the

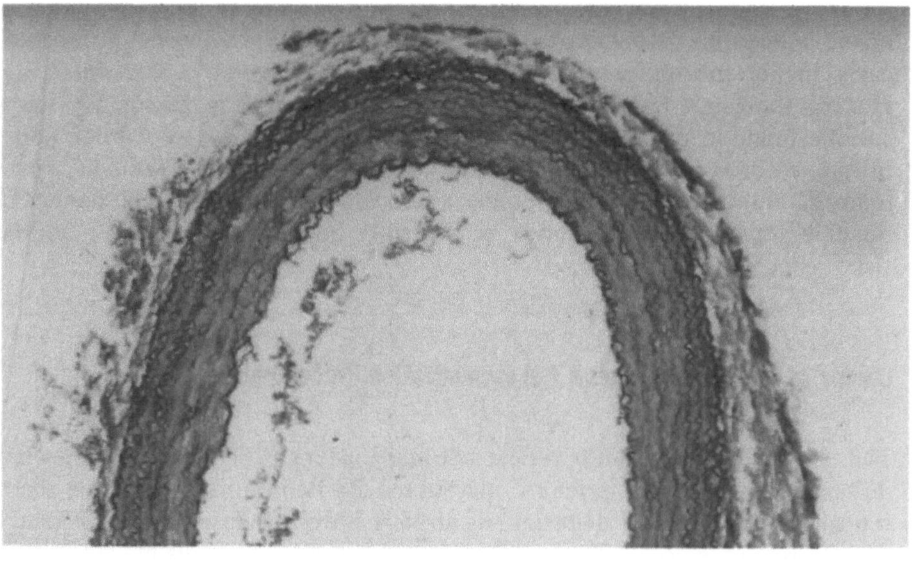

Fig. 5. Microscopic view of an internal thoracic artery which is a vessel of the elastic type. It is still not fully understood why the internal thoracic arteries are less prone to artherosclerosis

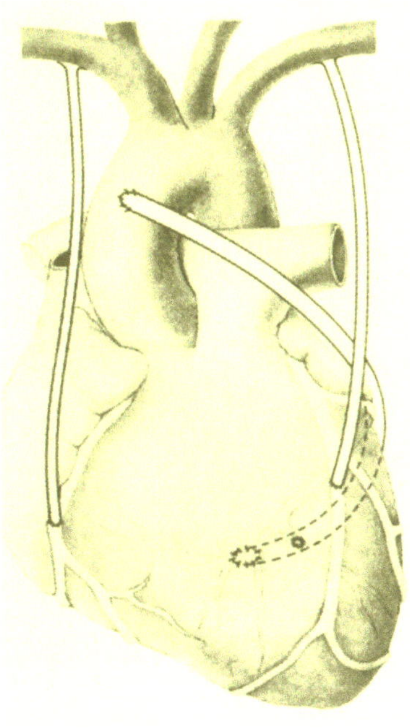

Fig. 6. Optimized coronary artery revascularization procedures include one or two internal thoracic artery grafts in combination with saphenous vein grafts

other hand, one must consider that in the immediate perioperative period the internal thoracic artery provides less flow than a vein graft, and that the former needs a few weeks to develop its full capacity to deliver blood to the myocardium. As a result, a widely patent vein graft supplying a large myocardial area should not be replaced with an internal thoracic artery alone [26, 40]. Hence, if still available, a proper combination (Fig. 6) of one or two internal thoracic arteries in conjunction with complimentary saphenous vein grafts is recommended to be used (or reused) for repeat coronary artery revascularization [12]. Additional length of the internal thoracic artery to reach more distal and/or multiple coronary sites can be achieved by using this conduit as a free graft. For the latter procedure, some authors have, however, reported long-term results similar to those achieved with saphenous vein grafts [17].

Various other arterial grafts can be used if the internal thoracic arteries are no longer available, and/or if no adequate venous grafts can be found. The right gastroepiploic artery is probably the most widely used arterial graft after the internal thoracic artery [20, 22, 29, 33]. The vessel wall of the gastroepiploic artery is of the muscular type (Fig. 7), and as a result this artery is more prone to spastic reactions. Furthermore, artherosclerotic lesions are also encountered more often in this vessel [8]. This finding is not surprising as abdominal angina due to occlusion of visceral arteries is a clinical reality. Considering the well-known anatomical varieties of the

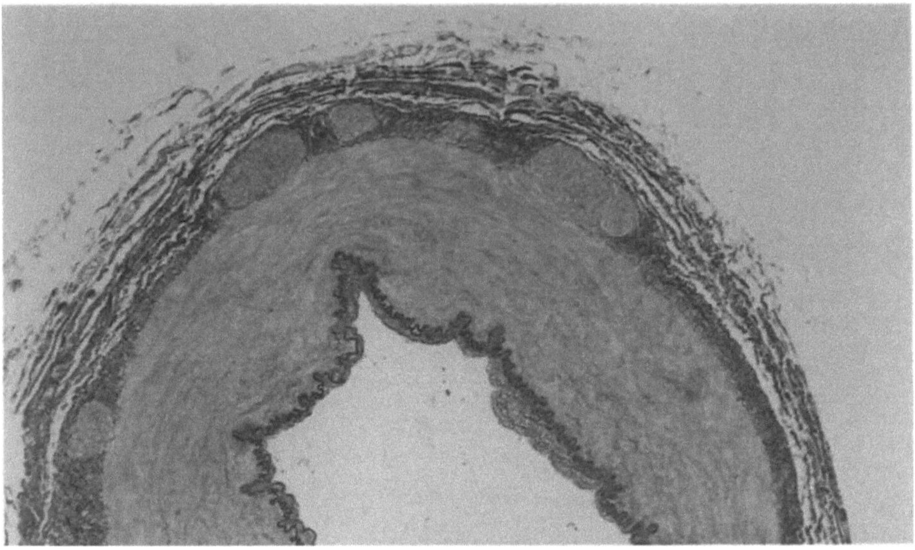

Fig. 7. The right gastroepiploic artery is a vessel of the muscular type. Hence, spastic reactions are more common and more severe than with internal thoracic artery grafts

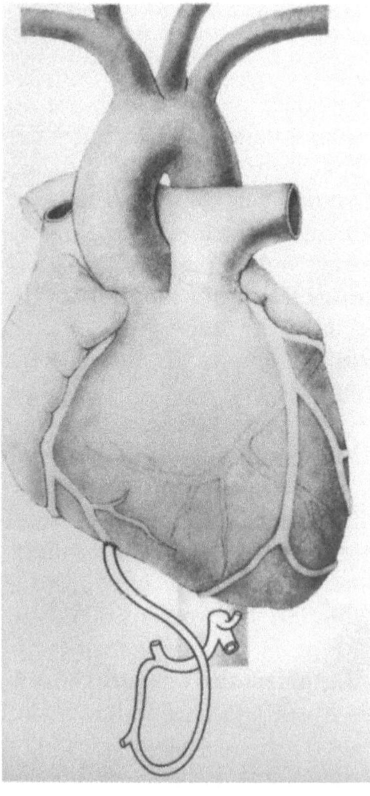

Fig. 8. The posterior descending coronary artery can be revascularized with the right gastroepiploic artery

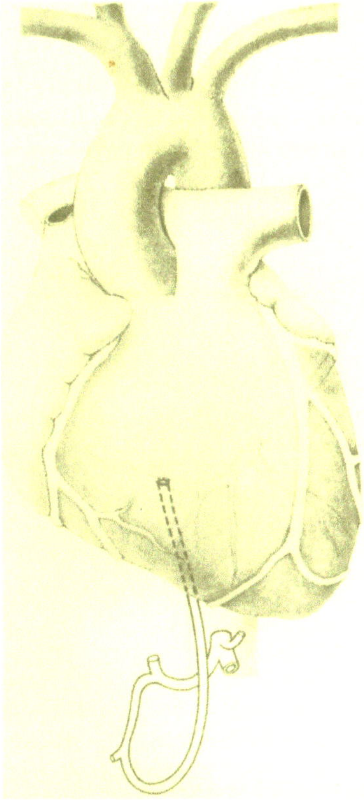

Fig. 9. The right gastroepiploic artery can also be used for revascularization of marginal branches

branches of the celiac trunk, preoperative angiography is strongly recommended. If a suitable right gastroepiploic artery is found, it can be routed ante- or retrogastrically through the diaphragm onto the distal right coronary artery or to the posterior descending coronary artery (Fig. 8). More complex but also more delicate revascularizations can also be carried out the branches of the circumflex artery (Fig. 9). Despite the fact that series of 200 patients receiving a right gastroepiploic artery graft have been now reported [34] no long-term results are yet available, and some concern remains with regard to the devascularized stomach as well as the potential problems in the event of major visceral surgery later on. Another conduit that has been used for myocardial revasularization is the epigastric artery. Only sporadic reports are available about its superior part, which is used in a pedicled fashion [38]. The inferior epigastric artery can be used only as a free aortocoronary graft and seems to be more suitable for myocardial revascularization [28]. As with other free grafts, the aortic anastomosis is the main problem with this type of graft. Specific problems with the inferior epigastric artery can occur in cases with previous use of internal thoracic arteries where necroses of the abdominal wall have been reported.

A number of other arterial grafts [42] have been used in the past, including the radial artery, lateral thoracic artery, subclavian artery, splenic artery, and others. Although there may be a place for such conduits in specific situations, there are as yet no long-term results in larger studies availaible except the radial artery, which has proven to be prone to early stenoses.

Surgical Techniques for Repeat Revascularization Procedures

In our experience, a systematic approach to repeat coronary artery revascularization as outlined in the following section is of major help in optimizing not only the repeat procedure per se but also, and even more importantly, the final outcome.

Evaluation of Conduits

Careful evaluation of the potentially available conduits is performed routinely in patients scheduled for repeat coronary artery revascularization. Following inspection of the remaining veins, phlebography is performed if questionable material is expected. Subclavian and internal thoracic artery arteriography is routine for patients undergoing coronary catheterization in-house. As reported by Bauer et al. [4], up to 26% of surgically significant anomalies can be recognized preoperatively. In this study angiographic visualization of the internal thoracic artery resulted in modification of the surgical strategy in 4% of the patients. Some information about internal thoracic artery flow can also be obtained by Doppler studies, and we take advantage of these techniques in patients coming to surgery without internal thoracic artery angiography. Likewise, the celiac trunk and right gastroepiploic artery are visualized during cardiac catheterization in patients in whom this conduit is likely to be used. The inferior epigastric artery and celiac trunk and its branches can also be studied with Doppler techniques.

Opening of the Chest

Some years ago resternotomy was a major problem because of the sometimes extremely tight scar between the heart and the sternum. However, this has been greatly simplified with the introduction of the oscillating saw, and injury to the heart and great vessels are now exceptional. Although the groin is still prepared for potential use during the procedure, i.e., cannulation of the femoral artery or intra-aortic balloon insertion, this site is now rarely used before sternotomy. After careful sternal division and atraumatic mobilization of the posterior sternal wall on both sides, the innominate vein must be freed before initial spreading of the sternum. An alternative approach to avoid reopening of the median sternotomy is the left thoracotomy, as suggested for reoperative bypass procedures by Ungerleider et al. [36]. Although suitable coronary artery anatomy and coronary lesion distribution limit the number of patients who can be revascularized completely, this route has been used successfully in 23/1176 repeat procedures, as reported by Uppal et al. [37].

Harvesting of Conduits

Parallel to the saphenous vein harvesting, if performed, one or two internal thoracic arteries are taken down in the usual fashion. Sometimes, there is an important amount of scarring tissue that makes this procedure more difficult. If the internal thoracic arteries have not been used or damaged during the first procedure, and this should be known from the preoperative screening examinations, these vessels are the conduits of first choice. Furthermore, right gastroepiploic and/or epigastric arteries are prepared as deemed necessary. It is of primary importance to have adequate bypass material prepared to choose from before the revascularization procedure itself begins. Exact operative tactics are decided from the knowledge of flow rates in prepared conduits and from the estimated amount of necessary flow after implantation (myocardial mass at risk).

Freeing of the Heart, Cannulation, and Identification of Target Vessels

Exposure of the anterior surface of the heart and ascending aorta are carried out progressively, and early cannulation is recommended. For this purpose the ascending aorta must be carefully evaluated to avoid atheromatous lesions. Previous cannulation sites may be of unpredictable wall thickness and are best avoided. If it is difficult to find an adequate cannulation site on a crowded ascending aorta, the arch or the descending thoracic aorta may be more suitable. Alternatively, a special thin-walled aortic cannula designed to be introduced with Seldinger's technique may be placed through the innominate artery, an aortic site with Teflon felt residues from previous procedures, or the femoral artery. Handling of previous grafts is a controversial problem. Basically, the no-touch technique is used as long as the heart is beating, and early ligation of diseased grafts is recommended thereafter to avoid distal embolization of debris. However, retrograde embolization into the aorta or, worse, the carotid arteries of clots coming from occluded grafts must also be avoided. Exact knowledge about the previous procedure is of significant help, as new grafts can be implanted distally from previous grafts and the latter can be identified due to their tendency to provoke adhesions. In some cases the previous grafts are not where they are supposed to be, and proper identification of the coronary arteries can be extremely difficult. When very dense adhesions are encountered, the aorta is cross-clamped, and cardioplegia is applied; freeing of the heart is greatly simplified with flaccid nonbeating heart.

Myocardial Protection

Adequate myocardial protection during repeat coronary artery revascularization procedures is a major issue. In our hands, combined antegrade and retograde techniques with blood cardioplegia have provided the best results in cases with vein grafts and/or occluded internal thoracic artery grafts. However, in patients with patent internal thoracic artery grafts these now classical techniques may be inadequate even if the internal thoracic artery pedicle was controlled and clamped. Hence, in some cases with patent internal thoracic artery grafts, adequate standstill of the heart can be achieved only if profound hypothermia is used [38]. Alternatively, warm heart surgery with continuous blood cardioplegia can be used even if the internal thoracic artery flow cannot be interrupted. Under these circumstances, however, the blood cardioplegia supply must be maintained continuously. In cases requiring relatively simple procedures directed to the anterior descending, right, or posterior descending coronary arteries the revascularizations may be performed in the fibrillating heart without aortic cross-clamping. This approach is not recomended for revascularization of the branches of the circumflex coronary artery. Isolated procedures directed to the latter vessels are better performed through a left thoracotomy [37].

Repeat Revascularization Procedure

Purposeful, expedient revascularisation reaching main vessels (≥1.5 mm) supplying large myocardial mass is performed. As mentioned above, final selection of grafts is determined by the quality of the conduit material available.At least one internal thoracic artery should be used whenever possible. Also in repeat procedures internal thoracic artery grafting can be performed safely if the new graft provides additional flow to the revascularized myocardium. If the new graft is a substitute for a patent previous graft, it is recommended to select a conduit providing at least as much flow as the one to be replaced. Flow measurement, either volumetric or with flowprobes (electromagnetic or ultraconic), helps to reach adequate decisions. Low arterial graft flow can be improved in many cases by hydrostatic graft dilatation using diluted papaverin solution. One must consider here that in the early phase a proper saphenous vein graft provides 2.7 times more flow than an internal thoracic artery. These comparative measurements were made for the same coronary artery bed by Flemma et al. in 1975 [10]. Therefore, if available, saphenous vein grafts also have a place in repeat procedures and especially in critical repeat procedures. All other types of arterial grafts described above are used mainly if proper internal thoracic artery and/or saphenous vein grafts are not available in sufficient quantity and/or quality.

Adequate Reperfusion and Monitoring

Adequate reperfusion before and after removal of the cross-clamp is as necessary as careful hemodynamic monitoring in the postoperative period. Doubtfully revascularized areas can be identified very early by graft flow measurements, transesophageal echocardiographic studies with or without contrast media, or thermographic methods. If inadequate graft flow is detected, immediate restoration of coronary artery flow is mandatory to prevent disasterous consequences [40]. Maintenance of acceptable arterial pressure during the weaning process and the postoperative period is important not only because driving pressure is the main component determining arterial graft flow but also because complete revascularization cannot always be achieved in repeat procedures, and therefore some myocardial areas may remain dependent on collateral flow.

Results of Repeat Revascularization Procedures

Experience at Zurich University Hospital

Patients and Methods. Over a 10-year period (1982–1991) we performed at our institution a total of 3706 consecutive coronary artery bypass procedures. During the same period 148 patients (139 men, 9 women) required repeat revascularization procedures. The secondary revascularization procedure was performed as outlined above and as previously reported [38].

For this study the patient charts, surgical protocols, and data obtained by systematic follow-up were analyzed retrospectively and completed with the information achieved with an questionnaire that was sent to the patients and/or their current physician. The results found are expressed as the proportion of patients with complete data. Perioperative myocardial imfarctions were diagnosed if two or more of the following criteria were present: creatine kinase more than three times normal and myocardial fraction more than 10%, significant Q wave in ECG and impaired ventricular function in postoperative echocardiography, angiogram, or isotope study. Long-term follow-up was analyzed in actuarial fashion (life table analysis).

Results. The mean age of the reoperated patients as the time of the secondary procedure was 58.4 ± 7.5 years (range 36–76 years), and the mean interval between primary and secondary procedure was 8.0 ± 4.3 years (range 1–21 years). The following risk factors were identified for these patients: smoking in 36%, obesity in 29%, hyperlipidemia in 22%, arterial hypertension in 17%, and diabetes mellitus in 5%. Over 50% of the patients (77/148) had at least two risk factors. Prior to reoperation the patients were classified by the New York Heart Association system (NYHA) as follows: functional class I 2/146 (1%), II 17/146 (12%), III 92/146 (63%), and IV 35/146 (24%). There were 2.7 ± 1.2 distal anastomoses established at the primary procedure, and 2.5 ± 1.0 vessels were revascularized at the reoperation (mean cross-clamp time 51 ± 29 min). The primary venous grafts were used exclusively in 133/141 (96%), and only 8/141 (5%) received arterial grafts. Arterial grafts were used whenever possible at the second procedure; at least one arterial graft was used in 120/141 patients (85%) whereas 15% of the patients with critical hemodynamic condition or unavailability of arterial grafts received only vein grafts. Mortality (30 days) was 6/148 (4%). The most important complications included excessive bleeding in 14/148 (9%), necessity of intra-aortic balloon pump in 13/148 (9%), myocardial infarction in 13/148 (9%), and infection in 12/148 (8%). NYHA classification at early follow-up revealed functional status class I in 60/132 (46%), II in 60/132 (46%), III in 11/132 (8%), and IV in 1/132 (1%). Hence the mean functional class of the reoperated patients was 1.6 ± 0.6 after surgery compared to 3.1 ± 0.6 before surgery ($p < 0.0005$). During the follow-up period of 51 ± 31 months (range 7–120 months) an additional 16 patients died, resulting in a total mortality of 22/148 patients (15%) over

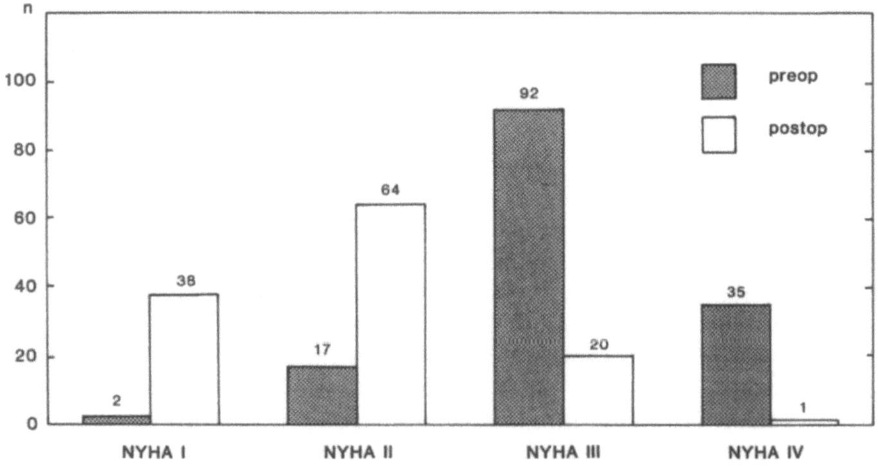

Fig. 10. NYHA functional class before and after repeat coronary artery revascularizations ($p < 0.0005$)

the study period of 120 months. Actuarial analysis showed a cumulative survival rate after repeat coronary revascularization of 93% after 1 year, 88% after 5 years, and 84% after 10 years of follow-up. Actual functional status in terms of the NYHA classification at the time of the last follow-up (51 ± 31 months after reoperation) was I in 38/123 (31%), II in 64/123 (52%), III in 20/123 (16%), and IV in 1/123 (1%; Fig. 10). Hence at this time the mean NYHA functional class of 1.9 ± 0.7 was still significantly better than before reoperation (3.1 ± 0.6; $p < 0.0005$).

Review of the Literature

Mean Interval Between Primary and Secondary Revascularization. Compared to earlier studies there are now increasingly higher intervals between primary and secondary revascularization procedures reported. The mean interval of 8.0 ± 4.3 years observed for our patients compares favorably to the figures reported in the literature. Accola [1] reported a mean interval of 5.3 years for first reoperations, 4.9 for second reoperations, and 4.7 for third reoperations. An interval of 8.2 years, very similar to ours, was reported by Cameron et al. in 1988 [5]. In the study of Lytle and colleagues [21] the interval increased from 50 ± 36 months for patients operated upon between 1967 and 1978, to 72 ± 44 months in the period between 1979 and 1981, and finally 84 ± 47 months for the period between 1982 and 1984.

Early Mortality. A large variation in perioperative mortality is reported for redo coronary artery revascularization procedures. Lytle et al. [21] observed a mortality rate of 4.6% between 1967 and 1978 compared to 3.4% between 1982 and 1984. Very similar results were achieved in our hands, where 30-day mortality was 4.0%. However, a perioperative mortality rate of 7.5% was reported by Accola et al. [1] for the third and fourth procedures whereas 4.7% was reported by Cameron et al. [5] for the second operation. Ivert et al. [13] reported a 6.0% mortality rate while Galbut et al. [12] reported 6.8%. Considering these figures, there can be no doubt that mortality in repeat operations is higher than that in primary revascularizations procedures, where the figures of 2.4% are given by Cameron [5], and we observed 1.8% [38].

Rate of Myocardial Infarcations. Occurrence of perioperative myocardial infarction is more difficult to compare in the studies reported in the literature as the criteria for diagnosis are not standardized. In our hands and using the same criteria, we noted a 9% rate in secondary revascularization procedures compared to 3% in primary operations. Lytle reported a 7.2% myocrdial infarction rate in reoperation procedures for the period 1967–1978 and 8.0% for the period 1982–1984. Other authors have observed an even higher incidence of perioperative myocardial infarction for repeat revascularization procedures; Ivert et al. [13] reported 13%, and Accola et al. [1] reported 11% for multiple reoperative grafting.

Late Results. Late cumulative survival rates for patients undergoing repeat coronary artery revascularizations have been computed by Cameron et al. [5]. In this study, with internal thoracic artery grafts in 71% of the reoperations, the survival rates at 5 and 10 years for the reoperation group were 86% and 82%, respectively, and for the initial operation group 89% and 78%, respectively. Deaths from any cause were included, as in our study, where we found a cumulative survival rate in reoperated patients of 88% at 5 years and 84% at 10 years. Galbut et al. [12] using bilateral internal mammary artery implants at reoperation found among the hospital survivors (100%) a survival rate of 85% after 5 years. Lytle et al. [21] reported, again for hospital survivors only, a survival rate of 90% at 5 years and 75% at 10 years.

Conclusions

Repeat coronary artery revascularization procedures are an effective treatment for recurrent myocardial ischemia following primary myocardial revascularizartions. Excellent long-term results can be achieved if the patients undergoing such revascularizations procedures are carefully selected. However, repeat coronary artery revascularizations are much more demanding surgical procedures, and mortality and morbidity are significantly higher than in primary procedures. Hence, the primary objective must be to avoid repeat revascularizations. For this purpose, complete coronary artery revascularization and systematic use of the best grafting material available, i.e., the internal thoracic arteries, at the primary procedure as well as secondary prophylaxis with regard to all identified risk factors is recommended.

References

1. Accola KA, Craver JM, Weintraub WS, Guton RA, Jones EL (1991) Multiple reoperative coronary bypass grafting. Ann Thorac Surg 52:738–744
2. Acinpura AJ, Rose DM, Jacobowitz IJ et al. (1989) Internal mammary artery bypass grafting: influence on recurrent angina and survival in 2100 patients. Ann Thorac Surg 48:186–191
3. Attum AA (1987) The use of the gastroepiploic artery for coronary artery bypass graft. Another alternative. Tex Heart Inst J 14:289–292
4. Bauer E, Bino MC, von Segesser LK et al. (1990) Internal mammary artery anomalies. Thorac Cardiovasc Surg 38:312–315
5. Cameron A, Kemp HG, Green GE (1988) Reoperation for coronary artery disease: 10 years of clinical follow-up. Circulation 78 [Suppl I]: 158–162

6. Coltharp WH, Decker MD, Lea JW IV et al. (1991) Internalmammary artery graft at reoperation: risks, benefits, and methods of preservation. Ann Thorac Surg 52:225–229
7. Cosgrove DM, Loop FD, Lytle BW et al. (1986) Predictors of reoperation after myocardial revascularization. J Thorac Cardiovasc Surg 92:811–821
8. Domeisen H (1992) Ausmass der Arteriosklerose der Arteria gastroepiploica dextra und der Koronarien. Thesis, University of Zurich
9. Fiore AC, Naunheim KS, McBride LR et al. (1991) Fifteen year follow-up for double internal thoracic artery grafts. Eur J Cardiothorac Surg 5:248–252
10. Flemma RJ, Singh HM, Tector AJ, Lepley D, Frazier BL (1975) Comparative hemodynamic properties of vein and mammary artery in coronary bypass operations. Ann Thorac Surg 20:619–627
11. Fox MH, Gruchow HW, Barboriak JJ et al. (1987) Risk factors among patients undergoing repeat coronary artery bypass procedures. J Thorac Cardiovasc Surg 93:56–61
12. Galbut DL, Traad EA, Dormann MJ et al. (1991) Bilateral internal mammary artery grafts in reoperative and primary coronary bypass surgery. Ann Thorac Surg 52:20–28
13. Ivert TSA, Ekeström S, Peterffy A, Welti R (1988) Coronary artery reoperations. Scand J Thorac Cardiovasc Surg 22:111–118
14. Jones EL, Weintraub WS, Craver JM, Guyton RA, Cohen CL (1991) Coronary bypass surgery: is the operation different today? J Thorac Cardiovasc Surg 101:108–115
15. Jülke M, von Segesser LK, Schneider J et al. (1989) Ausmass der Arteriosklerose der Arteria mammaria internal bei Männern im Alter von 45–75 Jahren. Schweiz Med Wochenschr. 119:1219–1223
16. Lehmann KH, von Segesser LK, Müller Glauser W et al. (1989) Superior results with internal mammary-coronary artery anastomoses due to better preservation of the endothelium. Thorac Cardiovasc Surg 37:187–189
17. Loop FD, Lytle BW, Cosgrove DM et al. (1986) Free (aorto-coronary) internal mammary artery graft. Late results. J Thorac Cardiovasc Surg 92:827–831
18. Lüscher TF, Diedrich D, Siebenmann R et al. (1988) Difference between endothelium-dependent relaxation in arterial and in venous coronary artery bypass grafts. N Engl J Med 319:462–467
19. Lytle BW, Loop FD, Thurer RL, Groves LK, Taylor PC, Cosgrove DM (1980) Isolated left anterior descending coronary artery artherosclerosis: long-term comparison of internal mammary artery and venous autografts. Circulation 61:869–874
20. Lytle BW, Cosgrove DM, Stewart RW et al. (1987a) Right gastroepiploic artery: alternative coronary bypass conduit. Circulation 76:351–354
21. Lytle BW, Loop FD, Cosgrove DM et al. (1987b) Fifteen hundred coronary reoperations: results and determinants of early and late survival. J Thorac Cardiovasc Surg 93:847–859
22. Mills NL, Everson CT (1989) Right gastroepiploic artery: a third arterial conduit for coronary artery bypass. Ann Thorac Surg 47:706–711
23. Mills NL, Everson CT (1991) Technique for use of the inferior epigastric artery as a coronary bypass graft. Ann Thorac Surg 51:208–214
24. Moncada S, Vane JR (1980) Prostacyclin in the cardiovascular system. Adv Prostaglandin Thromboxane Leukotriene Res 6:43–60
25. Myers WO, Schaff HV, Fisher LD et al. (1988) Time to first new myocardial infarctionin patients with severe angina and three-vessel disease comparing medical and early surgical therapy: a CASS registry study of survival. J Thoras Cardiovasc Surg 95:382–389
26. Navia D, Cosgrove D, Lytle BW et al. (1993) Is the internal thoracic artery the conduit of choice to replace a stenotic vein graft? The Society of Thoracic Surgeons, 29th annual meeting, Jan 25–27 1993, San Antonio; abstract book 190
27. Predel HG, Yang Z, von Segesser LK, Turina M, Bühler FR, Lüscher TF (1992) Implications of pulsatile stretch on growth of saphenous vein and mammary artery smoth muscle. Lancet 340:878–879

28. Puig LB, Ciongoli W, Cividanes GVD et al. (1988) Arteria epigastrica inferior como inxerto livre. Uma nova alternativa na revascularizacao do miocardo. Erz Bras Cardiol 50:259
29. Pym J, Beown PM, Charrette EJP et al. (1987) Gastroepiploic-coronary anastomosis. A viable alternative bypass graft. J Thorac Cardiovasc Surg 94:256–259
30. Sergeant P, Lesaffre E, Flameng W, Suy R, Blackstone E (1991) The return of clinically evident ischemia after coronary artery bypass grafting. Eur J Cardiothorac Surg 5:447–457
31. Singh RN, Sosa JA (1984) The internal mammary artery: a "live" conduit for coronary bypass. J Thorac Cardiovasc Surg 87:936–938
32. Snyder SH, Bredt DS (1992) Biological roles of nitric oxide. Sci Am May: 28–35
33. Suma H, Fukumoto H, Takeuchi A (1987) Coronary artery bypass grafting by utilizing in situ right gastroepiploic artery. Basic study and clinical application. Ann Thorac Surg 44:394–397
34. Suma H, Wanibuchi Y, Terada Y et al. (1993) The right gastroepiploic artery graft. Clinical and angiographic midterm results in 200 Patients. J Thorac Cardiovasc Surgery 105:615–23
35. Tobjörn SAI, Ekeström S, Peterffy A, Welt R (1988) Coronary artery reoperations: early and late results in 101 patients. Scand J Thor Cardiovasc Surg 22:111–118
36. Ungerleider RM, Mills NL, Wechsler AS (1985) Left thoracotomy for reoperative coronary bypass procedures. Ann Thorac Surg 40:11–5
37. Uppal R, Mills N, Wechseler AS et al. (1993) Update: left thoracotomy for reoperative bypass procedures. Ann Thorac Surg 55:1275–6
38. von Segesser LK (1990) Arterial grafting for myocardial revascularization: indications, surgical techniques and results. Springer, Berlin Heidelberg New York
39. von Segesser LK, Abdesslam N, Schneider PA, Faidutti B (1986) La révascularization des artéres viscérales chez le jeune adulte: évolution de la tactique chirurgicale. Helv Chir Acta 53:95–99
40. von Segesser LK, Simonet F, Meier B et al. (1987) Inadequate flow after internal mammary-coronary artery anastomoses. Thorac Cardiovasc Surg 35:352–354
41. von Segesser LK, Lehmann K, Turina MI (1989) Deleterious effects of shock in internal mammary artery anastomoses. Ann Thorac Surg 47:575–579
42. von Segesser LK, Schneider J, Turina MI (1992) Les autogreffes artérielles. In: Kieffer E (ed) Le remplacement artériel: principes et applications. AERCV, Paris
43. Weinhold C (1988) The benefit patients derive from aortocoronary reoperation. Thorac Cardiovasc Surg 36:266–268
44. Zeff RH, Kongtahworn C, Iannone LA et al. (1988) Internal mammary artery versus saphenous vein graft to the left anterior descending coronary artery: prospective randomized study with 10-year follow-up. Ann Thorac Surg 45:533–536

Cardiac Transplantation for Ischaemic Heart Disease

M. Yacoub

Introduction

Coronary heart disease is one of the commonest causes of morbidity and mortality, particularly in the Western world. Although there have been efforts aimed at prevention, early diagnosis as well as medical and surgical treatment of the disease, these have been only relatively effective. A significant number of patients present with severe heart failure or other manifestations of the disease that are refractory to conventional treatment (e.g., bypass graft failure, unsuitable anatomy). The only effective therapy for these patients is cardiac transplantation. Much experience has been gained with this form of therapy in coronary heart disease, with ischaemic heart disease constituting the commonest indication for cardiac transplantation in most centres [1, 2]. This has resulted in a progressive accumulation of knowledge, which is now sufficient to guide rational decision making in the majority of patients. There are, however, several areas which require further research.

Indications

The classical indication for cardiac transplantation in ischaemic heart disease is refractory heart failure due to irreversible, diffuse damage to the myocardium, resulting in severe disability and compromising prognosis. In these patients, every attempt should be made to exclude a correctable mechanical complication of myocardial infarction, or reversible ischaemic myocardial dysfunction (hibernation). The mechanical complications which could be amenable to surgical correction include left ventricular aneurysm, severe mitral regurgitation secondary to localised lesions of the papillary muscle and/or surrounding left ventricular wall, or ventricular septal rupture. As these conditions may occasionally be associated with irreversible, diffuse damage of the myocardium that may determine prognosis, every attempt should be made to ensure that the amount of remaining myocardium is sufficient to sustain life with or without revascularisation.

Although the concept of reversible myocardial ischaemia has been known for a long time, recent interest in its definition [3, 4], its mechanisms at cellular and molecular level [5–8] and, most importantly, its diagnosis has been stimulated by the availability and increased safety of revascularisation [9, 10], transplantation or both [11] (heterotopic transplantation) for these patients. The diagnostic procedures aimed at defining reversibility of myocardial dysfunction depend on the viability, cell membrane integrity, metabolic activity (with particular reference to glucose metabolism by the myocardial cells [12]) and inotropic reserve (usually defined by echocardiogram [13]). The most commonly used methods include thallium scintigraphy [14], positron emission tomography [12, 15–17] and Dobutamine echo testing [13].

As the main limitation to cardiac transplantation today is a scarcity of donors, it has been argued that this form of therapy should be offered only to patients with poor prognosis in an attempt to improve survival [18], and that the goal of improving symptoms and thus the quality of life should be of secondary importance. This is an oversimplification as these two goals are closely linked and could be of almost equal importance to the patient; they should thus not be considered in isolation [19].

Recently, the introduction of several fairly accurate prognostic indicators has been of great help in this regard [19–22]. The prognostic indicators depend on evaluating cardiac function, exercise capacity (maximum oxygen consumption) neurohumeral activation (brain natriuretic peptide, BNP, or prohormone) and signs of impending organ damage due to hypoperfusion [20]. Another potential indication for transplantation in ischaemic heart disease is the presence of complex ventricular arrhythmias that are refractory to medical and/or surgical treatment. With the increasing understanding of the basic mechanism of these arrhythmias at cellular and molecular level, the development of safer, more specific, anti-arrhythmic drugs and, most importantly, the application of implantable cardiovertor defibrillators (ICDS) [23], there should be no need to consider these patients for transplantation.

A particularly difficult, but fortunately rare group of patients who are sometimes referred for cardiac transplantation are those who have intractable angina and relatively preserved ventricular function, who have already had multiple unsuccessful operations and/or interventions due to bypass graft failure, and in whom the coronary vessels are judged to be unsuitable for any further interventions. Cardiac transplantation should only be considered on prognostic grounds if the coronary anatomy or other prognostic indicators warrant such a consideration.

Mechanical Support as a Bridge to Transplantation

Patients with advanced heart failure who are unresponsive to medical therapy, including maximum inotropic support and vasodilator therapy, with impending or actual renal and hepatic dysfunction can be helped by mechanical support while awaiting a donor organ. The most commonly used method is intra-aortic balloon counterpulsation, which is adequate in a proportion of patients. Patients with more advanced circulatory failure require the use of ventricular assist devices [24, 25]. For this purpose, extracorporeal left or biventricular pneumatic sac devices can be used for periods of up to 5 weeks. Support for longer periods of time have been achieved using pusher plate implant devices, either pneumatically or electrically powered (TCI and Novocor) [25]. Left ventricular support is usually adequate; however, about 20%–30% of the patients will require at least temporary biventricular support, usually due to either right ventricular infarction or a degree of elevation of the pulmonary vascular resistance. If strict criteria for accepting patients on mechanical support for transplantation are adhered to, the longer term result of transplantation is similar to that achieved in other patients. This is particularly important because of the scarcity of donor organs, which, arguably, should be used for patients who will derive the most benefit.

Technical Considerations

The most commonly used technique used for cardiac transplantation is the orthotopic technique. This usually entails removal of the heart with preservation of the posterior walls of the right and left atria, as originally described by Brock [26], Lower and Shumway [27]. This technique facilitates insertion, but could interfere with the electrical and mechanical function of the atria. We, and others, have introduced and used a technique of preserving the atria with separate anastomoses for the atria and pulmonary veins (Fig. 1) [28]. This results in a better contribution to ventricular filling. The exact effect of this technique on long-term function has not been determined.

Another technique used in these patients is heterotopic cardiac transplantation [29], which usually entails the use of the donor heart as a left heart bypass (Fig. 2). The advantage of this technique is that it makes maximal use of donor hearts, as smaller hearts can be made use of in larger recipients. In addition, this technique can be used in patients with moderate-to-severe, reversible pulmonary vascular disease and ensure that survival is not dependent on the donor heart. One of the main disadvantages of this technique is the fact that the recipient heart's function progressively deteriorates with failure of the aortic valve to open or develop continuous aortic regurgitation [31]. This could have an adverse effect on clinical outcome. In an attempt to prevent this and to maximise clinical benefit, we have used electrical linking of the two hearts to allow a system of counterpulsation, with each heart ejecting during the other heart's period of diastole. This brings improvement in cardiac output and metabolic benefit to the hearts

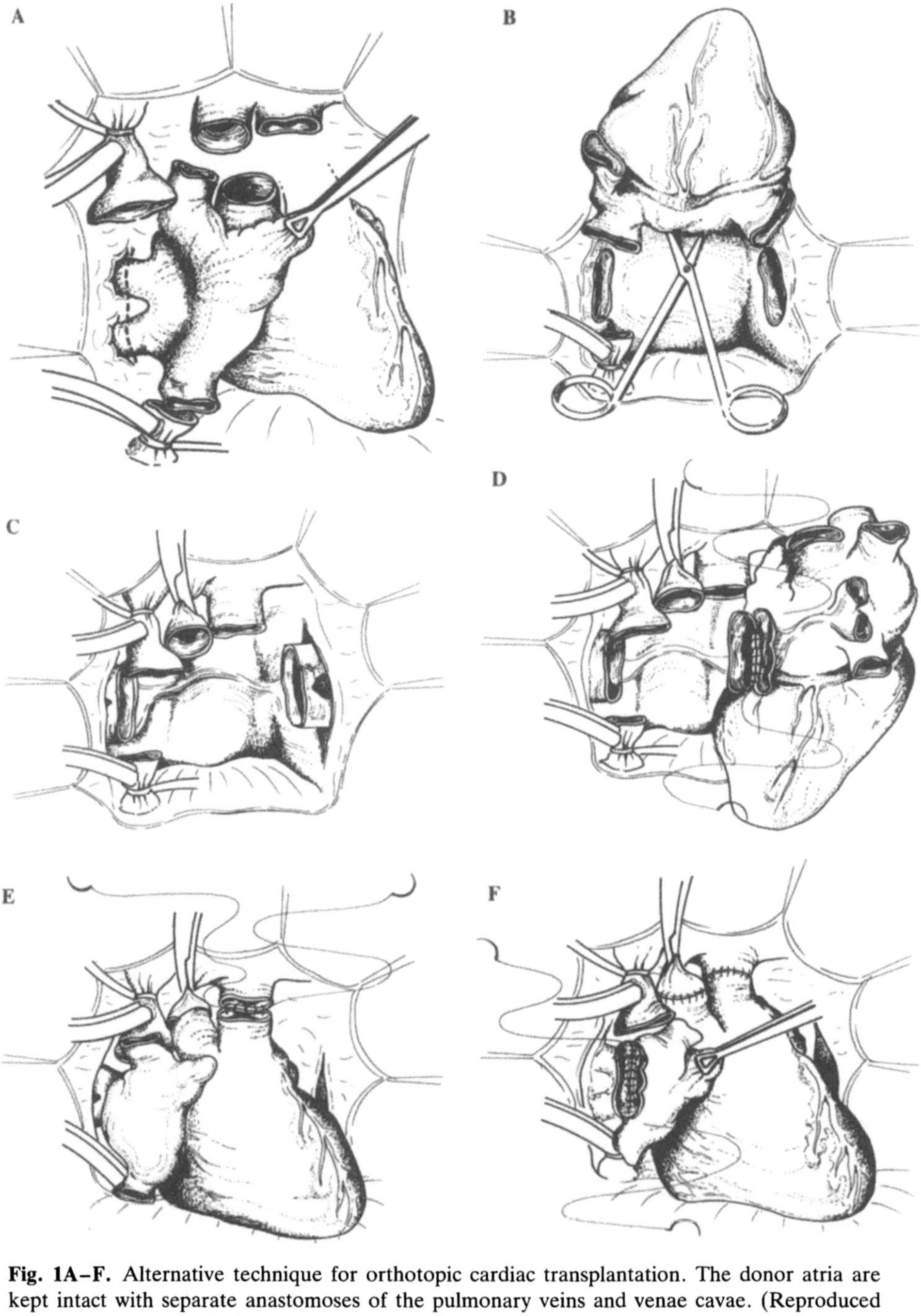

Fig. 1A–F. Alternative technique for orthotopic cardiac transplantation. The donor atria are kept intact with separate anastomoses of the pulmonary veins and venae cavae. (Reproduced with permission from [28])

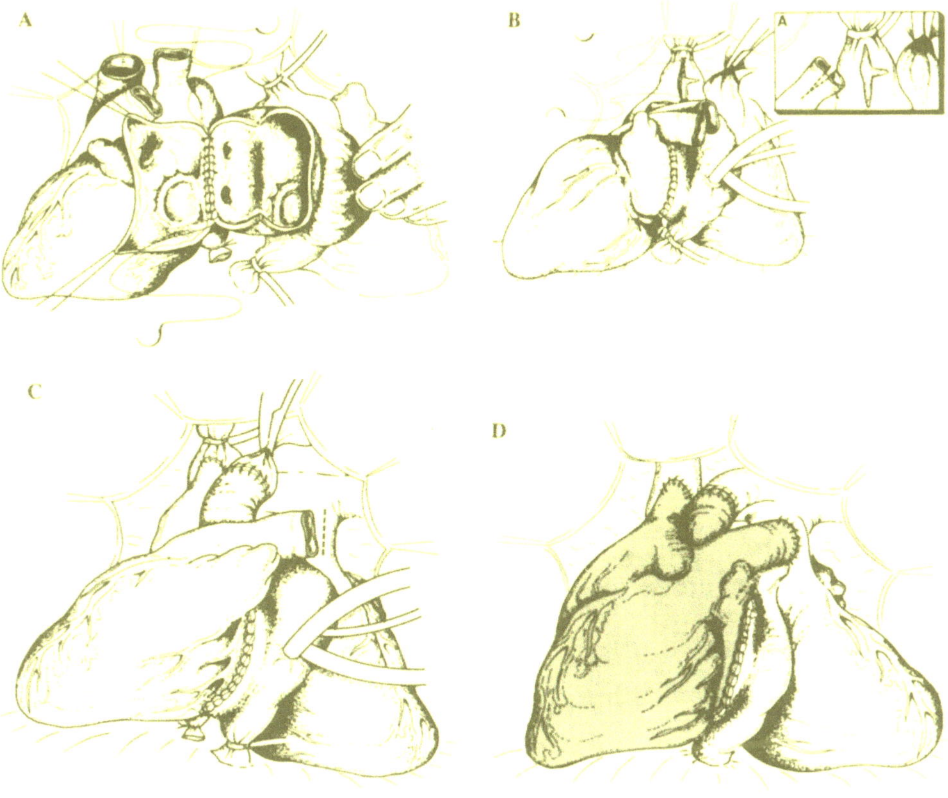

Fig. 2A–D. Technique for heterotopic transplantation. (Reproduced with permission from [28])

[32]. Heterotopic transplantation is commonly combined with excision of left ventricular aneurysm and/or myocardial revascularisation [11].

Immunosuppression

Immunosuppression is usually started just before or during the transplant procedure. The most commonly used drugs are cyclosporin, steroids and azathioprine (usually in combination as triple therapy) with regular monitoring of blood levels [33, 35]. Stopping or tapering the dose of steroids to 0.1 mg/kg per day is advisable because of their well-known side effects. The Harefield policy is to stop steroids as soon as a therapeutic level of cyclosporin is reached [34], usually within the first 3 –5 days. Routine steroids are only used in patients who develop more than three rejection episodes within a period of 6 weeks. In our experience, by the end of the first year, two-thirds of the patients are on no maintenance steroids. Induction therapy with polyclonal (rabbit or horse anti-thrombocyte globulin) or monoclonal antibodies (anti-CD3, OKT3) has been used in some series with the hope of preventing early rejection and possibly inducing a state of partial tolerance to the graft [35]. As these two agents, particularly OKT3, have been shown to increase the incidence of viral infection and possibly lymphoproliferative disorder [36], their use is usually limited to high-risk patients or for treatment of resistant acute rejection. A newer formulation of cyclosporin [37] has been shown to have more predictable pharmacodynamics with better absorption and, therefore, could have an impact on long-term results by maintaining an adequate predictable level of immunosuppression at all times [38]. Newer immunosuppressive agents such as other macrolides [39] (FK-506 and rapamycin) and mycophenolate mofetil (RS61443) [40] are currently being used for clinical trials. Some of these have several advantages – including anti-B cell activity – and thus could be useful in preventing antibody-mediated damage to the graft [40].

Induction of specific immune tolerance has not been achieved clinically in spite of the inspiring early work by Peter Medawar [41] and Houssak. Several avenues are currently being explored [42].

Monitoring of Acute Rejection

Early detection of acute rejection is essential to prevent damage to the graft, ensure reversibility, and prevent over-immunosupression. Currently, percutaneous transvenous endomyocardial biopsy is still regarded the gold standard for diagnosis of acute rejection [43]. Other non-invasive methods of monitoring include [44]: (a) left and right ventricular function (both systolic and diastolic, particularly the latter) by cardiac echocardiography or superior vena cava flow [45]; (b) cellular changes (either infiltration or damage to the myocytes) [44]; and (c) structural changes such as an increase in thickness or echo density [45].

Survival

The pattern of survival after cardiac transplantation for ischaemic heart disease depends largely on the clinical state of the patient prior to transplantation particularly in relation to the presence or absence of multi-organ damage. The risk of death is highest in the first year, with the 1-year survival being 75%–90% [2] (Fig. 3). After that, there is a constant hazard function for death of 2%–5% per year. The main causes of death are continuing immunological damage to the organ and the side effects of immunosuppressive

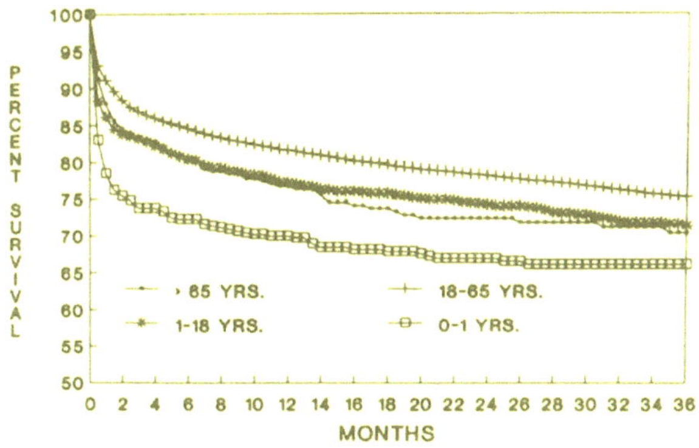

Fig. 3. Actuarial survival: hearts, 1984–1992 (Reproduced with permission from [68])

agents. Human leukocyte antigen matching has been shown to have a definite beneficial effect on survival [46–48], a fact which has stimulated efforts to institute prospective matching. The use of more effective, safer immunosuppressive agents or induction of specific immune tolerance in the future should improve long-term survival.

Physiology of the Transplanted Heart

The donor heart is subjected to potential damage by the process of brain death, long ischaemia and reperfusion during transfer and insertion, as well as effects of the cardioplegic solution itself [26]. Following that, the heart is subjected to immunological damage. In addition, the heart is denervated at insertion and, up until recently, was thought to remain denervated in humans. The influence of these factors has been extensively studied by a variety of tests, which have shown that inotropic state and reserve is preserved with minor changes in diastolic function [49–50]. The lack of sympathetic and parasympathetic innervation results in slow acceleration during dynamic and static exercise [50, 51] coupled with slow deceleration during recovery. In addition, post exercise tachycardia has been reported [51].

The loss of afferent supply (deafferentation) can also result in abnormal reflex changes. The secretion of atrial natriuretic peptide appears to be increased at rest, with an exaggerated response to exercise [52]. Immunocytochemical studies have demonstrated specific changes in the number and neuropeptide specificity of nerve fibres and ganglia in the heart after transplantation [53]. Recent evidence of at least partial sympathetic [54] and parasympathetic [55] reinnervation has been reported. The functional implications of reinnervation are currently being evaluated.

Complications

Following cardiac transplantation, continued non-specific immunosuppression and/or rejection result in a variety of complications which include bacterial or viral infection [56], systemic hypertension [57], renal dysfunction, lymphoproliferative disease and an increased incidence of different types of malignant tumours [59]. Although acute rejection can occur at any time, it is rare after the first 3 months. The most important, long-term complication is a specific form of coronary artery disease (transplant vasculopathy or accelerated coronary sclerosis).

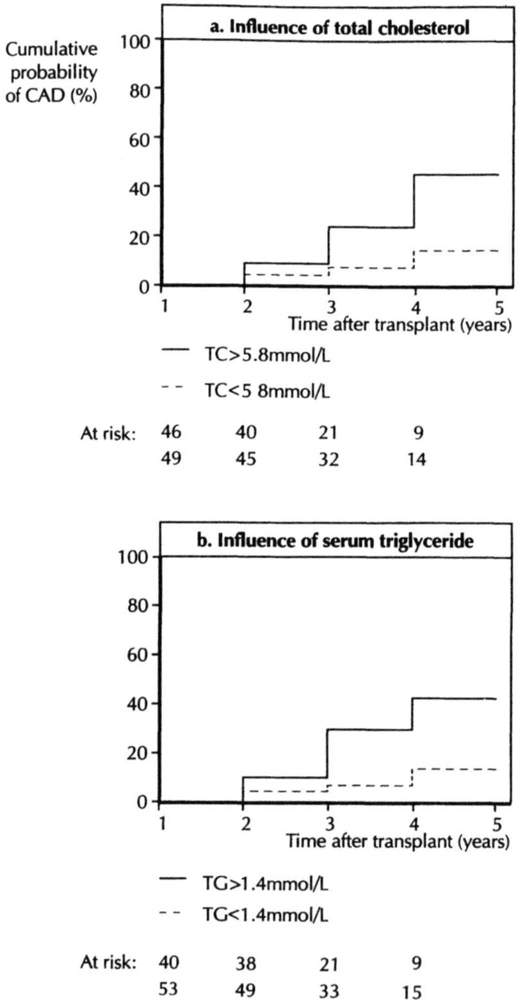

Fig. 4a,b. Influence of total cholesterol (**a**) and serum triglycerides (*TG*; **b**) on risk of coronary artery disease (*CAD*) at 1 year. (Reproduced with permission from [60])

Accelerated Coronary Sclerosis

The form of coronary disease known as accelerated coronary sclerosis has emerged as one of the most important determinants of long-term results of cardiac transplantation for ischaemic heart disease, both in terms of morbidity and mortality, with a progressively increasing incidence of up to 48% by 3 years (Fig. 4). The pathogenesis, clinical features, diagnosis, prognosis as well as avenues for preventing or treating this condition have been recently reviewed [60]. Several of the risk factors for *non*-transplant-associated or "classical" coronary disease have emerged as important risk factors for accelerated coronary sclerosis, particularly Lp(a) [61] and hyperlipidaemia [61]. The initial endothelial injury is almost certainly immune mediated, and could be cellular or antibody mediated (Fig. 5). Another clue to the causation of accelerated coronary sclerosis comes from a recent study by Drinkwater and his colleagues, who reported an increased incidence of the disease in patients in whom the University of Wisconsin Solution was used for cardiac preservation [62]. As this solution contains a high concentration of potassium (120 mcEq/l), it is possible that this helps to produce further endothelial damage, particularly as previous studies have shown that cardioplegia solutions containing a concentration of more than 20 mcEq/l of potassium may reduce the capacity of the endothelium to secrete nitric oxide in response to serotonin [63].

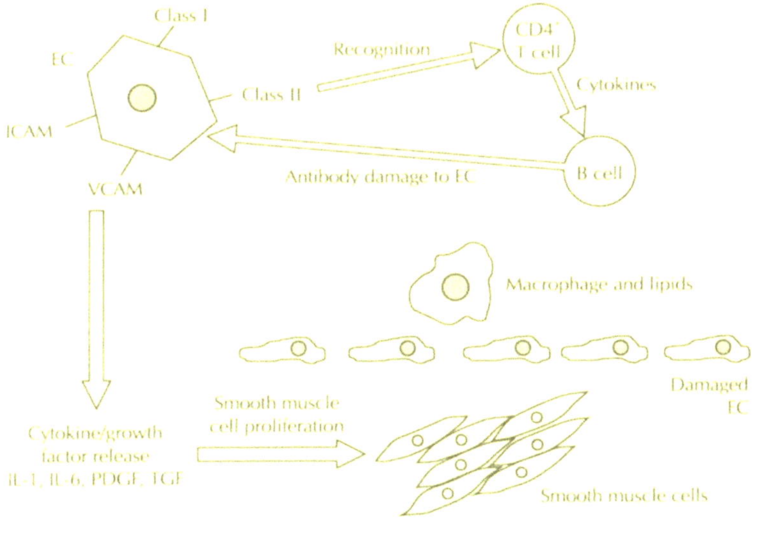

Fig. 5. Interactions between endothelial cells and the immune system lead to the development of accelerated coronary artery sclerosis (*ACS*; *EC*, endothelial cells; *ICAM*, intercellular adhesion molecule; *IL*, interleukin; *PDGF*, platelet-derived growth factor; *SMC*, smooth muscle cells; *TGF*, transforming growth factor; *VCAM*, vascular cell adhesion molecule). (Reproduced with permission from [60])

Our group has identified an endothelial-specific antibody with a molecular weight of 58–60 kDa in the serum of patients with accelerated coronary sclerosis which could play an important role in the pathogenesis of the disease [64]. Although up until recently calcification was thought to be rare in this form of coronary disease, a recent study using ultrafast computed tomography to quantify calcification has shown that calcification is not uncommon in accelerated coronary sclerosis, and its presence correlates to the coronary narrowing diagnosed by angiography [65]. Further research is urgently needed to establish the cause of the disease, which in turn will help us to develop rational forms of prevention and therapy.

Rehabilitation and Quality of Life

Although exercise testing shows subnormal exercise capacity and abnormal responses [51], it is possible to modify these parameters by an active programme of rehabilitation [66]. Similarly, abnormal skeletal muscle function and metabolism persist after transplantation [67]. Whether this can improve with time and/or rehabilitation remains to be established. Several quality of life studies have shown marked improvement in most of the parameters studied. These studies served to identify definite problem areas which also need to be addressed.

Conclusion

Cardiac transplantation has an important role to play in the treatment of a specific subset of patients with advanced coronary heart disease. This form of therapy is currently limited by the scarcity of donors, a problem which needs to be addressed by making use of all available potential human donors and developing techniques for the use of xenografts [42]. The medium-term results of cardiac allografts is good; however, the long-term results depend on evolving safer forms of immunosuppression and/or induction of specific immune balance.

References

1. Yacoub M (1987) The place of heart transplantation: the British experience. Eur Heart J 8 [Suppl 1]:37–38
2. Kriett JM, Kaye MP (1990) The registry of the International Society of Heart Transplantation: seventh official report. J Heart Transplant 9:223
3. Rahimtoola S (1989) Hibernating myocardium. Am Heart J 117:211–221

4. Bolli R (1993) Myocardial stunning in man. Circulation 86:1671–1691
5. Ferrari R, La Canna G, Giubbini R, Pardini A, Coletti G, Berra P, Alfresi O (1994) Hibernating myocardium. Annu Cardiac Surg 7:28
6. Ross J Jr (1991) Myocardial perfusion – contraction matching: implications for coronary heart disease and hibernation. Circulation 83:4076–4082
7. Bristow JD, Arai AE, Ansclone CG, Pantely GA (1991) Response to myocardial ischaemia as a regulated process. Circulation 84:2580–2587
8. Marban (1991) Myocardial stunning and hibernation: the physiology behind the colle-qualisms. Circulation 83:681–688
9. Rahimtoola SH (1985) A perspective on the three large multicenter randomised clinical trials of coronary bypass surgery for chronic stable angina. Circulation 72 [Suppl V]:123–125
10. Califf RM, Harrel FE, Lee KL, Rankin JS, Mark DB, Halten MA, Muhlbaier LH, Wichsler AS, Jones R, Oldham HN Jr, Pryor DB (1988) Changing efficacy of coronary revascularisation: implications for patient selection. Circulation 78 [Suppl I]:185–191
11. Ridley PD, Khaghani A, Musumeci F, Favaloro R, Akl ES, Banner NR, Mitchell AG, Yacoub MB (1992) Heterotopic heart transplantation and recipient heart operation in ischaemic heart disease. Ann Thor Surg 54:333–337
12. De-Silva R, Camici PG (1994) Hibernating myocardium definition and detection by positron emission tomography. Annu Cardiac Surg 7:33–40
13. Cigarroa CG, de Fillipi CR, Buckner B, Alvarez LG, Wait MA, Grayburn PA (1993) Dobutamine stress echocardiography identifies hibernating myocardium and predicts recovery of left ventricular function after coronary revascularisation. Circulation 88:430–436
14. Dilsizian V, Bonow RO (1993) Current diagnostic techniques of assessing myocardial viability in patients with hibernating myocardium. Circulation 87:1–20
15. Bonow RO, Berman DS, Gibbons RJ, Johnson LL, Rumberger JA, Schwarger M, Wackers FJT (1991) Cardiac positron emission tomography. A report for health professionals from the committee on advanced cardiac imaging and technology of the council on clinical cardiology. American Heart Association. Circulation 84:447–454
16. Eilzman D, Al-Aouar Z, Kanter BL, Von Dahl J, Kirsh M, Deeb GM, Schwarzer M (1992) Clinical outcome of patients with advanced coronary artery disease after viability studies with positron emission tomography. J Am Coll Cardiol 20:559–565
17. Bonow RO, Dilsizian V, Cuocolo A, Bacharach SL (1991) Identification of viable myocardium in patients with chronic coronary artery disease and left ventricular dysfunction. Comparison of thalium scintography with re-injection and PET imaging with 18F-Fluorodeoxyn glucose. Circulation 83:26–37
18. Mancini DM, Bisen H, Kussmaul W, Mull R, Edmonds LH, Wilson JR (1991) Value of peak exercise oxygen consumption for optimal timing of cardiac transplantation in ambulatory patients with heart failure. Circulation 83:778–786
19. Mudge GH, Goldstein S, Addorizio LJ, Caplan A, Mancini D, Levine B, Rilsch MR Jr (1993) Task force 3: Recipient guidelines/p terisation. JACC 22:21–31
20. Borer JS (1989) Prognostication strategies in heart failure and valvular heart diseases: Current concepts and their support. In: Yacoub M (ed) Annual of cardiac surgery. Current Science, Philadelphia, pp 115–124
21. Cohn JN, Rector TJ (1988) Prognosis of congestive heart failure and predictors of mortality. Am J Cardiol 62 [Suppl]:25A–30A
22. Stevenson LW, Tillisch JH, Hamilton M, Luu M, Chelimsky-Fallick C, Moriguchi J, Walden J (1990) Importance of haemodynamic response to therapy in predicting survival with ejection fraction ≤20% secondary to ischaemic or nonischaemic dilated cardiomyopathy. Am J Cardiol 66:1348–1354
23. Klein H, Trapper HJ, Feigirth HG, Nisam S (1993) Prospective studies evaluating prophylactic ICD therapy for high risk patients with coronary artery disease. PACE 16:564–576
24. Rokitansky A, Walner E (1989) Total artificial heart and assist devices as a bridge to transplantation. Int J Artif Organs 12:77–84

25. Hill JD (1989) Bridging to cardiac transplantation. Ann Thorac Surg 47:167–171
26. Cass MH, Brock R (1959) Heart excision and replacement. Guy's Hospital Reports 108: 205–290
27. Lower RR, Shumway NE (1960) Studies on orthotopic transplantation. Surg Forum 11:18
28. Yacoub MH, Mankad P, Ledingham S (1990) Donor procurement and surgical techniques for cardiac transplantation. Semin Thorac Cardiovasc Surg 2:153–161
29. Barnard CN, Losman JG (1975) Left ventricular bypass. S Afr Med J 49:303
30. Galbraith TA, Yacoub M (1987) Heterotopic heart transplantation: operative technique and results in heart transplantation. In: Myerowitz DP (ed) Futura, Mount Kisco, NY, pp 155–168
31. Akasaka T, Lythal D, Cheng A, Yoshida K, Yoshikawa J, Mitchell A, Yacoub M (1989) Continuous aortic regurgitation in severely dysfunctional native hearts after heterotopic cardiac transplantation. Am J Cardiol 63:(20)1483–1488
32. Thurgood JM, Cowell R, Paul V, Kalsi K, Seymour A-M, Ilsley C, Mitchell A, Khaghani A, Yacoub MH (1994) Haemodynamic and metabolic effects of paced linkage following heterotopic cardiac transplantation. Circulation (in press)
33. Lindholm A (1991) Therapeutic monitoring of cyclosporin: an update. Em J Clin Pharmacol 41:273–283
34. Yacoub M, Alivazatos P, Khaghani A, Mitchell A (1985) The use of cyclosporin, azathioprine and antilymphocyte globulin with or without low dose steroids for immunosuppression of cardiac transplant patients. Transplant Proc XVII (I):221
35. Renlund DG, O'Connell JB, Bristow MR (1990) Strategies of immunosuppression in cardiac transplantation. Semin Thorac Cardiovasc Surg 2:181–188
36. Swinnen LJ, Costanzo-Nordin MR, Tischer SG, O'Sullivan EJ, Johnson MR, Heroux AL, Dizikes GJ, Pifarre R, Fisher RI (1990) Increased incidence of lymphoproliferative disorder after immunosuppression with the monoclonal antibody OKT3 in cardiac-transplant recipients. N Engl J Med 323:1723
37. Ghada M, Eadon H, Leaver N, Yacoub M (1994) The use of Neoral in heart transplant recipients. Transplant Proc (in press)
38. Lindholm A, Kahan BD (1993) Influence of cyclosporine pharmacokinetics, trough concentrations and AUC monitoring on outcome after kidney transplantation. Clin Pharmacol Thor 54:205–218
39. Schreiber SL, Crabtree GR (1992) The mechanism of action of Cyclosporine A and FK 506. Immunol Today 13:136–142
40. Allison AC, Engui EM, Sallinger HW (1993) Mycophenolate Mofetil (RS-61443): mechanism of action and effects in transplantation. Transplant Rev 7:129–139
41. Billingham RE, Brent L, Medawar PB (1953) Actively acquired tolerance of foreign cells. Nature 172:603
42. Yacoub M (1994) Transplantation in the third millenium. In: Newsom-Davies J, Weatherall D (eds) Health policy and technological innovation. Chapman and Hall, London, pp 37–48
43. Billingham ME (1982) Diagnosis of cardiac rejection by endomyocardial biopsy. J Heart Transplant 1:25–30
44. Valantine HA, Hunt SA (1993) Clinical and non-invasive methods of diagnosing rejection after heart transplantation. In: Rose M, Yacoub MH (eds) Immunology of heart and lung transplantation. Edward Arnold, London, pp 219–231
45. Lythal D, Gibson D, Swanson K, Mitchell A, Ilsley C, Yacoub M (1990) Quantitative analysis of myocardial echo amptitude–a useful marker of cardiac rejection. Circulation 80 [Suppl II]:677
46. Yacoub M, Festenstein H, Doyle P, et al. (1987) The influence of HLA matching in cardiac allograft recipients receiving cyclosporin and azathioprine. Transplant Proc 19: 2487–2489
47. Opelz G, Wujcoak T (1994) The influence of HLA compatibility on graft survival after heart transplantation. N Engl J Med 330(12):816–819

48. Morris PJ (1994) HLA matching and cardiac transplantation. N Engl J Med 330(12):857–858
49. Borow K, Newmann A, Arensman F, Yacoub M (1985) Left ventricular contractility and contractile reserve in humans after cardiac transplantation. Circulation 71(5):866–872
50. Banner NR, Yacoub MH (1990) Physiology of the orthotopic cardiac transplant recipient. Semin Thorac Cardiovasc Surg 2:259
51. Banner NR, Lloyd MH, Hamilton RD et al. (1989) Cardiopulmonary response to dynamic exercise after heart and heart-lung transplantation. Br Heart J 61:215–223
52. Singer D, Banner N, Cox A, Patel N, Burden M, Buckley M, MacGregor G, Yacoub M (1990) Response to dynamic exercise in cardiac transplant recipients: implications for control of the sodium regulatory hormone atrial naturellic peptide. Clin Sci 78(2):159–163
53. Wharton D, Polak J, Gordon L, Banner N, Springall D, Rose M, Khaghani A, Wallwork J, Yacoub M (1990) Immunohistochemical dimensions of human cardiac innervation before and after transplantation. Circ Res 66(4):900–912
54. Wilson RF, Christensen BV, Olivari MT, Simon A, White CW, Laxson DD (1991) Evidence for structural sympathetic reinnervation after orthotopic cardiac transplantation in humans. Circulation 83(4):1210–1220
55. Banner NR, Khaghani A, Mitchell AG, Radley-Smith R, Lockwood P, Lloyd MH, Yacoub M (1987) Haemodynamics and lung functions one year after combined heart lung transplantation. Br Heart J 57:87 (Abstract)
56. Dummer JF (1990) Infections complications of transplantation. In: Thompson ME (ed) Cardiac transplantation. Davis, Philadelphia, pp 163–178
57. Ozdogan E, Banner N, Fitzgerald M et al. (1990) Factors influencing the development of hypertension following cardiac transplantation. J Heart Transplant 9:548
58. Thomas JA, Crawford DH (1993) Biology of lymphoproliferative disease in transplant patients. In: Rose M, Yacoub M (eds) Immunology of heart and lung transplantation. Edward Arnold, London, pp 243–260
59. Sheil AGR (1988) Cancer in dialysis and transplant patients. In: Morris P (ed) Transplantation: principles and practice. Saunders, Philadelphia, pp 603–618
60. Yacoub M, Rose M (1994) Accelerated coronary sclerosis. Annu Cardiac Surg 7:80–89
61. Barbir M, Kushwaha S, Hunt B, MacKenna A, Thompson GR, Mitchell A, Robinson D, Yacoub M (1992) Lipoprotein (a) and accelerated coronary arterial disease in cardiac transplant recipients. Lancet 340:1500–1502
62. Drinkwater D, Rudis E, Laks H, Marino J, Stein D, Ardebali A, Aharon A (1994) UW versus Stanford cardioplegia and the development of allograft coronary arterial vasculopathy. J Heart Lung Transplant 13(1–2):S47 (Abstract)
63. Mankad PS, Chester AH, Yacoub MH (1991) Role of potassium concentration in cardioplegic solutions in mediating endothelial damage. Ann Thorac Surg 51(1):89–93
64. Dunn MJ, Crisp SJ, Rose ML, Taylor PM, Yacoub MH (1991) Detection of anti-endothelial antibodies by Western blotting – positive correlation with coronary artery disease after cardiac transplantation. Lancet 339:1566
65. Barbir M, Bowker T, Ludman P, Mitchell A, Wood D, Yacoub M (1994) Ultrafast CT scanning for the detection of coronary disease in cardiac transplant recipients. Am J Cardiol (in press)
66. Kavanagh T, Yacoub M, Mertens D, Kennedy J, Campbell R, Sawyer P (1988) Cardiorespiratory responses to exercise training after orthotopic cardiac transplantation. Circulation 77:162–171
67. Stratton JR, Kemp GJ, Daly RC, Yacoub M (1994) Effects of cardiac transplantation on bioenergetic abnormalities of skeletal muscle in congetive heart failure. Circulation (in press)
68. Kaye MP (1993) The Registry of the International Society for Heart and Lung Transplantation: Tenth Official Report – 1993. J Heart Lung Transplant 12(4): 543

Subject Index

Springer-Verlag and the Environment

We at Springer-Verlag firmly believe that an international science publisher has a special obligation to the environment, and our corporate policies consistently reflect this conviction.

We also expect our business partners – paper mills, printers, packaging manufacturers, etc. – to commit themselves to using environmentally friendly materials and production processes.

The paper in this book is made from low- or no-chlorine pulp and is acid free, in conformance with international standards for paper permanency.

FSC
www.fsc.org
MIX
Papier aus verantwortungsvollen Quellen
Paper from responsible sources
FSC® C105338

If you have any concerns about our products,
you can contact us on
ProductSafety@springernature.com

In case Publisher is established outside the EU,
the EU authorized representative is:
Springer Nature Customer Service Center GmbH
Europaplatz 3, 69115 Heidelberg, Germany

Printed by Libri Plureos GmbH
in Hamburg, Germany